ME AND MY PAIN

The Challenges of Living with Chronic Pain

ABBEY STRAUSS MSW, MD

Copyright © 2009 Abbey Strauss

All rights reserved.

ISBN: 1-4392-3863-4
EAN13: 9781439238639
LCCN: 2009903993

Dedications and Acknowledgements

To all those many people, who through their pain and suffering, trusted me enough to enter their worlds, and in doing so, taught me about the reality of their lives.

And in particular, a special thanks to my wife, whose experience was the ultimate fountain of great insight and strength for all of us.

Table of Contents

Introduction – Is this book for you?
1. A bit of history and an overview 4
2. How the pain started 20
3. A typical case 24
4. Do doctors understand what life is like for the 28
chronic pain patient?
5. Well, you've got to learn to live with the pain 53
6. Pain and personality changes 67
7. Addiction, iatraddiction and pseudoaddiction 96
8. Punishment for what the doctor can't fix in patients . 124
with unfixable emotional problems
9. Lying 142
10. Sleep 156
11. Relationships 161
12. Why medications work one day and not the next . . . 189
13. The victim becomes the perpetrator 210
14. What is pain? A medical perspective 217
15. I had a friend who got better 264
16. Doctor shopping: it looks like an addict but it's just . . 265
looking for help
17. Under treatment and mistreatment 275
18. Suffering 295
19. What the psychologists see 309
20. That word 'addiction' 333
21. Pain in the dying versus pain in the living 361
22. The extended pain patient 370
23. Pain patients have to be perfect people 384
24. Insurance companies 393
25. Epilogue and recommendations 430
26. References 461
27. Index 487

Introduction:
Is this book for you?

This book comes from people who personally suffered from some aspect of pain. The pain may have been within their own bodies, or it may have been the emotional suffering that comes from living with someone in pain.

I belong to both these groups. My wife, now a hospice nurse, endured a terrible period of pain that nearly took our lives away. Then I suffered incredible neck pain. Fortunately surgery took away most of our pains, yet the experiences of living with the pain, and of the incredible struggles to get pain relief, indelibly marked our lives.

This book has even another keystone: I am a physician. So I have three platforms from which to speak: as a physician who treated pain, as the husband of a former chronic pain patient, and as a former pain patient myself. This three line saying captures my resume on chronic pain:

> *I've seen the elephant,*
> *and I've heard the owl,*
> *and I've been to the other side of the mountain*[1]

This is not a book on how to treat specific aliments. Indeed, the world of pain treatment is now a welcome and ever-so-rapidly improving part of our technical world. This is good.

This book, however, looks at how to live with the common problems of pain. It examines the issues of suffering when pain is managed, properly and improperly, by both patients and doctors.

The pain treatment world now has a good momentum. Real change is happening. Laws now allow physicians to treat chronic pain patients without as much fear of regulatory persecution. Many doctors know how to properly treat chronic pain. Quality of life issues are becoming more important than mere dosing issues. The terrible attitudes and the wounds that all these older problems once caused are less common.

> *The Hebrew word 'tikkun' best captures what is happening; 'tikkun' means to heal, repair and transform. 'Tikkun' is our purpose.*

But the progress is far from enough. Occasional horror stories still appear about unscrupulous doctors who claim to be treating pain, but are in fact only maintaining addictions. These repugnant events literally hijack the good work of honest pain management practitioners. Insurance company and regulatory hurdles still exist, but bit by bit they are being overcome.

The stories and emotions captured in this book are real. They came from my experiences with countless pain patients and their families. This book, therefore, is a convention of ideas, explanations, and suggestions to help us all grasp the facts of pain and the world into which it puts its victims.

> *The suffering may be within you, but you may not be the cause of the suffering.*

Some sections in the book are scientific and technical, some are expressions of what patients report, there are many stories about people in pain, and some are essays about the roles and history of suffering. The book ends with suggestions of what can be done to energize and support efforts to hopefully make things better.

Is this the book for you?

Yes, if you, or someone close or important to you, suffers from chronic pain and one or more of these applies.

Do you feel?
- That the medical community is misunderstanding you.
- That you are basically a psychologically normal person without any emotional, social, or monetary benefit from the pain.
- That you are waiting to be seen by a specialist or are being unsatisfactorily treated for your pain, or that you have been told by doctors and clinics that your pain is untreatable even after aggressive trials of the most current treatments have been made, and you feel hopeless and endlessly suffering.
- That you have been told that your primary problem is a psychiatric problem or an addiction, and the pain is not real or as bad as claimed.
- That you have to work too hard to get access to adequate pain relief.
- That you have given much thought and struggled to find some reason for, and a place for, the pain in your life.
- That at times life is too hard to live because of the pain and what it has done to you and your family.

Say yes to any of these and this book should offer you some emotional and intellectual relief as well as assistance.

This book is about the daily reminder of what it is like to live with pain. It is about that uniquely personal relationship between "Me and My Pain."

CHAPTER ONE
A bit of history and an overview

This book writing project began 1996. Then it slept for over a decade because many things seemed to begin to change for the better. But too many problems in the management of pain still exist, so it was time to re-start the project. One major on-going problem is the under-treatment of suffering.

Impressive technical improvements have nourished important clinical and way of thinking shifts. Now there is a deeper and wider-spread recognition that pain is often under-treated, and that treating with opiates is safer than once thought. Wonderfully rigorous scientific research is underway. The professional literature has even advanced to the degree that it speaks of such intriguing differences in such areas as how genetically based stress point patterns could affect how sensitive or resistant a person is to pain.[2] Pain is not always just in one's head.

New non-opiate treatments now exist such as ziconotide (Prialt®), pregabalin (Lyrica®), milnacipran (Savella®) tapentadol (Nucynta®, which acts as an opioid and non-opioid), and duloxetine (Cymbalta®). Anticonvulsant use for pain control has become quite common. Surgeons and anesthesiologists also have better interventions, devices and corrective techniques. Transcranial magnetic stimulation (TMS) is approved for the treatment of depression; the technique uses electromagnetic pulses to alter brain activity, and while still experimental, work thus far shows it may be helpful with chronic headaches, shingles, fibromyalgia, and peripheral neuropathy.

Neuroimaging can now show blood flow changes in response to pain.[3] We are beginning to use our distinctive genetic patterns to individualize and improve treatment success. This is known as pharmacogenetics.[4] A newly discovered protein, known as p11, may be pivotal in treating both depression and pain.[5] The roles in pain played by glial cells and neuronal growth factors, such as BDNF (brain derived neurotrophic factor) in the central nervous system are now being aggressively studied. More doctors now use the term "treat to effect", which means treating until there is a good response. And very importantly, but certainly far from the bottom of the list of changes, are the fantastic, robust and vigorous patient fueled advocacy groups that force the world into more realistic attitudes towards pain. These are all very good developments.

Pain affects about 20% of the population. It burdens all life's realms. As a result, the business aspect of pain treatment has become a popular, in-vogue business. Sadly, too much pain treatment comes out of questionable clinics that seem all too ready to treat people with questionable medical needs.

Another distributing trend is that physicians are moving too much of the pain experience into medical models and away from the psychological models. The call to treat the 'suffering aspect of pain' is still too restrained. Many will disagree with me on this point, yet the mental health aspects of living in pain are too quickly given off to other professionals. In doing so, the primary physicians fail to realize that many of the mental health issues of being in pain are caused by, and therefore might be lessened, by the nature and style of a physician's choice of pain treatment actions. For example, many patients frequently report that many pain management doctors self-infuse themselves with a hero quality. Many doctors rebut that they have to protect themselves from unsavory patients, and so somewhat of a police-like, authoritarian quality exists in many of their practices. A patient said that a "cop on patrol flavor" moved into many pain management offices. It is troubling that the world of 'pain management' *expects* to have unsavory patients knock on their doors. This lowers the bar down into a cynical and odd ecosystem. These are a serious topics that later will be extensively and bluntly discussed.

Another problem is that many patients feel doctors are too quick to make negative psychiatric judgments when problems exist with them. Even psychiatrists have been known to mislabel pain patients.

> A 52 year old suffered a TMJ injury. Over many years, she had over a dozen surgical attempts to try to fix the problem. One psychiatric evaluator, hired by her insurance company, and who saw her only one time, said she suffered from Munchausen's disorder (a psychiatric condition in which there is no bona fide medical illness). He clearly did not care to listen to the details of her story. In a score of years, I spent over 1000 hours with her. She hated her pain, and she always fought additional surgery as much as possible. The insurance doctor was very wrong.

> Another insurance psychiatrist pejoratively claimed that her great concern with her facial appearance stemmed from vanity issues. The truth is that she was bothered for years as she watched her chin disappear. The same examining doctor discounted the effects of her exposure to a FDA recalled TMJ implant known to cause deformities, and that she was quite comfortable with her appearance before the injury and implant. So he labeled as vanity what she saw as frightening changes in the shape of her face. Though this doctor was wrong, his opinion

worked its way into her file as if it was a basic psychological truth about her.

This type of problem will be discussed in much detail later.

A nursing journal report in June 2008 said that one of the most common nursing frustrations was when physicians prescribed either too little or the wrong pain medication. [6]

Then this appeared in the New York Times in 2008: [7]

> "There is on undeniable fact about chronic pain: More often than not, pain is not treated or undertreated. A survey done last year by the American Pain Society found that only 55 percent of all patients with non-cancer related pain, and fewer than 40 percent of those with severe pain, said their pain was under control. But it does not have to be this way. There are myriad treatments – drugs, devices and alternative techniques – that can greatly ease chronic pain, if not eliminate it. Chronic pain is second only to respiratory infections as a reason that patients seek medical care. Yet because physicians often do not take a patient's pain seriously or treat it inadequately, nearly half of chronic pain patients have changed doctors at least once, and more than a quarter have changed doctors at least three times."

Other writers and patients equally lament about the pain treatment problems.[8] Patients often tell me what they feel about many of the pain management practices they've used. One patient re-named his new pain management doctor as "the-guy-who-is-trying-to-manage-my-whole-life-cause-he-doesn't-trust-me-doctor…" I repeatedly learn that patients hesitate, or even fear, talking to their doctors about their real dosing needs, or that they underplay their needs so not to offend the doctor. They dread being absolutely honest about their medication needs for fear the doctor will drop them as a patient. One very astute patient observed that "the lab tests I have to take aren't being used to make sure I have a good enough blood level of meds to control my pain. No, those lab tests are there to see if I am telling the truth about what I swallow. What an atmosphere!"

> "I've come to realize that prepositions are all about tones. I wish I could talk 'with' my doctor. Instead we talk 'to' each other."

Problems tend to emerge from what can be labeled as the *behind the gas station or strip mall pain clinics*. These dispensaries time after time pop up and are frightfully widespread. Just look at the ads in the newspapers usually available for free outside of take-out restaurants. One has to wonder if or how they service legitimate patients.

These questionable clinics seed our uncertainties that these are no more than walk-in medication mills, like easy take-out pharmacies for those with for less than genuine pain needs. Horror stories from these clinically indifferent pain clinics chill the entire profession and galvanize the regulators into panic. Some who claim to be hierophants (that is, someone who is supposed to help humanity; physicians are supposed to be hierophants) are actually just ethically detached cash businesses. Florida Statewide Prosecutor William Shepherd labeled these doctors as "signologists" – "corrupt physicians who provide no treatment and merely sign-off on prescriptions. In 2007, "110 people in Florida died from heroin, while more than 2,100 died from prescription opioids." [9] This same article reports other cases of doctors who never saw patients yet prescribed medications for them. A key quality is that within the signology clinics, the patient's connection to the medication is usually stronger than is the relationship with the physician. They should be at least equal.

> The husband of a pain patient said: "My opinion of some of those pain clinics – they plunder the weak and take advantage of their illnesses just like someone whose interest in their own profit is so rationalized that it removes any sense of moral responsibility. It is the criminal, and too often the corporate mindset, to sell a product, usurp their customer's fragilities, and earn money regardlessly. There is none of the traditional, sacred quality that saw medicine as a non-brutal profession. Shame on them."

But honesty requires that we see the another side to some of these clinics: Many of these clinics serve the uninsured, or those whose emotional needs are so intense that a 'real' clinic or average practice would not give out medications with the ease and 'turning away of the other cheek' as they get in these cash and carry clinics. And should one of these clinics take insurance, then the effect further reduces the burden on other community medical resources. Many of these pain clinics appear seedy because they appear to be servicing a 'seedier', more troubled group or just a poorer crowd. A troubled person in real physical pain is in as much pain as a non-troubled person in pain, though the later is more likely to have corollary support mechanisms, such as money, family or better insurance. I've heard people say some that of these pain clinics are but a notch away from the methadone clinics in that they are in reality treating addictions. This is a good point. The methadone clinic is more upfront because their clients admit to problems with narcotics. Indeed, the methadone clinic may offer more of a respectful and therapeutic flavor than do the pain management clinics. The essential question is why one would choose a pain clinic versus a methadone clinic for an opioid supply? I suspect it is that the methadone clinic is more highly structured and demands a more rigorous level of patient responsibility than do the walk-in pain clinics. I would also suggest that the users of the pain clinics do not seek to control their addictions in the same manner as do those who go to the methadone clinics.

There is an agonizing and dreadful disappointment when doctors exploit the business opportunity granted to them by their medical licenses. In 2007, the US FBI specifically mentioned 'pain management and associated drug diversion' on their monitoring list for Medicare and Medicaid fraud.[10] These are the awful pain management stories that get into the media. The truth is that these are not real pain management stories; rather they lean towards criminal stories about criminals who use pain management tools to perform their crimes. The reaction to these tales makes for a backwash that too often lives in the idea that taking away the tools will prevent the crime. That, of course, is wrong. Preventing any crime is done by removing the motivations or needs for the crime. There are so many points of intervention. Start by getting rid of the bad doctors. Then force the drug seeking patients into good rehabilitation. The interventions list is long.

Another spillover is the pollution that these stories release into the community's thinking. It is as if some understated, but real danger and impropriety exists when treating pain patients.

This is an enormously complex issue. In 2007 the *New York Times Magazine* further explored the problem.[11] Among the many poignant statements in the article are two compelling comments about the doctor-patient relationship. The first comment chills. The second comment warms.

> 1. "In addition to medical considerations, real or imagined, there is another deterrent to opioid use in the doctors' mind: fear."
> 2. "The basis of the physician-patient relationship is trust. Trust is especially valued by pain patients, who often have long experiences of being treated like criminals or hysterics."

We will return many times to the doctor-patient relationship issues.

Other developments are enthusiastically welcomed. Attention is now being given to children with pain.[12][13], to teachers who have to manage chronic pain students in their classrooms,[14] and to adequate pain control in the elderly.[15][16] It's sad because these areas should not have needed special attention. What logic lead to such long held thinking that children ought not to be given pain medications? Giving proper pain control to everyone ought not to have ever been an issue. Many of these valuable changes grew out of the hard work done by the pain advocacy groups.

> The Mayo Clinic in Minnesota ran a pediatric pain rehabilitation program for adolescents with chronic pain. It was a three week hospital based program. They report that 15% to 20% of children and adolescents have chronic pain, with 5% of all children being so handicapped

> by the pain that they cannot function. "Life with a child who is experiencing chronic pain often spirals into serious family stress." Many of the children needed less medications by the end of the program. The children are in the program 5 full days a week for 3 weeks. Their parents are in classes about 20 hours a week. [17]

By the same token, a tragic story from Seattle reported that a 15 year old autistic child died after the dentist gave him inappropriate pain medications following dental work. The case caught the attention of the Health section of the American Bar Association's Journal.[18] The case speaks to the issue that too much pain management is done by those who do not understand the process of proper management. In the Seattle case, the hospital changed its policy such that now pain management specialists must approve such prescriptions.

The Veterans Administration, in a policy known as the '5th vital sign,' now requires VA medical personnel to ask about pain.[19] Once again, it boggles the mind to think that medical personnel had to be mandated to ask about pain in their patients. State governments have also recognized that appropriate pain treatment is a patient's right. In 2001, the California courts forced doctors to seriously examine how they treat pain patients. Indeed, in 1994, the Medical Board of California sent pain treatment guidelines to all physicians in the state, and in 1997, California passed the Pain Patient's Bill of Rights. California also began to require pain management training as part of physicians' on-going education.[20] Much of this work was spearheaded by the quiet Sacramento based Harvey Rose, an internist who served as a mentor to me and others in pain management. His work was a central impetus for the California Intractable Pain Act. He died recently.[21] All in pain should know about, and offer their thanks, to Harvey.

In 1999, the Health Care Financing Administration (this was the Federal agency that ran Medicare. It is now known as CMS, or the Center for Medicare and Medicaid Services) ruled that patients must be informed of any rights they have under state law to make decisions concerning pain treatment. In essence the Federal government was taking an interest in how pain was treated.[22]

Finally, doctors were considered negligent if they failed to treat pain.[23] [24] In 2001, the Joint Commission on Accreditation of Healthcare Organizations (commonly known as JCAHO) adopted a set of pain assessment and treatment standards that required agencies to monitor their pain management operations.[25] [26] In 2008, Medicare ruled that hospice patients must "have greater rights to effective pain management." [27]

In 1989, an article appeared on how 'pain management' could be an 'alternative to euthanasia'.[28] The article remarked that "the fear of addiction in terminally ill patients would be laughable if it had not caused so many patients to endure needless pain." How true, how sad, and how embarrassing that it took almost 20 years before Medicare and other agencies changed their rules and attitudes about this.

> "I kept asking my doctor if any of the agency heads or Congress people would stop being so afraid of pain management if one of their family was in as much pain as was my aunt before she died."

Yet even with these wonderful moves, so many problems in pain management still exist. Look around. Why do the major media still need to write about inadequate pain treatment? Why did a 2007 article in Oncology Nursing[29] report that in 2002 "approximately 28% of Hispanic patients received analgesics that were insufficient in strength to manage their pain and that physicians under estimated pain severity in 64% of Hispanic patients." Why in 2004 were 50% of Hispanic and African American patients still under treated for their pain?

> The Hispanic group revealed four problematic themes: a lack of communication about under medication, that patients presented with the qualities of macho and adnegada (Spanish for being unselfish), that family is more important than cancer pain, and that their illness or the medications made them feel like prisoners.

Too many of the old problems and attitudes still breath and are still active.

Many patients continue to report that they need more medication than their doctor is comfortable prescribing. This is a tricky situation. The discrepancy may stem from the doctor's own philosophy and policy towards pain relief and prescribing, or perhaps it reflects the doctor's own discomfort with unusual situations, such as might exist in a particular case. Sometimes the problem is due to trepidation that the doctor may cause harm, or feed into, a psychiatric problem. Doctors often fear being cleverly duped by the patient.

A central diagnostic impediment in pain management is that pain is just as subjective to those who report it as it is to those who measure it.

> "I know it seems odd to compare pain to love, but they are feelings, and each of us knows it differently within our souls and so each of us lives with it differently. You can't quantify my

measures of love. Even my actions may belie my level of love. The same goes for pain. I can love or be in pain and still function. My functioning reflects my other needs and my ability to deal with adversity. It has nothing to do with my pain or love. I just want to love more and be in pain less."

Psychiatric patients who also suffer from chronic pain can be complicated. They may live under layers and layers of different operating variables. But by the same token, having a psychiatric problem does not automatically complicate their pain management needs. If the emotional and pain treatment needs do complicate each other, then the doctor may have to work 'out of the box' if the patient's clinical needs don't fit inside the standard treatment box. Many doctors are not comfortable in this clinical corner. Many non-psychiatric professionals talk of and speak to the psychosocial aspects of a patient's life, but this is often just veilleity. (Velleity is a 'stated intent to do something', but the inclination to do that 'something' is in point of fact weak, rudimentary, or non-existent.) "My doctor spoke of my life issues, but it was just talk. He never went past mentioning it, like that was somehow enough. I got the feeling he didn't want to touch it." Later in this book we look at how a doctor's own style and personal comfort with complex cases can impact someone's pain.

I know a psychiatrist who admits he is afraid to prescribe medications outside of FDA accepted doses. He is not known for treating complex cases. I know another psychiatrist who has a boutique practice. She shows no shame announcing that she refers out all the really complicated cases. I had the fortune of treating one of her failures; the patient only needed higher doses of medication along with a higher dose of psychotherapy. This paradigm applies to complex pain patients as well. Clinical success is, time and again, often just a matter of giving the patient what they 'truly' need.

Too many pain patients have doctors who are unlikely to adjust a dose to match the patient's real needs. This may come from 'opioidphobia,' which is the aversion to the use of opioids. It is particularly evident if an unusually high opiate dose is needed. This phobia is often based more on a personal philosophy than science. Many patients do quite well with high doses: this too will be discussed later in the book. Patients don't know what a new doctor's dosing philosophy is until after they've entered treatment. Should the doctor be the only one on their insurance list, then the patient might be stuck in a bad situation.

It's hard to imagine that debates even occurred with regard to the safety and appropriateness of treating cancer pain.[30] This has changed. For a long time, many people believed that it was even inappropriate to give high doses of narcotics to the dying. Doctors who treated the dying were thought to be inappropriately practicing medicine, and for a while, it rose up to the level that some form of criminal activity might be placed against a doctor who aggressively treated the dying with narcotics. This is from Ann Alpers in 1998: "How is the growing awareness of dying patient's pain and the willingness of prosecutors to charge physicians with crimes connected? Pain at the end of life is frequently treated with narcotics, prescription drugs that are closely regulated by state and federal law. That complex web of laws and a growing fear of legal sanctions deterred physicians from prescribing controlled substances." She addressed the "actions brought against physicians for care, particularly pain control, at the end of life." [31]

Fortunately the debate on how to treat end of life pain is finally much less of an issue. Now the passionate focus has moved to how to treat the pain coming from nonterminal conditions. The hospice movement is credited for many of the improved pain control strategies for people who suffer pain while dying; we need a similar movement to focus on the pain for the non-dying patients. One impressive project involved with the hospice and palliative care movement is known as 'EPEC' – Education in Palliative and End of Life Care.[32]

> "My wife had tumors all over her body. I found a doc who treated her quite well as an outpatient, but when the infection hit, and she needed hospitalization, the hospital doctor cut her pain meds way back. I went crazy! I fired so many doctors over that....and in the hall I told one of them that I'd be just fine if we detox her in the grave, but until then, give her the meds. He didn't, and she died real fast. I think she died from the pain as much as the disease. She gave up. We never had a chance to get to hospice..."

A collective wish lives within pain managers to move away from narcotics. Though opioids control pain, they do not fix the cause. And while safer – in the right contexts – than many other interventions, opioids are not without side effects. The World Health Organization has a step-wise protocol of pain medication use that begins with the non-narcotics. But sometimes narcotics are simply needed. Using them is not a sign of failure, indulgence, or incompetence.

A lot of good science is being devoted to finding new pain controlling interventions, but we cannot forget that while the research is underway, patients sit in pain. Not controlling the pain means a life is being wasted.

Proper pain management was once a mission. Now it is a lucrative business. In the past there were generally two broad classes of pain management doctors: those who really cared and fought to convert a bad situation into a good one, and those who saw an economic window through which to sell pain medications, with an eye more on their own profit than on real clinical improvement. The horror stories that came out of this second, for-the-profit-group, raucously smacked the problems of seedy pain management right into the center of the public media arenas. When responsible media looked at the first group of doctors, the really-caring-ones, they saw how this small group of missionaries was indeed seeking to mend the ailing. But despite the articles and comments on proper pain management, the second group of doctors sold more newspapers.

Many pain patients do get adequate treatment. But too many don't. The public literature, such as the two *New York Times* pieces already referred to above, attest to the incredible level of inadequate pain treatment. An internet search of the responsible media sources will further support this. This problem lies as much within the doctors as it does within the patients.

Furthermore, consider that only as recently as in September 2008 did the US House of Representatives pass the "National Pain Care Policy Act of 2008" (HR 2994). The disquieting twist is that in the year 2008 there still needed to be a bill to improve pain care. Such a bill should not have even been necessary. Why do we, as medical professionals and a society, need an act of Congress to improve pain management? Here are few words from the bill: "Despite the fact that pain affects more than 76 million Americans – more than diabetes, heart disease and cancer combined – it remains woefully under treated and misunderstood. All too common are stories of patients in the grip of pain, who are left to consult multiple care providers before their pain is properly diagnosed and managed, if it ever is. Not only is unmanaged pain emotionally and physically debilitating for patients, it also places a heavy burden on family and caregivers..."

Managing that burden required the creation of new programs by the FDA and the Centers for Disease Control and Prevention. One program addressed the surge in accidental opioid (and other) overdoses.[33] By January 2009, the FDA reported that unintentional poisoning was the second leading cause of unintentional death, with 23,618 such incidents in 2005. Approximately 95% were due to drug overdoses, and half of those were associated with prescriptions. The new focus became on how doctors could safely prescribe controlled substances for proper pain management. One goal was to develop more objective and reliable methods to assess pain. We agree with that goal. An American Medical News article on this same topic supported the FDA-CDC program. [34]

*　*　*

It's terribly sad that a medical condition needed a process similar to the civil rights movement to force our community to transform its attitude towards those who suffer from the condition known as pain. Part of the problem was that the medical community did not know how to reliably categorize, interact with, and treat these patients. It was, unfortunately, also a medical arena much too open to abuse and exploitation.

This is a *person in pain* book that looks at these issues, and in doing so, hopefully it will invigorate, explain, soothe, exonerate, and empower anyone who suffers from pain.

CHAPTER TWO
How the pain started

Several years ago my wife needed surgery.

The type of surgery is not as important as is the fact that it failed. She was left with unbelievable and constant pain that brought all our lives to a complete stand still. What had been an active and vivacious woman become someone unable to live a life of her own choices. Following the surgery she had to always listen to the pain.

The pain controlled her. It kept her from sleeping. She needed large quantities of pain medications to reduce the pain just so she could eat. Her weight dropped. She became prone to infections. She stopped menstruating. And we began to fight.

The children watched their mother slip backwards. Friends and family did not understand such turmoil. People accused her of being an addict and of being irresponsible. She fell into a deep depression and required psychiatric care.

Some people never doubted her pain, but we felt they doubted its intensity. Why, she and I would ask, would good friends be so doubting?

Life was a tortuous merry-go-round. She had the pain in and of itself; she had the fear that she might never get better; and she felt the awful emotional anguish that came when some people began to doubt her.

Even I at times, in the midst of anger, fatigue, and complete frustration, could not understand how severely she suffered. We spoke of some dreadful things to each other during the months of pain. There is no pride in how low the pain brought us. But there is pride in that, little by little, we found ways to live with it. We used every resource we could find. It exhausted us emotionally, socially, and financially.

There was no shame in asking for help or changing doctors as we looked to so many people for help. We began to mature into the "chronic pain patient and family." Unfortunately, not all our friends matured with us.

Doctors' told us that she 'could not be in so much pain.' She would reply that there was certainly nothing to be gained by being so ill; her time in bed was never enjoyed. She hungered to be a normal mother and wife. Her anger at the medical system grew dark and vile as we spent thousands and thousands of dollars for treatments that did not work. I once said that our lives were under the microscope because of how people looked at us. Later I realized it was more like being under a big gun because of how other people doubted us. Sure, some doctors believed in her pain and pathology, but oh how quickly and happily they left the pain management to others.

Finally, we found a doctor who could correct the basic damage. He was able to remove well over 99% of the pain. He was the 26th doctor that we consulted. We know how fortunate we were. It took a medically radical and permanent procedure to help her, but she is lucky in that the deficits from the corrective procedure are minor. So we are lucky, very lucky. But the good fortune is a tempered by the fear that the pain might return. We were told that it might. Now, even little pains trigger the most awful fears. We are both fighters, but honestly, we don't know if we could sustain another battle.

She, as a nurse, and I, as a physician, now approach pain patients with a new attitude and empathy. She presently functions in management levels of a hospice. She even started a program for the palliative care of children.

Both of us, each in our own ways, have been wounded by a disbelieving system that far too frequently took large amounts of our money, that claimed to be experts in pain control, that would not risk themselves to help us, and that so comfortably came to inaccurate, premature, and unsubstantiated presumptions about our motives. This all caused pain in its own style. And the psychological price tag for all this is still a long way from being paid off.

So what is pain?

Pain is a 'warning sign that something is wrong.' Pain's purpose is to trigger mechanisms to reduce, correct, or remove the problem. Biopsychosocial homeostasis is the goal. This means that pain wants itself to be removed from your body and your world. Pain screams "get rid of me!" It wants you to get back to a comfortable balance in life. But until it gone, pain controls in so many ways. It is then so disheartening when the sufferer begins to pick up the static and standoffs in the pain management system. The patient quickly learns how much is wrong both with his body and the pain management treatment systems. Many quickly learn that getting proper pain care is as much a financial and political process as it is a clinical one.

Pain is an 'emergency to the body, mind and soul.' Chronic pain means that our body's 'repairing skills' can't resolve the emergency causing the pain. Unending pain is not natural. Its on-going presence keeps the person from homeostasis. Uncontrolled pain can overwhelm the psychological ability to adapt. Proper pain management, therefore, pleads for more than medical interventions. Good treatment requires a personalized tool set that is compounded from the sum and product of a person's medical access and the evolving attitude towards one's fate and the quality of life. Making the tool set can be difficult.

CHAPTER THREE
Different but typical cases

A young lady sustained a minor facial bone fracture. It initially seemed like a minor injury, but it threw her into a 30 year odyssey of failed surgeries, pain worsening implants, pain clinics, biofeedback, psychotherapy, diagnostic procedures, lost of her job and marriage, needing lawyers, living on disability, and having to go through numerous consultations that never corrected the injury nor removed the layers of psychological trauma and pain.

Her life became a standstill. The better part of her day was spent warding off pain. Her need for medication was very high. She knew her own pain cycles: some of them were so bad that no amount of medication could stop the pain. She called these her 'pain attacks.' Many of her doctors said there is no such thing as a pain attack. She knew they were wrong.

In all fairness, there were also times when she needed less medication. But she could never be without it.

She called herself the 'weather lady' because she could feel barometric pressures go up and down. The capsules around the surgically invaded joints had became unusually thick, so when the outside air pressure dropped (perhaps from an incoming storm), the capsules stretched. And that hurt. The normal biological process of releasing the inside pressure was blocked, leaving her with an "over-stuffed balloon inside me" that caused pain. She called it the 'soon-to-rain pain.'

She hated her medication. It symbolized everything wrong in her life. It also symbolized the anger at what had happened to her. It was a constant reminder of how limited she'd become, of how she must never leave the house without first checking her medication supply, and of how she no longer could be spontaneous and be away from home for unplanned periods of time. She equated how her relationship with medication was the same as a dialysis patient's relationship is to the dialysis machine. But unlike someone who cannot be away from a dialysis machine for more than 1 or 2 days, she cannot be as far away from her medications. "I don't even have those 1-2 days. Kidney failure would be better than this pain."

> *Her body's pain control system can't manage the pain, so as the dialysis patient needs a machine, she needs pharmaceuticals to keep her alive.*

She waits for things to get better. And she refuses to give up hope that someday, somehow, something will put an end to her odyssey. "I'm the 'three-some-lady' – some-day, some-how, some-thing." She described her malady as a 'pain illness'.

Before the adequate dose of medications was found, she often fell into nasty pits of desperation. She remembers how many nights she would scream with pain. "Death would have been ok, but I really didn't want to die." Her pain was marked by hours of "hot ice picks going up through my face." Even with the better medication doses, the pain attacks still occasionally "got past the fence and came to visit me…..I began to wonder why I was being stalked and punished….."

What unraveled and aggravated her, in ways and with feelings so big it was beyond her ability to put them into words, was how easily people called her an addict. She told me "I need narcotics to survive. No such label is put on people who need dialysis to survive."

She often pondered if she could draw a line between the mere 'existence of life' and a 'quality of a life.' "I exist but without quality. Where is there real joy? I don't know." She wondered if an artist sketched her, how could he reference her quality?

Her 'pain illness' eventually developed complications from other illnesses. She suffered greatly. But her spirit never faulted. She spent years reaching out to other pain patients, trying to teach them what she had learned about surviving the battles with the pain. Those contacts, with the 'thank you's' that followed, were the roots that fed her soul. She rarely credited herself with any legacy, but her humility blurred her own vision to the good she left inside the souls of others.

Many other cases are not as dramatic as hers, but the sufferings are nonetheless similar. I have seen people with post-injury pains, clear-cut disease causing pains, and even some can't-be-explained pains. One lady had a sciatic type pain which defied all neurological diagnosis. A middle aged man had incredible neuropathy in both feet. A hard working woman's knees challenged her every day with ruthless arthritic pain. A 40 year old woman was thrown by an accidental electrical shock that left her with cruel shoulder pain. A lawyer could not find relief from pitiless migraines. A former motorcyclist suffered severe and daily post-injury pain. Another lawyer's pain came from collapsing vertebrae. The list is endless, yet it has a common and sturdy dominator: they all hate their pain, their lives were good before the pain, aggressive treatment and medication use enhanced their lives, and they had journals and journals of tales of how hard they had to fight to get effective treatment.

Patients Who Lie to Doctors

A few patients have lied to me.

I suspect I was tricked and deceived about 3-4% of the time. I attribute this low rate to the resolute infusion of psychiatry into my pain management. Looking back, I see that two people definitely conned me. I must say, however, they did so both to me and others in a masterfully criminal manner. Indeed, their criminal skills would make for a good movie. But their schemes failed.

Only a very few number of patients altered prescriptions or acted such that I had no choice but to discharge them from my practice. But the vast majority patients, some of whom did fudge or connive a little, but who stuck with me, and me with them, got better. They learned to be honest with themselves. It was not always a smooth process.

Those with whom we had to part clinical ways clearly suffered from such large concurrent problems that, for a sundry of reasons, I could not address. I wonder that if resources had been different, then perhaps some of those people would have been graduates rather than expulsions or drop-outs.

Those who lie to doctors are frequently labeled as doctor shoppers. They go from doctor to doctor asking for prescriptions. Various states are trying to stop doctor shopping by using central computers to monitor all narcotic prescriptions. If a pattern of duplicate prescriptions is detected, then the doctors are notified and the prescriptions will not be automatically filled. Other sanctions may occur. This may not eliminate the dishonest patient who sees only one doctor, but it will curtail the ability to go from office to office, like a honey bee, gathering prescriptions to be filled at several drug stores. Electronic prescription writing software reduces also fraud and alterations since the patient is never handed a written prescription.

Many states are beginning to limit the use of web based, on-line pharmacies by insisting that the patient needs to have a legitimate script based on a real relationship with a prescriber. Though possible, it's harder to lie when face to face with the doctor.

CHAPTER FOUR

Do doctors understand what life is like for the chronic pain patient?

It's astonishing how many patients feel that their doctors do not understand them.

It is getting much better, though. Many doctors are trying to understand, and they are trying to show a richer concern to their patients. But patients and doctors live in different worlds, and the gaps between them are so large that it may never be easy to bridge.

Some doctors chose not to open themselves to what life is really like for their patients. Doctors have their own sense of where they draw the limits of their own professional responsibility. And the patient's own expectations may not match how the doctor chooses to practice medicine. Understanding these differences will often explain the riddle as to why a better doctor-patient relationship might not exist.

The doctors who keep an emotional distance from their patients might be explained as a means to protect themselves from their own emotional reactions to an endless exposure to human misery. But maintaining this distance could effectively deflate and suspend the creation and positive use of empathy with the patients' suffering. Many doctors may not realize that maintaining this position uncouples them from their patient, and it may additionally serve to help them deny their own unique roles in their treatment failures.

Though callous, the fact is also that some doctors don't care about their patients as people. A patient might be no more than a customer. One patient said that his doctor's vocabulary is limited to the word "next...!"

> "I got the feeling he was probably a good guy in parts of life, but medicine was a business to him, and he was quick and superficial and I was just a machine needing repair. No more, no less. He didn't need me to survive, but I needed him. He didn't talk to me! Asking for more time with him was like taking food away from his kids.... he smiled, he nodded, but his karma said he wasn't interested."

Many pain management doctors deal better with pain if it is limited to an intellectual event. This is why they chose professions that did not require honed psychiatric skills. Pain is a straightforward situation that they try to relieve. Many may radiate an acknowledgement of the emotional aspects of endless pain, but they pass the care of those problems to others.

Pain is both an emotional and physical event to its sufferers. Patients therefore don't usually reject their doctor's psychological referrals, but they often say that they would like "at least little of that balm to come from their primary doctors..."

The emotionally disruptive aspects of pain ought to dissipate if the pain is relieved. But the 'pain disruptors' are very much alive when the pain is not gone. *Pain is an omnipresent exasperation to its sufferers.*

One patient captured this notion this way: "Suffering dwells in the pain. It is the parasite. I am the host..."

It is amazing how often professionals advise patients that their 'reported pain is in excess of the pathology.' This comment tacitly suggests that the patient gets some pleasure or secondary gain from being in pain. This is often far from the truth. It is an unforgivable insult to even suggest it. But it reflects how the doctor interprets the patient's reports. One patient asked if I knew "what my pain management doctors really thought about me?"

> She saw the second opinion doctor for one hour. His questions were clearly written by someone else, and he didn't encourage unsolicited extra information. He wrote the insurance company that in his professional opinion the patient was malingering. She subsequently called the IME doctor to ask what facet of non-genuine professional medicine did he follow. That so irritated him that he then amended his report to say she was also hostile.
>
> She asked me where his attitudes came from. I couldn't offer any of his personal history, but I could say that he didn't seem to want to open the gate to the rest of her life.
>
> By the way, her lawyers had a field day with him.

Another problem is that so many medical team members are too reckless when they consider constant pain complaints as ploys to get narcotic medications. The larger problem is that the mere allegation of this can flush like a tsunami to blemish a legitimate patient's clinical records. Such a slapdash attitude and remark can destroy any clinical trust in both directions, from doctor to patient and from patient to doctor. Later in this book are suggestions on how to re-build that trust level.

> A man was hit by a train. Numerous bones were fractured and he could not thereafter walk or use his hands as he could before the injury. At deposition the opposing lawyer used questions

from an insurance company physician, suggesting pre-existing injuries following a minor tricycle accident when he was 4 years old and that now he only wanted his pain meds and money. The patient lost his sensibility but did so with precision, saying that he did fall off his bike as a child but between then and the current accident he lead a perfectly normal life. He asked the lawyer to ask their physician to explain these intervening 43 years. The case soon settled for the patient's benefit.

After the settlement, the patient told me: "What got to me is that the other lawyers wanted to give my doctor some doubt about me being real. They scared my doc a little. So he and I had a real good talk. I began to feel that he began to wonder, maybe even doubted me, and then I began to doubt him 'cause our sessions felt more distant, kinda less comfortable,' if ya know what I mean. I wanted him to trust me. After we talked, 'cause he's a good guy, he said he always wanted to trust me too, but he was scared he missed something, because of the hoopla about addicts and all. Anyway, we'd fixed the cracks in the wall and we both feel better...."

It is sad, but even well intended and honorable doctors are not immune from being lied to by patients. As such, every doctor has to approach new patients by being doubtful and tough. No one has sufficient radar to always perfectly gauge another person's honesty.

A patient may not know of his new doctor's fears. So it may appear safer in the beginning for everyone, doctor and patient, to doubt more than trust, despite the chilling effect it can have on the first rounds of a relationship. But unfeigned integrity and assurance will emerge over time.

These are some concerns and observations:

> Some of a "doctor's defensive attitude" can come from how patients act. Most every doctor has heard comments such as "Hey thanks doc, but I forgot my check book, but don't worry, send me the bill and I'll personally see that you get paid, and thanks for the script, by the way," but the bill is never paid.
>
> Or: "Gee doc, I really wanted something else from you, so I'm not coming back. And you can forget ever getting paid from me. Your staff has a bad attitude too, and I'm calling the medical society on you."
>
> Or: "Wait, I don't think Medicare should pay you for that. I'm reporting you as fraudulent just like it tells me to do on the paper that comes with my Medicare check."
>
> Or: perhaps a doctor gets a letter from the medical board suggesting he is not treating a patient in an appropriate way. But the patient is an extraordinary case! The investigators start with only limited information about the case, so the doctor effectively goes 'on trial', needs lawyers to defend him, and risks being scolded or sanctioned because he made the treatment fit the disease. Only after much costly legal bantering might the full dimension of the case be finally reviewed. (This assumes the doctor

did treat in a defensible manner.) Because this situation happens to even good doctors, it results in many doctors being frightened to do things which might raise 'flags.'

Some doctors, as with any profession, are unquestionably in business only for the money, but fortunately the great majority just want a reasonable courtesy, a working doctor-patient relationship, and reasonable payment for their work. They want to trust their patient's motivations and honesty. They enjoy and want to help their patients. They want an easy and productive practice style.

Another issue among doctors is the result of the climate of their training. Patients are not aware of how this infuses predispositions in many doctors. Many doctors have a very difficult time admitting to errors. Patients often see an arrogant quality if a treatment course is questioned or fails. Doctors train to be good decision makers but they are not as good at selling their decisions to uncertain and inquiring customers or with dealing with failures. Sometimes the frustration is also a function of the limited amount of time that a doctor can afford to spend with any single patient. Doctor's are rarely, if ever, trained on how to admit and correct errors, diplomatically manage their frustrations, etc.

> A man brought his wife to the hospital. She was obstreperous and the doctor was losing his patience. So the husband of the lady in the adjacent bed, a retired successful salesman, and who could not have ignored the energetic neighboring conversation, said to the doctor: "Let me do your work, doc, give me a few minutes." He spoke to the unruly patient, with good success. He accomplished what the doctor had failed to do.

Most medical training tends to overplay those patients who 'might' be misusing drugs. One cannot fault the schools and books for making note of this possibility, but it is often discussed in a fashion which hints that patients who fail to respond to 'reasonable' treatments are predominantly 'drug seeking.'

Doctors don't like to be called gullible or foolish. So treating subjective pain often introduces reservations about clinical precision. As noted elsewhere, it is so much easier to report than to measure pain. Exploring for an explanation and motivation for drug abuse is incredibly complex. Most non-psychiatrists have limited or no patience for it. Non-psychiatric physicians don't see this problem as one they want to solve.

Another frequent grievance is how often treatment teams seem to place the reason for treatment failure onto the patient. This is especially so in chronic pain management. Many patients report this feeling! The blame, however, rightly rests with medical science for not yet being able to resolve either the physical or emotional problems causing the pain.

Patients long for the doctor who will hold their hands while saying "I'm sorry too, I know how hard this failure must be..." If the pain cannot be fixed then the doctor ought to treat the suffering. Patients can accept that a mechanical technique or medication falls short. Patients cannot accept when doctors fall short of being human.

But why does this happen? It happens because the treatment of suffering requires a shift from being an *objective* clinician to being a *subjective* human being. The doctor has to move back and forth from the objective to the subjective. It means subjectively extending emotional energy to patients, or sitting for long periods of time with someone who is suffering. Then they also have to be equally skilled with the hard science objective skills. This aspect of medical care – to be both skilled and compassionate – is so wanted by patients. TV medical shows, such as *Gray's Anatomy*, are all about this.

Too many doctors consider the subjective as soft science. It is also a risky immersion into ministering for which many are untrained or with which they are personally uncomfortable. Doctor's tend to prefer being the mechanical (procedural or pharmaceutical) heroes from which the basic improvements emerge. They shy away from the comprehensive emotional part of the healing process; it is not the heroic role they want. But it is so unbelievably impressive and heroic when a doctor spends a little time in this arena! We tend to let physicians slip away from this role, assigning it to the nurses, clergy, social workers and others. Doing so suggests that doctors have grander and more critical scientific skills that excuse them from the emotional aspects of a patient's life. This is wrong, so very wrong. The special skills needed to heal human emotions is too often not part of the physicians' self-selected tool kit.

The patient's unswerving heroes are often the therapists, nurses and others with whom they commiserate, vent, touch, and share their lives. They give the hero labels to those who sweat with them, or are up at night with them, share being scared with them, and who understand what it is like not to be able to eat, travel, have sex, or just to sit in a movie theater. It means having someone with whom to unhurriedly share a destroyed, out of control, or markedly handicapped life. It means time to ponder and explore fears, or just feel some genuine emotional support. Interestingly, patients do not routinely expect much of this from their doctors, so when it happens, even for only a few moments, the effect is profound. Patients know a doctor may not have the time to be a therapist. But getting even a little time and 'touching' from the doctor is water to a thirsty person.

Many doctors chose not to use this type of medical model. It is too akin to psychotherapy. So they shy away. Might this mean that many doctors *are afraid* of their patient's real lives?

> A medical staff committee accused a doctor of getting emotionally involved in a female patient's care. "I have never seen a doctor be so concerned! It looks like there is some over-familiarity here," said one of the committee members. When confronted, the doctor argued back that his 'emotional concern' was only human and proper clinical advocacy and decency. But this concern was misinterpreted as if he was not being totally professional with his patient. Yet his style of concern allowed him to better know her, which ultimately made for a quicker and more successful treatment. Nonetheless, many of his colleagues still labeled him as non-professional.

Life, for those chronically in pain, has to be built around the pain producing handicap. But why do so many good people in chronic pain have such a difficult time building this existence?

> "How can I say it more? The damn pain is with me all the time, just all the time. There is never a free moment, never. I'm a slave, bound to a master who hates me...teach me how to be different! It sucks all the energy out me. And I don't have the money to hire cooks and shoppers and house cleaners. How do I change?

In court the lawyer asked me why I wasn't suing for lack of consortium. I said I can live without sex. I can't live in a dirty house, so I am really suing for lack of vacuuming! The jury laughed because they knew I was right. "

Pain treatment is complicated. Pain is not always the same from moment to moment, and what are tolerable levels of pain for one person may not be tolerable for another. The sum of these patterns, blended with the countless lists of a person's life's variables, becomes the '*signature of a pain patient*'. To understand a person is to know their signature. Similar signatures also exist for every pain treating professional, and these configurations can be called the 'signature of a professional'. This will be discussed later in much greater detail.

A person's cultural background is one very powerful signature variable. Bates wrote an excellent book on the topic.[35] "Therefore," she said, "if one is raised in a cultural environment which accepts and encourages (or on the other hand, prohibits and discourages) an outward emotional expression of pain, or in one that defines focusing attention on the pain as either an appropriate or inappropriate response, these culturally acquired patterns not only may lead to certain types of reporting, but also to different levels of perceived pain intensity."

We all need to be keenly aware of our own psychological projections. Doctors need to therapeutically engage and intermingle with the unique biases and cultural aspects of their patients' worlds. They also need to know what biases and cultural aspects they bring into their medical practices. The need for this type of insight applies to patient and doctor.

It is interesting to compare pain threshold tolerances. A general consensus exists that some eastern European groups better tolerate pain than do Westerner's. It may be a matter of attitude or pride. Perhaps they are more embarrassed to show pain because it implies some moral or spiritual shortcoming. It may also be that they have some genetic qualities which can better resist or ignore pain.

Happier and more content people are not necessarily better able to handle pain. Certainly a vivacious or peaceful life may reduce the impact of pain, but it does not eliminate it. In fact, to understand a pain patient requires that a treatment team know what the person was like before the pain started.

Depression is different. It can heighten pain. Depression also wears many faces, and not all depressions are biologically based and so they may not respond to medications.

> "I went to my daughter's recital. Everyone thought I was in less pain because I was obviously enjoying myself so much. But such 'emotional raptures' live more in the memory than in real life, and I will gladly suffer the aftermath pain to have a nice memory of her on the stage. But once at home, honestly, there was no way I could maintain that frame of mind. The doctor wanted me to take a mood lifter pill. No, it's not needed. I'm not depressed. But I'm sure disappointed in where life is taking me..... but then he said the mood lifter pill might also reduce pain transmission – so I tried it. But I'm not depressed."

People who 'tough it out' when they choose to use less medication too often set an unrealistic and poorly grounded standard for everyone. It is as if the person who needs less medication is somehow superior, stronger, less blemished, or less psychologically flawed than someone who needs more medication. Let's ask three questions before we bestow some special quality on those 'those who need less medication':

> Are their pains equal?
>
> Are their biological systems equal?
>
> Are their psychological, social, economic or religious bridles equal?

The core question is 'how does any particular person respond to the pain?' A whole host of problems pop up because a 'response to pain' is subjective. Furthermore, the actual report of pain can be flavored by the atmosphere created by those who ask about the pain. It is known as the halo effect. This is an interesting concept:

A 'treatment response' is typically 'fashioned' by the patient's background character, culture, etc. So a treatment response report may not be what is truly happening because the doctor and patient have not developed working understandings of each other's biases, etc. This is where many doctor-patient problems are born. For example, it can be a matter of how one makes or reads facial expressions. Facial expressions are telling indictors of emotions. One recent book devotes a chapter to the facial expressions of pain.[36] A stoic facial expression may be interpreted as a good treatment response since pain expressions are not being seen, though the pain truly exists. The patient might feel they have to appear stoic when they feel the opposite because they fear being honest. The reason for that fear can emerge for many reasons, and they have to be explored for a proper doctor-patient relationship to exist.

To fashion a response is a very common human event. Just because someone can psychologically 'shape' a response is not necessarily positive evidence that the patient is 'shaping' the pain as well. This rather convoluted notion is best explained by examples:

> A patient complains of pain. Part of the description of the pain is based on the patient's character: does he whine, does he laugh, is he strong, is he weak, etc. These psychological characteristics paint the patient's signatures, and it is with this data that a doctor measures the effect of pain treatment.
>
> Another patient may not want to alienate the doctor, so he may shape his reports to the doctor by downplaying the pain's intensity. The doctor considers that 'veneer' as valid evidence of deep and good pain control. A patient's anticipation of the doctor's attitude also shapes how the patient reports his response to the treatment. This may keep the treatment alive, even if it is suboptimal, because the doctor is happy and "she will still treat me." Shaping the response does not necessarily mean that the person is lying or faking about the core problem. This predicament is usually resolved if the doctor spends enough time to really get to know his patient, and the patient feels safe enough to be honest.

These are all parts of a patient's pain signature.

One patient felt he was in a contest to see who can tolerate the most pain. The contest came from his Biblical upbringing about the role of pain in life and the honor bestowed on those best able to tolerate pain. The mastering of *physical pain* was a powerful tool because it is assumed to lead to *emotional or philosophical pain;* this pain, in turn, would (in his world) mature into wisdom. Pain, therefore, was beneficial. The more pain he suffered, the closer he would get to purer levels of religious illumination, explanation, and consecration. Should a doctor hold similar beliefs, and so expect this of his patients, then the atmosphere of his practice will accordingly contour the style, limits, expectations, and allowances of his relationships with his patients. These beliefs can grow into spoken and unspoken guidelines about how to treat, what to expect, how to approach failures, and how to show gratitude for treatment.

This is not a minor problem, even among psychiatrists. Even bipolar disorders are often misdiagnosed if clinicians rely on their own "theoretical orientations" rather than adhering to established guidelines."[37] Studies report that it may take years before a correct psychiatric diagnosis is made. Might this also be a problem in pain management circles? Must a patient fit the doctor's orientation? How is the patient sure the doctor is offering objectively correct treatment?

Let's track the thought a bit more. Countless times a day non-addicts needing chronic pain medications are labeled as 'addicted.' We suspect many of those professionals who do this labeling are doing so to protect themselves. I've seen many professionals claim their diagnosis was correct, and they stick to their argument by insisting on the validly of their criterion, even when the data shows differently. Maybe they do this because they are simply biased, naïve, or, as some people feel, they do it to show off their own self-declared and overconfident clinical acuity.

'Addict' is as pejorative a word as one can use. Put that word on a medical chart and it will never go away. The flawed assumption is that the doctor who wrote it down truly met the proper clinical standards to support the diagnosis. The standard of diagnosis properly demands a detailed look at the person, the reasons for the drug use, etc. But to far too many people, just because a professional wrote it down is taken to mean that the conclusion is correct. In reality, the assumptions leading up to many of these chart 'addiction' notes are often untested, or even flawed. These 'opinions' are converted to the status of 'facts.' Such conversions are dangerous.

In all likelihood, most non-psychiatric physicians could not spontaneously give a fully defensible definition of addiction. (We will later do so.) The term is too cavalierly tossed about without consideration of its impact. Imagine the hurt of inappropriately being called an addict!

The 'first words' spoken about someone can leave hard to erase scars. The scars can become unfounded legacies. Weigh in to the differences suggested by the notions of 'addict' as compared to a label that says the patient is 'medication dependent secondary to untreatable or chronic pain.'

Now we move to the 'hunt.' I've seen it many times. Many deny that it exists, but it is quite real. The hunting doctor wants to be smart enough to find the truth that no one else could find. The social reward of the hunt is that "the unexplained has been explained….and I was smart enough to find it!" This is a spin-off of the competition felt by doctors-in-training.

Many doctors faced with treatment failures or unresolving, troubling challenges will begin the hunt. Many times the hunt produces a label that uses ill-described psychiatric conundrums to explain why the doctor and his skill set cannot be the reason for the failure. It can be posted as a short 'label', such as 'the patient is manipulative," or it can live in the subtle but real tenor of their chart notes.

The hunt confuses subsequent professionals because it fails to honestly report the real complexity of the case.

Chart data may be written in a way to filter and support the hunt and its conclusions. Hard clinical data is polluted with editorials. Good forensic evaluations and lawyers always want to know what was not written in a chart. Remember that every chart is slanted because the writer chooses what data to include or exclude. We assume the chart is always scientifically objective. It is not.

So 'a hunt' is an effort to rationalize. It is a defense mechanism on the part of the treatment team as they face failure.

Hunters often use a psychiatric diagnosis as the reason for the treatment failure. But isn't it so disquieting that the "psychiatric" diagnosis slipped by when the patient first started treatment, despite a supposingly thorough initial diagnostic work-up. One has to wonder why it was missed at the start.

Some doctors don't employ the hunt. They just discharge the patient from their practices.

> Joe suffered a rapid onset of terrible elbow discomfort. Repeated evaluations found no hard pathology but those around him agreed he was in enormous distress. He appeared in pain, and no psychological reason for this existed. He tended to be a hypochondriac as well. He read about every side effect to every drug he had ever been prescribed, and he often refused a treatment because of his fears. In truth, that made him so annoying to so many. Some nurses wanted to tell him "get a grip," "don't worry so much," or "get over it." Of course that only inflamed the situation on both sides. Little by little his attitudes offended so many doctors that his chart reflected his saga with comments such as

"he is crazy, unrealistic, spoiled, too difficult, and non-cooperative." Notes of this obsessive preoccupation did not exist in the intake summary at the pain clinic. But the chart was riddled with such notations during the last few months of affiliation with the clinic. Finding a new pain management team was difficult because the chart notes from the former doctor "made me look more psychiatric than pain. Those notes never reflected that all I needed was some time with the doctor to work with the doses slowly. And if I got better, I'd be different too. Part of my behavior was because the pain wasn't being controlled. I think they really just wanted me out of there."

Eventually a sophisticated psychologist began to work with him. He needed to have his hand patiently held at the same time he was being kicked in the toosh. But he learned to be less fearful, and a new pain treatment team began to work well with him.

There are some nasty spin offs from the hunt. Too often people get a diagnosis of malingering or of a borderline personality disorder. Patients may be told that they are addicted to the sick role, or that they are accused of manipulating the system for money gain. The diagnosing health care team is often just plain wrong more commonly than we want to count.

Chronic suffering can produce a demanding person. Doctors don't like demanding patients. The question to be asked is this: why is this person so demanding? A doctor's professionalism lies not so much in remembering to ask this question, but in the ability to sift through the answers and arrive at a genuine list of motivations so a proper treatment can be developed.

Multi-approach pain clinics are becoming more popular. Some are very good, yet so many pain patients do not get their treatment in such clinics. Instead they see general practitioners or go to walk-in clinics. Typically most patients have no well trained mental health professional to provide on-going psychotherapy to explore and modify the unrelenting existence and reality of their suffering. If these mental health efforts do occur, they are often too brief, and stop when the insurance ends. But by the same token, not all mature pain patients need psychotherapy.

> "The first clinic had a psychology guy and he was good but he didn't have the grit to tell the doctor I needed more meds. The second clinic had no psychology people but I got all the meds I needed, even with less time in the office. That didn't feel right, so the third clinic hit the spot but it was like hitting a concrete wall – a dead stop when the insurance said no more. The doctor said he would fight for more time if I paid for his time to write the letters. Ok, I understand he needs to be paid for the work, but I can't afford 30 minutes of his time that insurance won't pay for. I said, hey, let's do the letter in a session! He said okay, but his sessions were only 10-15 minutes, and that wasn't enough time, so I got charged for the doctor's extra time. I'm on disability. The insurance company said no to the appeal and they wanted the doctor to appeal again! But it was again at my cost, and the doctor told me I best see a lawyer 'cause he felt a fight was brewing. I then went to my

> general MD who gave me only one month's supply of meds until I found a new doctor. Lord, doctor's have the power to take the pain away with only a prescription if someone pays for it. I don't understand. I'm sinking here, I don't understand. And ya know what, I am paying for it in pain because they won't pay for it in money! I'm holding it back, but one hell of a nasty attitude is growing inside me."

This clinical scenario is far too common. A financial stalemate forces a transfer to a doctor who is comparably under-skilled, ill-equipped, or too afraid to carry on with adequate treatment of the chronic pain patient. The result is that the patient falls into a middle land between no or inadequate care.

Many doctors feel sympathetic but do not act on that sympathy. This is often not an issue if the treatment is straightforward, ordinary and successful: patient's comfortably put up with less than engageable treatment team personalities when things work and there is reduced pain and suffering.

On the whole, pain clinic doctors are mechanics. This is fine since someone must do the invasive procedures or dole out medications. (Some psychiatrists act this way as well. Medications are their 'procedures.') If these doctors avoid the non-procedure related or medication controlled emotional problems in their patients, it is not a fault, per se, but merely a description of their chosen philosophical positions.

One particularly annoying label is that 'the patient's pain has a supra-tentorial component'. This is not an official label. Instead it is a slovenly opinion that the pain is not real and that it is only imagined by the part of the brain which lies above the tentorium (the tentorium is a sheath in the brain, above which is the cortex where many of our thoughts are generated.) In simple terms, this translates to this: "I doubt if the pain is as real or as bad as she is reporting." This attitude infuses doubt about the pain's origin. It's an implied psychiatric diagnosis.

Many doctors would probably be more aggressive in their treatment if they weren't so fearful of legal sanctions. Doctors are overwhelmed with regulations and insurance impositions. They have to act according to a 'cook book' of medicine – this is sometimes called 'evidence based medicine'. On the whole this may serve some safely purpose because it insists on at least a minimum standard of care. But people and their needs are not consistent. Exceptions have to be allowed. Consultations and documentation may support the need for unusual or expensive treatments. The problem lies in the time, commitment, and money needed to do all this work.

The methods by which doctors are expected to work, given similar situations, is known as the community standard of care. A doctor who treats differently, or out of the 'standard of care', will often see his work 'reviewed' with the objective to protect patients from dangerous or dodgy treatments. Even good clinical outcomes, with superb documentation and appropriate consultations from other doctors can place a doctor into an excruciating and bottomless jeopardy because with unusual cases, the standards of care are often more subjective than not, since what is questionable science today may be good science tomorrow. This problem can have political aspects as well, since so many people judge by the headlines and not the details of a story. The emotional and financial costs to assemble a defense can be overwhelming, so doctors often refuse to risk themselves even if the clinical base is warranted.

> The standards of care are not an absolute list of criterion. In March 2008, Trescot wrote about

treatment guidelines: "These guidelines are based on the best available evidence and do not constitute inflexible treatment recommendations. Because of the changing body of evidence, this document is not intended to be a 'standard of care'." [38]

Another problem is that all the doctors in the community are not equally skilled. The best are often pulled down by the worse. In court the worse and the best doctor may both get the same stamp of "an expert." A lay jury often cannot appreciate the subtleties of differing clinical opinions and skills.

"My brother and I have the same arthritis. But we have different insurance companies. So we have different pain doctors. He is doing great – which pleases me to see him like that! But I am doing just ok. I bring his treatment protocols to my doctor, but I'm told he doesn't believe in such aggressive treatment. So I switched to my brother's. We'll just had to accept the out of pocket costs.

And I am better, thank you."

Several years ago it was considered outside the community standard of care to give high doses of a medication for panic disorders. Doctors who did so feared reprimands and accusations of fostering addiction or of covering up the 'real' causes of the panic. Pharmacies were reluctant to dispense high doses of medications. Insurance companies refused to pay for these higher doses of medications. But psychiatrists knew that patients were getting better on the higher doses, so to provide these patients with effective treatment, the doctor's continued their non-standard treatments. Now, higher doses are well established, and it can be outside the standards of care not to use them. The same occurred with pain control – it is now outside the standard of care to under treat a pain. In short, what was once considered dangerous is now considered appropriate and wise.

The "standards of care" for non-terminally ill patients once centered more on the technical aspects of care than on the moral or ethical aspects. I saw a case in which a pain management doctor said that they will not give high dose pain medications to a non-terminally ill patient. Yet in this same case, other experts felt that using higher doses of medications was appropriate. So where is that elusive, but so powerful and commanding, ultimate standard?

> A committee reviewed a doctor's care plan for a non-terminally ill pain patient. One committee doctor, considered a basically a good person, who otherwise tried to provide very reasonable medical care, reviewed the case. He noted that the side effects of the pain medications were serious and "given what's happening to this woman, wouldn't you rather let her suffer the pain than add all these other problems stemming from the narcotics?" He chose to overlook the suffering in favor of what, in his mind, was the lesser evil in a high risk patient for whom there was basically no quality in life unless someone took the risk of treating her horrible pain. The patient's husband asked the doctor why he thought that way. He then found another hospital for his wife.

Too often the medical community chooses to focus on the danger of the pain medications but not on the danger of the pain itself. That second danger is known as suffering. When doctors cannot cure the pain, then they should at least address the suffering. Not doing so is human cruelty.

But remember too that doctors are only people, who by training are well educated, but who still host all the known varieties of human emotions, fears, logic, and illogic. Don't give them more credit or authority then they deserve. Some are angels who help as much as possible. Some are trained but simple mechanics, and some are just business people running retail therapy shops.

...Thought...

> Why are people cruel to each other? The beginnings of this might come from a Biblical theory about the origins of violence. Cruelty appears when people do not recognize in another that which is the essence of their own being, and so they can turn away from others and do not have to hear their pain. People try to protect themselves from knowing other's pain by believing that these "other people" are not really human beings just like themselves. It is therefore possible to turn their backs on others' pain without moral difficulty.

...Thought...

> "Me and my wife, we're not fancy folks, no, not fancy at all. But she's a fine woman and got's a heart'n soul big as they come. Couple months back she took a fall, broke her leg and been into and out of hospitals since. That leg is bad, real bad, and she limps worst than a sick horse, if ya know what I'd be meaning.

We went to a Doc hereabouts and he did his best, bless his soul, but he'd said this is too complex a problem for him, so off we went to the university. Had to get my boss to give me some time off, and my wife, she wouldn't go until she finished some chores 'cause that's the way she is. I knowed it hurt her bad to do those chores, but she made a promise and a promise is her way.

So we went up to university and, oh, what a big place! The people were all kinda nice, mostly, and the doctor looked and touched, and looked and touched some more, then he said she'd need an operation. So okay, she had it done and 'bout a week later we came home. But the pain never did go away. We'd call him and at times we had to be so childish, but we'd have to beg the man for help 'cause the pain was bad and all she'd do is sit in the chair and I could see it on her face that she weren't right. She and my son would be fighting more than usual, and I'd hear her up and down all night. Broke my heart, it just broke my heart cause the doctor wouldn't give no pain meds. That went on for a couple weeks, and I could see she was losing her mind, but she was losing it all by herself. She's a proud woman and ain't going to give in easy, so she kept that outside face up real good, but I know my lady's eyes, I do, I do, and I saw her loosing it inside. So off we go back to university. And the doctor, he'd look and touch and look and touch again, and then he said there ain't nothing wrong! Why, I don't think my mouth and eyes could open any wider! Nothing wrong? Nothing wrong?

I said, doc, you got this all wrong, all wrong. And he said no, he did not, and then he asked a social worker to talk to us. And I'll never get over it, but she asked if our marriage was good! She asked if we were planning to sue the man who owned the sidewalk where she fell. She asked me if sometimes my wife would put on acts to get her way! Never. Just never.

So I got a bit madder than I ought to have. I also got a bit loud too, of which I ain't proud. But they was wrong, so wrong.

So I went out and found that doctor again. And I cornered him, being loud but polite, ya know, trying to keep decent, but he wouldn't listen. And then I told him about my father's words to me, that when something is broken, ya keep trying to fix it, and if it's a person, ya never give up trying to fix it. This doctor, well, his notion was that when ya can't fix it ya just forget it. Now, this old man had been watching me talk to the doctor. He was sitting 'cross the hall. He spoke like he was from England. He come up to me after the doctor took off, and said to me that he was eavesdropping, and I said that's okay, and then he said there's a doctor nearby who would help us. I told the man he was angel and we called the other doc to make a time for a visit.

I told my wife what all had happened. She just smiled at me like she does and said we'll find a way. And that new doc, he did help. Just a few pills a day and my wife is back. Bless him and that guy from England."

CHAPTER FIVE
Well, you've just got to learn to live with the pain

Imagine hearing that!

Does this mean nothing further can be done to help with the pain? Does it mean the doctor will withdraw his care? Does it mean access to other medication trials are over? These words conjure up fears of a very scary future.

For many doctors, this is the statement of an end point: his clinical struggle failed. To the patient and family, this is the worst of all curses. An endless struggle now faces them, and they wonder if they must do it all alone. Far too often the patient has a sneaky and demoralizing inkling that the reason the doctor is "giving up" is because the doctor is at his 'personal' clinical limits rather than at the 'real edge and limits' of science.

> The death knoll also rings for family and friends. Such a declaration is the end of what had been, for at least a while, some promise of a normal life for those involved with the patient. It is the return of a most horrible curse. People get angry, scared, confused and even not sure if the doctor's opinion is truly accurate.

Ending treatment often leaves patients with this gut question: has everything indeed been tried? One patient felt his trust in his doctor collapse after he heard that other patients, with equally complex conditions, got into unique clinical trials. A patient must not feel that "If the doctor can't fix it, then he forgets it..."

How different and therapeutic it is when a doctor says "we'll keep your medications well supplied and monitored until something else comes along."

All of us live with some pain. Most of us accept this as one of the inevitable burdens of life. But severe, disabling pain is different. And yet, as terrible as pain is, the loneliness is worse. Being told to 'live with it' is a banishment into isolation. That feeling of 'deportation' is often the unspoken secret of living with pain. To be in pain is to be solitary. It cannot be physically shared. It can only be reported. At best others can acknowledge it. Patients are supposed to be able to communicate their pain with their doctors. Pain that is under control allows people to reach out to life. It's delightful to see this happen. In fact, one key to understanding the pain patient's real personality is to observe what they do with their lives when the pain is under control.

Pain patients are great at sharing their experiences to other pain patients, but in the end pain is a very private, unfriendly, personal, often shrouded, and a staggering experience.

> "You do really know what I mean, don't you!"
> said she to he. "Yes, oh yes, I do!" he responded.

Brain cells fire in such a pattern that we call pain. If we could ignore these patterns of cellular activity, like the way we ignore temporarily hunger or cold, might we also ignore the sensory pattern which is pain? They seem to be similar neurological events. The answer is simple – yes, we can ignore pain. But just for a short while. Not paying attention to hunger or severe cold will ultimately result in death. So too is it with pain, though death from pain may be more in the psyche than in the body.

Pain is not designed to be unending. It is intended to identify a problem that needs to be fixed. Once fixed, the pain leaves. *By nature we are not supposed to live with permanent pain.*

Pain disrupts lives. It's an alien within us that won't leave. That is why it is so hard "to learn to live with it." It is not a natural way of life to live with aliens. So asking a pain patient to 'learn to live with it' is asking them to live in an unnatural way.

> This is where many problems begin. Many books about pain have introductory comments about the role of pain in our lives. The first role of pain is when, as infants, we cry out because we need help or we are uncomfortable. The implication is that pain is a call for help and that pain is a device to get people to take care of us. This may be partially true and accepted at that stage of life, but danger lurks if we too glibly assume that pain is also used this way in adulthood. There may be cases when pain is indeed an infantile regression, but this event cannot be automatically generalized.

A wise chronic pain patient made a study of attitudes towards pain. He said:

> "Listen. I was in church. The preacher spoke of the seven deadly sins. Sunday he spoke about sloth. It was first considered the sin of sadness or despair, depression, of no joy in life, and being apathetic too – they called it acedia. It's kinda like me 'cept I don't have the apathy, but I sure get the despair.
>
> Then the preacher used the word 'tristitia', which is Latin for being unhappy with one's

station in life. This made me think, and you gotta go slow as I tell you this – I had to be like a snail the first time I thought it through.

Apparently once tristitia was thought by Dante, and some modern folks too, to mean a failure to love God with every part that is within a person. Now, the preacher then said that 'sloth' means that we are not being as honest with ourselves and not living up to our potential. He said if we failed to use our talents, and if we did not achieve our potential, then we are sloths. It sounded like being a sloth was because we were lazy or sick. He also used the word 'indifference', which is an unwillingness to care or really try. Being a sloth sin was number 4 on the sin list, not the worse, not the least. So I did some reading. What got me is that the punishment for being a sloth was to be thrown into the snake pits. All this made me do a lot more thinking.

Now, I love God but since I've been in pain, I kinda wonder if He loves me. But back to the point here – I wonder if the people who judge me on 'my pain' hold some feeling that there must be some sloth features in my makeup, that I don't want to work, or I'm holding back on my potential out of a deliberate choice. I can see how someone with the street addict problem, who doesn't want to do things, may be slothful. Or maybe someone has a depression and they appear slothful. I can't say. The key is this: does God think I'm a sloth?

The few days after that sermon I was glued to the awareness that some of those old judgments from other people are still alive. Yeah, at times over the pain years I even touched on feelings that I, too, was wrong to complain so much about the pain. But now I look back at those thoughts and I see that they came from me feeling like I was defective, or that I was something akin to being sinful. Maybe those old value judgments are still more alive even in me too – maybe more than I've realized.

I try my best to overcome what the pain has done to me, but when I ask for more or different meds, it's ain't the sloth talking. It's the anti-sloth forces in me crying for endurance supplies.

Here's a scheme for you. I cut my life up into epochs. There's the kid epoch. Then there was the teenage and college epoch, and then the young adult gun-ho, early career epoch. But now I'm in the pain epoch. I also call these my 'pain years.' I gotta trust that this epoch will also someday end."

Millions of people learn to live with handicaps. We watch many of the handicapped and sit amazed at how strong and resilient they are. They become our heroes because of their determination and ability to beat the odds. Unfortunately, though, we tend assume that their levels of pain or disability are the same as everyone else's *and* that this same extraordinary ability to fight must also exist in others. Mastering hardships gives us an excellent role model, but to automatically use these heroes as criteria for 'what all people should be like' can badger and be unfair to the more average pain patients. A friend of mine calls these perfect and heroic folks the "phantom perfect patients."[39] Could someone who became a swimmer despite a malformed hip be able to do the same if their joint pain was extremely bad? It is hard to make comparisons and conclusions without including all the unique details of each case.

Untold dangers lie in the uncontrolled use of comparisons. Remember that comparisons need to be made between equal variables. Too often comparisons are made without enough consideration to the overlapping of all the tiny details within the cases being compared. Sometimes the real data in a case is 'carved and re-shaped' until it fits a category: this process is known as jiggery-pokery. In short, the patient is made to fit the disease or treatment as defined by the professional and not necessarily the real clinical situation. This can also be related to the notion of the hunt.

There is no harm, and in fact there may be a lot of good, when successful people are used as models. We see them fight against their handicaps, and we rejoice in their successes. But terrible problems appear when such representations become idols. Doctors and patients must understand *all* the details about the person who became the hero. Is the hero's pain completely gone, or can they function now only because a balanced set of medications are being used? What else happened to make the person into a success story? How different it is when someone gets better because they can financially afford treatment!

A patient told me this:

> "I went to the doctor because there was a lump in my throat. After the x-rays they told me I had a tumor, so I then went to a surgeon for a biopsy. A week later I had the surgery. It was

terribly painful, and I told them in advance that I was always very sensitive to pain. When the nurses gave me the pain medications, I often said that the one dose wasn't high enough. Little by little I know I had become a nuisance to them, and little by little I got the feeling they began to consider my personality as a weak and drug-seeking. I even heard several nurses talking outside my room about how impolite I had become. Imagine the arrogance of thinking no one could hear them—how stupid!

Day by day I heard bits and pieces of conversations, and day by day I got cooler and cooler feelings from them. I was being cast into something I was not. Only one nurse actually sat with me—she was sweet—and we reached an understanding. She assured me that I was correct in my requests, she tried to buffer me from the other nurses, she was timely with the medications and I looked forward to her shift. The other nurses, I felt, saw me only me as a person with distinctive needs that, unfortunately, were a bit out of the ordinary."

How many times has a legitimate pain patient felt he was labeled as deficient or morally weak because he couldn't do what someone else did, namely, live with the pain?

Several years ago this was broadcast on a South Florida television station:

A television news report talked about how a nurse with bad migraines had fallen into the overuse of a pain medication. The video scenes then depicted how successful she was once she finally stopped the narcotic use, but there was no mention of the current state of her headaches. Perhaps she was using another medication for pain control, perhaps she is now happily married, won the lottery, or who knows what? The implication was that solely removing the narcotics made her into a happy person.

One of my TV watching, headache suffering patients felt this story suggested that medications are bad. There was no real material in the story about the levels of pain in the nurses life. The focus was narrowly concentrated on the fact that she no longer used medications. "Great," said my patient, "but how was the headache fixed?"

The story is unfair and ill-fitted to the average headache sufferer because the details are too sparse. But the implication is treacherously plush. This news report was more a sermon than a dispatch. Such 'editorial bents" are not seen that much anymore, but years of such stories bequeathed attitudes and philosophical trails that remain. Too many people doubt the reality of someone else's pain.

When pain cannot be controlled, the task then becomes to build up as much of a life for the patient as possible in areas that the pain cannot touch. This means there has to be a diluting out of some of the bad in their lives with good events. This can be difficult. But often it is the only route. The chore may demand a lot of the psychological, religious, and philosophical pillars in a person's life. The task is to build mental attitude sets which accept that the pain will continue to exist but which will seek to reduce the pain's effect on the person's life. It may be, in reality, a partial capitulation that allows the pain to have its own cycles, but there has to be the attitude and skills to rapidly fill in the times of less pain with as much joy as possible.

The Mature Pain Patient

When someone has lived in pain for a long enough time, they eventually come to accept their life style and limitations. For lack of a fancier term, let's call this the *'mature pain patient.'*

This is how a mature pain patient develops: Someone new to unrelenting pain may find themselves fighting and trying to discount the pain. There may follow an overzealous use of medications in a desperate brawl with their reality. They don't know how to control the pain! This can be emotionally exhausting.

This grows into what can be called a 'giving up stage.' It can produce many behavioral and emotional problems. A great deal of personal alienation might occur as well. It is, in every sense of the word, the same as mourning the loss of a loved one, except that in this case, the lost one is one's former self.

At times this battle seems to be impossible to win. Pain becomes a quiet, unavoidable intruder. Patients try to understand why fate brought pain into their lives. Some even consider the pain to be a punishment from an offended deity. Even many non-religious people might wonder if there is some truth to the punishment factor.

This pattern will season the person to their reality, and they 'mature' as they accept the true dimensions of their life. They also begin to more melodiously seek opportunities to improve the stable sources of quality in their lives.

> "I know I'm not the perfect person, but I can't figure out for the life of me why I'm afflicted like this. I've come to accept so much of it. I'm the wiser

man of pain now. But something is still wrong...I need to find a balance, so I'm looking."

It seems confusing that some people try to stand tall and want to show off how much pain they can withstand. This would suggest some pride in being able to tolerate the punishment for being bad. To a very few, the pain is cleansing.

Though physicians have replaced priests and the shaman as the primary health care givers, the hearty interest in supplications for healing from the God's continues. Priests once asked the God's for information about which behavior was offensive. Once known, corrective actions, incantations, exorcisms, and sacrifices were made to convince the God's to 'undo' the painful curse. It was a noble task to conquer pain and disease. Hippocrates believed this: "it is divine to subdue pain *(divinum est opus sedare tiolorum)*."

Early Christian healers used faith and prayer to subdue pain. Many contemporary clergy also maintain that faith can heal or reduce pain. In fact, the oft seen sign or poster declaring "Get right with God" uses the same remedy as did the early approaches to pain removal. In some respects, the patient was asked to give into God's ways (e.g., to let go of any individual will and place their lives in God's hands). People were also asked to confess to one's sins and transgressions as part of this process.

The similarities between those older treatment strategies and those now used in contemporary psychotherapy are numerous. Looking at our own attitudes and souls, at what metaphors we use to explain and define ourselves, and learning how to deal with inexplicable tribulations, can be therapeutic. When modern medicine fails, we still turn to strategies that are hundreds of years old.

> ....what remains impossible to ignore is that many of those old strategies do help....

The oldest and most indispensable therapeutic strategy is to help the patient find a purpose and meaning in life. This cannot be understated. When 'meaning and purpose' become friends, adversities are less daunting.

It's also important to be sensitive to the cultural differences in how people approach suffering. There is a propensity for many cultures to prefer trials of spiritual healing before they go to physicians. The 'going to a physician' may be done reluctantly because it might suggest that they failed their culture's first choice for treatment. That 'failure' might taint them with a stigma. It may also tinge the presentation to the physician such that a depression may be suspected, but in fact the 'depression' is a 'disappointment.' Treating it as a depression might alienate the patient.

In 2009 Grant[40], at the Université de Montréal, reported that those who were trained in Zen meditation achieved remarkable control of pain. The quest, then, is to know if meditation changes the way someone feels pain. Perhaps the technique would allow for less pain medication use. They noted that slower breathing rates during the tests coincided with reduced pain. But is this a realistic option when the goal is to control on-going, treatment resistant pain? It does speak to the power of the mind over short, or acute durations, of pain. And this, of course, speaks to the importance of learning non-medical interventions in the challenge to control or reduce pain. All of this is part of the development of the mature pain patient.

One has to also wonder what would happen in the mind of a Zen master if his skills failed to control his pain?

The following questions need to be asked when pain is considered untreatable: Have all avenues of medical and psychiatric, spiritual or religious interventions been truly explored? Have the doctors driven to the ends of all those avenues, or have they stopped short because of their own needs, fears, insurance blockades, or other attitudes, rather than continue to fight for the patient's needs? If the local doctors cannot, or will not, do more, will they help to find new referrals to other doctors? And will treatment continue – at whatever level of success – as the search goes on? The treatment team must bridge all the recourses in a person's life. Failing to do so could undo whatever healing occurred, even if it is small. Sometimes the supportive connections have to be made to other patients. The patient can never be left to feel alone. And again, all these events leave scars that consolidate and toughen the sufferer, but we want a productive, not an unproductive, outcome.

> She often said her really bad days were less so if, on a bad day, she gave support and instruction to another, less mature, pain patient. On the phone or computer, she would speak to them about hope and failure. She would often keep her own despair quiet because she wanted her life coaching to be 'strong and sunny.' She told me that some of her doctors thought that "I only want to take medications to make me feel better. No, I really feel better when they give me the meds so I can give to others. Making me feel better means I can make others feel better. That makes for an awesome day. My job is to help people find and keep strength, better perspective and realistic hope."

Children and Pain

The leading cause of death in children under age 19 is cancer. The chance of getting proper pain medication tends to vary with the hospital or other ancillary factors, and not with the clinical need. Orsey[41] and her group published a paper in 2008 that of 1,466 patients with cancer under the age 24, only 56% of them received opioids during the last week of their lives. Those with private insurance received opioids 63% of the time, and those on Medicaid or other government plans received the same treatments only 52% of the time. Children under 10 years old or those with brain tumors trended to gets less opioid therapy. The author comments that we do not have good data on how many children die in pain.

> "I had a son who died from bone cancer. It was the biggest test of my life. I looked at that little boy and wondered where his smiles came from. I told him God existed and we'd all be together again, and I guess being a kid, there was no cynicism or religious doubt in his heart. Maybe his immaturity was good. We'd say "Do you hurt?" and he'd say "A little." But I looked to his eyes and saw there was pain. I'd sleep next to him – maybe as much for me as for him – and I'd feel it when he moved. His groans were screams to me. God, I used to say, God, please at least give him restful sleep.
>
> So my wife and I asked the doctor for pain meds, mostly to give him at night. He said no. I said what? He said it's not safe and we don't want to introduce him to narcotics. I asked him, as nicely I could contain myself, in what year did he go to school? He was plum insulted.

> My wife had some extra Percocet from after a tooth pull, and we gave it to him one night, and he relaxed and slept. I cried because he relaxed. So we told the doctor who then got mad at us. Well, we fired him right on. A nurse sent us to another doctor who must've come from the school of angels. He gave us good meds, and we say a God Bless and thank you to him every day.
>
> That last month of his life, when the tumor was so big, at least the pain was not so big. And then the hospice doctor was good about the pain meds. Then he passed, and we know in our hearts that the pain of our loss was a bit less knowing he did not have so much body pain.... that new doc, and then the hospice, didn't abandon us, they didn't let all of us agonize."

Many of the concepts in this book apply equally to adults and children in pain. Non-lethal painful conditions are horrible burdens for children as well as adults. Some forms of arthritis and headaches are two common pain childhood conditions. Treating children must be very individualized and aggressive! If a child will not die from the condition, then we cannot let them pass though and miss life because of our unwillingness to treat their pain.

No patient can be abandoned, for in abandonment are the seeds of an intolerable and emotional pain that is far worse than the physical pain itself.

CHAPTER SIX
Pain and personality changes

Pain changes people.

It changes how they view and interact with the world.

Too often, honest pain patients sense they are being accused of exaggerating their symptoms. They feel they are charged with the crimes of lying and of being less than totally honest.

Bad people experience pain to be just as brutal as do good people. But because of other issues in their lives, the bad ones face extra obstacles which challenge how others perceive their pain. Too often the 'bad aspects of their lives', whatever they are, are ranked as more consequential than the physical pain.

Pain can break up marriages, ruin careers, deplete financial resources, and destroy or markedly change what was once happy and normal in a person's life.

Many emotionally immature people become mature when faced with pain. Life in pain takes them on a trailblazing new hierarchy of revised values. One 26 year old pain patient said the pain experience 'renovated' his thinking styles. "I now live in a refurbished world. What was important is not that important anymore." Those who cannot mature may face delayed or decelerated clinical success.

Maturity may indeed foster new life values and styles, but it can also breed despair and death. Virtually all chronic pain patients at one time or another have considered suicide or euthanasia.

"I was really just a kid when my pain started. Then one of my doctors called me an addict, and being afraid that I might have slipped into depravity, and so scared that so many of the authorities were right that I was 'sick', I began doing what I always did when I needed to make sure that I was ok. I read books about people and studied myself! And lo and behold, I came to understand survival.

I saw two levels of survival: physical and emotional. My pre-accident life was fortunate. I never was sick before the accident. But like most everyday people, in my life, time and time again, my emotions had been attacked. These attacks hurt deeply, but I survived. I always survived. So I felt strong.

Until the pain, that is. Once the pain started I realized that it could kill me if I didn't master it. I tried everything. But nothing worked. I saw Chinese doctors, chiropractors, pain specialists, etc., and all they could do was reduce it a little – for which I was grateful! But little more could be done.

One weekend, during a rain storm, the pain was horrible. I had no more pain medications. The doctor on call for my regular doctor would not give me medications. He was 'uncomfortable' prescribing narcotics. I tried an emergency room, but all they offered were a few codeine tablets and ibuprofen. Interesting – I now think about the times when a girlfriend painfully slashed open my emotions. But the emotional pain from her was never a threat to my survival! Those girlfriend emotions hurt, but this physical pain could kill. That girlfriend pain went away. I suddenly understood how people do things for physical survival. I had to. I stole some narcotics from a friend. I never thought it possible for me to do something like that, but I never knew the need. And I began to deeply hate me, my life, the doctors, the government, and the idiot driver who hurt me!"

Violent outbursts of tremendous anger at one's fate are common. Outbursts typically focus against the person who caused the pain (e.g., the driver of the car, the doctor who made the mistake, etc.), to God, or to just bad luck and fate.

Sometimes the anger is at oneself for being foolish and doing something imbecilic, like diving into dangerous waters, driving while intoxicated, etc. Sometimes the anger is not at the cause of the pain (the cause of it might be accepted as a random act of bad luck), but is aimed at people who are supposed to understand and treat the pain. But the most common anger is towards the fact that there may be no end to the pain; this is the real suffering experience.

Pain is not silly. It slants and re-orients values. It is like the teenager who becomes a parent and suddenly realizes how demanding a child can be. A child is expensive and time consuming, and it is a responsibility which will not go away. For someone who lived a 'party' life, who floated into and out of events and tasks, who was indifferent to many of life's onuses, who had been demanding or fickle towards others, who was intolerant, who wanted the easier way in life, or who was an amateur with regards to life's woes — then unwanted and unrelenting pain may grow them up. The process may take some time, but it often happens. A silly person may become a serious one. But the opposite may also occur if the person lacks core skills to deal with adversity. That is when psychotherapy is needed.

Pain brings out the strengths and weakness of a character. Even the strongest person may waver or collapse after a long period of an unsuccessful contest against pain. A person may pass through disappointment, which may give birth to a depression.

> "My brother calls it a contest, and it is really a contest between my endurance and the pain. The difference is that I wear out, but the pain never seems to tire."

Countless articles discuss the presence and role of depression in pain patients. It is a major, often missed problem. About 50% of all depressions are un-recognized when people go to their regular doctors.

Many pain patients do suffer from depressions. But all pain patients are not 'clinically' depressed.

We need to study the cultural floor of a 'depression.' Many cultures may reject treatment. African Americans, Asian-Americans, American Indians, and Latinos have their own cultural backgrounds that can detour them from getting to the right mental health care (even in the context of pain management care). Adding chronic pain to a cultural picture may create a bigger hurdle than usual when it becomes necessary for someone to accept a referral for mental health care.

> In April 2009, Joe Neidhardt, told a group at a National Association for Rural Mental Health

meeting, that "We must meet our patients where they are." The theme was that the application of Western, evidence-based medicine must be applied, and let to rest within, the cultural context of the patients. Dr. Neidhardt said in the article: "Spiritual deprivation looks like depression, so it's important to address all those issues in the first diagnostic interview." For example, doctors must not accept that dreams can predict the future, but they have to respect that their patients may believe it. [42]

Some of this is also the worrisome quality of stigma. The U. S. Surgeon General Report in 2001 said that the problem of stigmatization is equal or greater in minorities than compared to whites. [43]

Stigma results in a lack of understanding and support from others. The definition of 'stigma' is a mark of disgrace or reproach, usually against one's reputation. An older definition is 'a point on the skin' that bleeds during certain mental states, as in hysteria. Long ago the word referred to a mark on the skin of a slave or criminal.

An endless battle with pain can bring on desperation and disbelief about life because life has become stuck on an unchangeable and bad course. This feeling can grow into a depression. Depression then, in and of itself, can worsen the pain because life is not good, and when one thing is bad, it may make other troubling things in life worse than they might actually be.

Many times doctors overplay the role of a reactive depression to a life situation in a pain patient's life. They assume when depression (or the situation) goes away then the patient will also not suffer as much pain. Of course this can happen at times, but it may not happen as well.

All the antidepressants in the world will not undo a purely reactive depression. But they might actually help reduce some of the physical pain via pharmacologic activity. But if an antidepressant fails to help, it might heighten the despair. "Look, another thing failed." The catastrophe of the core situation will only worsen. Reactive depressions need concurrent treatment with psychotherapy and patient advocacy.

One of the needed professional skills is that a doctor know the patient well enough so they know when to use antidepressants, other non-medical interventions, or more pain medications, etc., in order to keep some stable equilibrium in the patient's world. This is often not easy. Even the best doctors might fail to meet this challenge. Failures like this contribute to how a patient's personality may change. Such failures can erode the fiber of any emotional core.

A referral to a mental health professional, in theory, is a great move, but many mental health personnel are also too timid or untrained in the proper use of narcotics and other pain treatment methods. They are often not strong enough psychotherapists for someone in a basically unfixable situation. Good intentions are not adequate. We know that all professionals are not clinically equal despite the wearing of the same labels. And as noted elsewhere, one must also adjust the timing and manner of the mental referral to the patient's cultural expectations, financial realities, etc.

> "I can't tell you how loud my Dad got when he heard that the doc wanted me to see a shrink. He said no one in 'his' family couldn't manage

> pain or needed a shrink. Yeah, it wasn't the first time we fought over how differently we saw the world. How'd we settle it? I don't tell him about my counselor. When I get a good insight, I say "Hey Dad, I was thinking, and ya know….." So I bring it all home but in a different wrapper."

Often mental health referrals come too late. Delay can harden and complicate the patient's personality. Delay can make a once easy job into a hard one.

...Thought...

> Sometimes the patient or a family will resist the referral, as if the referral means the person has drifted off into a mental illness. This negative response can be avoided if the primary doctor discusses and involves some aspect of psychiatric care of the patient from the very onset. The doctor needs to early in treatment introduce the emotional aspects of pain. Doing it later on may follow the failure of the medical aspects, so bringing it up later might also suggest that the failure was the product of psychiatric problem. This is when people say things such as "I'm not crazy. Take the damn pain away and I'll be fine!"

> Some patients relish a psychiatric referral. It is a time of relief. They finally get to deal with their emotional issues. Many of these people might have quietly known they were not doing well but may have been afraid to admit it. That they did not ask for mental health help earlier may have been because they were too

embarrassed to do so. Having someone else suggest it removes some of the worry about it being their fault that they are still suffering. One might hear: "The doctor was right, I need help with this problem..."

Some patients ask for a psychiatric referral. These folks tend to know themselves better and are not afraid to ask for help. Quite often they show the best improvement. "Doc, who's a good person to see for pain and depression problems? I don't feel like I can handle this all by myself."

One of the major issues in pain control is the suspected overlapping of addiction with certain personality types. Addiction, in the common sense of the word, rarely occurs, but behaviors do develop which look like an addict. When these "look like an addict" situations are studied it becomes striking that the problem is twofold: (1) the patient is usually being under treated for the pain, and (2) there is only a weak, if any at all, trusting relationship between the doctor and the patient. Very often this situation is the fault of the doctor and the treatment team, not the patient.

One addictive-like behavior happens when the patient simply needs no more than a regular supply of pain relieving material. Too often this process escalates towards the pejorative and sensational picture of a' junkie' working to 'just get drugs.' This is especially so if the patient wants only quick visits with little talking, etc. But perhaps this is all that is needed. The patient merely comes in, maybe in somewhat a mechanical manner, and little more than a medication check is performed. Then the patient leaves. It still can be quite the legitimate matching of clinical services to the patient's actual needs. Not every chronic pain patient has dysfunctional emotional problems. Some people are amazingly strong and stoic.

Some can even joke a bit about their pain management needs. For example:

> A 45 year old nurse suffered a back injury. Fortunately a TENS unit was able to control the pain. Without the TENS unit she could not work, socialize, grocery shop, and so on. She always joked, but was actually dead serious that she would 'get crazy' if she didn't have extra batteries available.
>
> "People think I'm a battery junkie and I suppose I am. I always look at the clock and so I can always have my next electrical fix. I know I won't die and all I'd do is hurt, but honestly, without the TENS, I would be immobilized. Offer me an hour with any actor or a set of new batteries, and I'd first go for the batteries, because without them I'd be no good for the guy."

Two other deplorable labels frequently describe difficult to treat patients. They are 'manipulative' and 'borderline personality.' Both suggest a demanding, conniving and insatiable personality. The word manipulative is fairly well understood, but the term borderline is an intricate psychiatric concept. The borderline personality is a complex, difficult and serious personality disorder that often manifests itself in belligerent, overbearing, emotionally consuming styles. They actually often have fragile egos.

Similar behavioral characteristics are seen in those who are not manipulative and not borderline. In fact, these labels might follow and reflect more *how someone responds* to a situation. So the cause of a troubling behavior may be a source from outside the person. The source and cause of the problem may actually be the treating doctor's philosophy or personality.

Sometimes patients are considered pushy. For example:

> Patients who tell doctors how to treat them are seen as pushy.
>
> Patients who constantly ask for dose revisions are seen as pushy.
>
> Patients who complain about being ignored or kept waiting are seen as pushy.
>
> Patients who tell the staff that their case is different and 'please listen to what I have to say so the same mistakes aren't made twice' are seen as pushy.
>
> Patients who often bring new ideas to their doctors are often seen as pushy.

Pushy people present as manipulators. They try to get things done their own way. New treatment teams often forget that the chronic patient has spent years being a patient. So the patient knows their own history and needs quite well. The pushing is a demand that the treatment team get to know the real history and situation. One lady said that "the more the treatment team made assumptions about me, the pushier I got."

Bring into the picture a well-meaning, but inexperienced, biased, or unprepared (i.e., doesn't know the case well enough) professional. Is the new professional likely to come up with any innovative and meaningful ideas for a long term chronic pain patient? Probably not. Experienced and mature pain patients know this all too well. So they 'push.' One patient called it 'lobbying for my best care.'

Chronic pain patients have been though it all. Unless there is something distinctive to learn, then, in what might be a polite or impolite manner, they often explain that they won't repeat old treatment trials. They also want much more proof that something new has a sustainable and successful clinical track record before they try it. Such a position by the patient has been taken to mean that the patient is non-cooperative or trying to manipulate the system to get his own way. A mature professional, however, will see this merely as self protection on the patient's part.

A treatment team's emotional approach to such chronic patients has to be gentle, unhurried, reputable, and with an invitation to jointly individualize the care. Too often, especially when insurance is paying for the care, treatment decisions occur without the input of most important member of the team — the patient! Is it any wonder that patients become feisty or taxing when they are told about such third-party decisions, especially if they are not what the patients need? These responses all combine as part of the cumulative temperament inherent in the 'pain patient's signature'. Experienced patients demonstrate skepticism and wisdom towards many treatment plans because so many prior ideas have failed. These mature pain patients and their signatures grow from the accumulated acumen gathered during their firsthand experiences.

> "I've had this leg pain for 8 years. I've seen a hundred doctors. I've tried every drug and every therapy, and I've read everything there is to read about it, and I can deflate almost any

> plan a doctor proposes. I don't think they like me being so smart. Sometimes the insurance company gives me a new adjustor and they talk to the doctor about me, and then I'm told they will or will not approve a procedure. They never spoke to me! And, quite simply put, that makes me nuts. How's that strike you? And am I so difficult to work with? No, I just want to know who is doing what about me.
>
> But I can't walk out of the disability policy because I ain't got no other income."

Trust is destroyed when pain is under treated. The patient gasps for air while being told by an insistent professional that, according to the professional, they are getting enough air. Such insistence is a crime of the highest magnitude. It says that the treatment team doesn't believe the patient's pain level, and that the patient is allowed pain relief only up to the level allowed by the staff.

> A very hard working, honest, and mature man hurt his back. The various orthopedists told him that taking 4 to 7 pain med doses a day was too much. But the patient said that that dose worked very well for him for over a year. With that dose he was able to maintain a good job, there was still a little pain, and that the known risks of the medication were less than the known risks ascribed to more surgery. One doctor even said he should feel no pain "with that much medication." The patient quipped back that the doctor should have the same back injury.

Many patients go from doctor to doctor in search of pain medications. This looks exactly like an addict seeking drugs. But the real motivation for this behavior is customarily not understood. One patient said that after years of psychotherapy, TENS units, physical therapy, biofeedback, surgery, acupuncture, chiropractic, herbs, and on and on, that his going from doctor to doctor would stop immediately if he could find a single doctor who would give him enough medication to control the pain.

> "...it makes me feel like a thief or a criminal—I can't stand the deception. But the deception means nothing when the pain is killing me. It's not me, not the real me. I can't trust any single doctor because he'll think I'm just a junkie and I'm not following his directions—can't he see that his treatments are just, well, inadequate? But he's my insurance doctor and I can't afford to go anywhere else.
>
> I'm embarrassed to tell anyone. Imagine what type of character they must think I am! I know it's wrong, but all I want is someone to repair my elbow so it doesn't hurt anymore and that'll be the end of it, please God. And please God, forgive me for the times when I go to those walk in pain clinics that will give me some extra meds, even though it costs me so much money. I don't know what I'll do if they pass a law where some central computer knows about my extra supply source."

Severe pain can bring out the worst in a person. Knotty aspects of unsettled emotions can also amplify the pain and delay any growth into a mature patient.

Some patient's find that pain fits into their own self-image of suffering. Pain can reduce emotional suffering because it brings up another problem on which to focus. So not needing pain medications may mean the return to an older, and perhaps less controllable, emotional pain. This is indeed a rather small group of people with a complex psychiatric picture. Much denial may exist in these patients. Only a sophisticated psychotherapist should deal with these types of issues.

> A 43 year old woman suffered many deep psychological blows in her life. There was always an undercurrent of being the 'victim', and that she had no real luck in life. Many fears lived in her heart. She learned how to cover these fears with excellently developed deflectors. Her inside world was troubled and full of skepticism. Though she actually was loved by many, and had been successful in her career, she always felt it was an easily broken equilibrium, and that something could easily happen to abruptly take all the successes away. The pain did just that.

> This is her story. Two years ago she was the innocent victim of an auto accident. She developed headaches and severe damage to her hip. No amount of oral medication treatment seemed to take the pain away. Only intramuscular narcotics worked. She fought the pain and hated the medications. She looked at the needles as if they were the 'devil agents working for the pain.' Inwardly she felt that it was her 'lousy fate' to hurt. It made all her fears worse. But when she was finally and adequately medicated, the fears dropped as rapidly as the pain

faded away. For the first time in years she could once again function. The "drugs became my ticket to life. No doctor was going to interfere with this formula!"

The drive to 'fix' the bad hip became less of a strong motivator than was her insistence of keeping an on-going and adequate medication use. A close and trusted friend finally called her an addict when she told him the full story of why she was using the medications. That frightened and angered her, but it also made her think. In time she saw that the medication was both helping control the pain as well as reducing her emotional fears. She entered psychiatric help but could not have done so without the financial support of a brother who paid for it. The treatment helped. She finally dealt with the self-defeating aspects of her long and sad sense that she had to perpetuate her sense of being the victim.

Interestingly, in the course of this process many doctors called her an addict, which added to her weak self-image. That delayed her seeking psychiatric help. The comment from the friend was different because she trusted the friend, and it ultimately fueled the anger to get to know herself better

This case highlights the grueling and daunting task of how hard and important it is to know how much of the pain is psychological, if the medication is being used to calm physical versus psyche pain, what the person was like before the pain began, what effect the pain has had on the evolution of the personality, and so on. Professionals need to be perfectly clear about these areas before they make any statements about a personality. Being a pain treatment failure does not mean there is a subterranean psychological problem causing the medical fiasco. However, constant pain will change a personality into what might superficially be seem as an emotionally disturbed or lopsided person.

One dangerous assumption is that all people are fundamentally strong characters. This is wrong. More people are more fragile than one might suspect. People may have low pain or frustration thresholds and may have known it all their lives, but because of good fortune they have been able to avoid situations that test these limits. Many pain patients suffer more than they might if their tolerances, be they social, psychological, or even genetic factors, were tougher. By the same token, many, but not all, people can grow if given sufficient time and fitting assistance.

> "If I was tougher I know I'd handle this better. I guess I'm not what I thought I was. The pain pointed out the weaknesses in me. It took some time to accept that. Now the psychologist is helping me learn some good ways to handle this."

It seems too easy to say "let's make them into stronger personalities so they will suffer less from their injuries." It's unrealistic to maintain the misguided belief that all people have equal potential and that there are no limits to how much stronger someone can be made. Insisting on this process can itself cause incredible suffering, especially if the pre-pain personality lacked that aptitude. It can begin a whirlwind of failure and despair. Likewise, even if an inherent aptitude for change does exist, failure can still happen if there is not enough allowance given to how long it really takes for someone to change. Seasoned psychotherapists and physical therapists know that some conditions, and some people, take longer than others to get better. This is why it is so important to know what people were like before the pain entered their lives.

> "I know I could get better, but I just need more time. This treatment program is for 4 weeks only, and I can't afford outpatient care as intensive as I need, so I am afraid of failing. I was never a lion, so please give me time! I can't do it just the way or as fast as they want me to. I'm not that strong. I never was. I'll never have the spunk and will never be like the guy who lost his legs and now plays golf. It's a nice goal, but it's for younger people. Let me just be able to sit calmly and read again."

One question often asked is how soldiers endure so more pain than others. The answer may be quite simple: the personality of the soldier is to fight and be strong. They battle for a spirited cause. They train to resist some levels of suffering and pain. Their injuries are quickly tended to, and they receive an honorable badge because they suffered in the course of protecting others. Some of the ego gratifications are bottomless. Parents who are injured saving their children are very much like the soldier. But what about the 'injury' received in a non-noble ordeal, like being hit by drunken driver? Why are the resulting effects different?

The answer lies in the cultural and psychological significance of the injury.

> "Vietnam was no honor, but we were moving a bunch of kids before Charlie bombed what they thought was our fuel supply. I got hit, but it was ok because we were moving the kids. My leg – whoa, all messed up! And the pain now is just plain bad. But when it's bad, I know where it came from, and in that is the story I'm real proud of....so it makes it a little easier. I'd still like the VA to find a way get it fixed, though."

How different it is with this type of story:

> "My pain? You want to know about my pain! Man, it's that bastard who was too drunk to be driving and me, I was too unlucky not to be anywhere else in the whole damn world..."

One of the topics discussed later in this book is the old notion that pain is punishment. How many times do pain patients say: "I don't know what I did that was so bad to deserve this?" It makes the patient wonder if they are, or were, defective, bad, or somehow sinful. It makes them also fear that they must be weak characters because strong characters don't suffer so much. Consider a good man who was a fairly religious person; he was so badly hurt in an accident that he ended up with chronic pain. Week after week he prayed to God for help, but little help came. He saw his own life deteriorate as the pain increasingly controlled him. He began to lose his money, his job, his dignity, and so on.

His pleas for God's help did not ease the suffering. Imagine how his personality changed? How can one alleviate his interpretation that he must have been rejected or abandoned by his God? How do we reconcile that he was a honest and charitable person, and yet now he is cursed with such anguish? Then too, how should he react if other problems arise, such as insurance companies and doctors who complicate his life when he did nothing wrong? How does he face a lifetime of lost dreams that are eclipsed by a permanent indentureship to the new master called 'pain'? Indeed, how does anyone align themselves to the changes of such a harsh new reality? It is often very difficult.

The Bible does not make a very clear distinction between mental illness, physical disease, and being possessed by evil spirits. The Mesopotamians and Egyptians regarded illness as the end product of evil spirits; that is, the Gods were mad at the person and would no longer protect him. This allowed for the invasion by evil spirits as the explanation for the ailment. Pain, simply put, was punishment. As a result, treatment was often done by exorcists.

The Israelites saw health as a divine blessing, so disease indicated that a spiritual relationship had broken down between man and God. Disease to the Israelites may not always be the product of sin, but it could be a drifting away from God.

God became the only true healer, so doctors took on the role as God's helper. Ecclesiasticus felt God gave the gifts of healing to men. "The Lord created medicines from the earth, and a sensible man will not despise them." Jesus resisted the notion that each disease had a specific sin, and instead saw disease as a result of evil in the world as a whole. His power to heal sickness and forgive sins was a way of showing what the new kingdom will be like. James later said "Confess your sins to one another, so that you will be healed." However, until all things are better and the kingdom of God is established, people will continue to be sick, grow old, and die. Traditional Christianity teaches that when Jesus returns, these problems will disappear.

Long before Jesus, Hippocrates tried, in about 400 BC, to move medicine from mysticism and religion into a science and an art. But as history has shown, not all accepted (even to this day) Hippocrates's notions, which leaves religion and subjectivity still playing a major role in the approach towards illness and suffering.

An clergyman with severely painful arthritis grew angrier rather than calmer when he tried to use his religion and theology to explain his pain.

> "Listen, I've been a minister for 32 years and I saw so much suffering. Then it began to hit me — my horrible sin is that I doubted those pitiful souls who hurt so much, and 1 tried to console them only with words. I heard, but could not understand, their anger at God. Now I do understand because my arthritic joints taught me about those other people. I look at my hip and say thank you for what you taught me, and damn you for what you do to me.
>
> Here's the dilemma. Christ said that if we believe in God, then we can be healed. But then Christ left, promising to come back some day. In the meantime we have to suffer. I don't know why He left such a mess. If He is so merciful then why doesn't He come back now? Believe me, trusting someone gets thin when you're in pain. All the wonderful medicines in the world that exist and people still suffer—why? Maybe He won't return because of my sins. He will come back when there is no more suffering in the world — but can I wait for all the sin to be gone? I'll be dead, and for what gain?

Remember, His healing was a foretaste of what will be in the future. He seems to forget that I live now. Should I ignore the present on the promise of a future? It's rather difficult, at least for me. If I do nothing bad, but my neighbor does, then I suffer because there is still evil in the world. They are bad and I suffer. These are subtle, old, but still occurring attitudes in our community. And in my head too, I'm sorry to say.

Lord knows I've tried to undo evil and make good, but I can't be responsible for everyone, yet I am punished for anyone who is bad. Am I a bad clergyman because I didn't fix the world? Am I being punished for having human flaws? That makes me mad. I can also now see how, in the name of religion, people justify killing 'bad people' or beginning 'ethnic purification' policies— but I gotta calm down. Just the thought of that makes me quiver.

I would have to be God Himself to correct all the evil in the world. So for my pain to go away—that is, to be healed by God—do I have to have the strength of God? Do you see my logic here? If I want to get better then I have to be what I can't be. I cannot be God! I'm doomed. I can't be God and I can't correct all the sins in the world. The best deal I can get is that if I believe in God and Jesus, then I'll have a better life in the after world.

If my pain was mostly anxiety or apprehension, then that reassurance would sure make me feel better. But horrendous arthritis doesn't know of a promised good after life. Maybe I will be rewarded in heaven. I try to keep this in mind. But I've my doubts. So now, who am I to look for help? God? No, because He put the onus on all the sinners here. Me? No, because I honestly lived a good life. Everyone else? No, because then I'm liable for more than any mortal can control. Doctors? No, they are too afraid of sinning by making me an 'addict.' But, think of it this way, did you know how much they sin by making me suffer? So there is no way out. I know, I know, I know. There is no answer. I don't know anymore."

We have seen many 'religious' people say that there must be a distinctive reason for a pain or illness to happen. The problem is that quite often God chooses not to reveal the purpose. Hope lives in the soil of 'all will turn out fine in the end, so put up with the pain now because it's only a step to a better end.' It's wonderful when this belief works. It's an alarming hopelessness when it doesn't.

It's not fair to deflate a patient's hope. Maybe they feel that a hidden agenda exists for them, but many of those with these strong beliefs eventually wane and dwindle as time passes and no answers or relief appears. It is a devastating reversal for a person to give up hope. But it does happen. And it can change a personality. One person put it this way: "I never lost hope. I gave up hope. There's a difference. The hope is still in the closet. I'd be happy to take it out if I felt it could work."

Sometimes the loss of hope forces people to get angry enough to move through the pain. This can be beneficial. Perhaps the patient finally comes to the realization that nothing special or magical will happen, they can't wait any longer, and they have the choose to live within the limitations of the pain or die. Depending on many other personal, legal and ethical factors, many may try to argue that death is a disciplined, logical, wise, and brave choice. Death in such case is not a loss of the will to live. It is the realization that one cannot live without quality.

If disappointment digs deeply and fiercely enough into a person's soul, then the will to live may be lost. Part of the treatment team's dealings with any patient is to prepare for this day of reckoning, and provide as much internal strength and external support so he will choose the 'fight back and live' mode as opposed to the 'give up and die' one. [44]

There are times when being non-religious or a nihilist may be psychologically more comforting than believing in the usual religious doctrines. To many readers this will sound blasphemous and irreligious. But to see religion fail someone in 'innocent pain' can harden even the most pious.

Part of the psychology of being in pain is the psychology of being alone. Imagine feeling that neither doctors, nor friends, nor God Himself, can help. Can one fault the skeptic? To fully understand the pain patient one must understand loneliness.

The loneliness of pain is worsened by the sometimes overt, and sometimes subtle, suggestion that the patient is lying about his pain or that it is 'more mental' than physical. How can some share this anguish or be given help for this anguish if people doubt that the anguish really exists? Over time the pain patient withdraws into an inconspicuous isolation. Self-doubt grows, and unless someone emotionally rescues them, they drift further and further away into their own pain-ridden and unaccompanied existence.

Suicide is probably more common that realized. The French word 'ennui' means emptiness or boredom. In psychiatric circles it has come to mean indifference and a giving up, that is, there is no excitement or hope left in life. Durkheim used the word 'anomie' to describe why suicide is much more likely to happen when the meaning and stability of life has been erased, modified or weakened in unacceptable ways. Pain can do this to a life.[45]

Loneliness can change personalities. It is so hard to live by one self through such prolonged misery. We must let pain patient's show us their non-pain personalities. These patients must retain some control, certainty, and connection to life. Touching them is how we help them live. They, in whatever way possible, then rejoice by giving us something back in return. We make them into people and not merely patients. And that is what makes life worthwhile. And that is when we all rejoice. And that lessens the loneliness.

Life is so often tied to suffering that we must think about how to approach it. The philosopher Schopenhauer said suffering is essential to all life. Through suffering we increase our knowledge because, through suffering, we learn that there is something more to want in life. If a person can achieve what he wills (i.e., wants), then he would eventually feel contentment. But happiness can never fully exist because all our wishes can never be entirely fulfilled. It's the unfulfilled wishes that cause pain. Even the urge to procreate merely brings to life a new person who will later suffer and die. In fact, some say the shame of the sexual act is because it leads to procreation which will create another person who will suffer; as such, life and suffering are interwoven and inseparable cohorts.

Suffering is worsened when there is an intense will. The less we will, then the less we suffer. The proposed extension of this idea is that if one wills not to be in pain, then the pain will diminish. There is a small quality of truth here. But the strength of that quality varies vastly, from situation to situation and person to person, footing itself on a thousand variables. We must not overuse this notion.

Emotions are a series of three comparisons: of what we are now, of what we were, and of what we want to be. As such simply living reminds the pain patient of what life can be like without pain. These reminders burst out of hopes and memories. These hopes can be crushed as one compares oneself to the lack of limitations seen in those of the surrounding world.

Suicide removes the life force that calls up the will to live. As a result, the logic transforms into the sense that merely being alive causes the pain. Remove life and pain is also gone. This is such a dire circle of logic that every step must be made to prevent and remove it.

> "When I see what everyone else is doing in life, and I compare it to what I cannot do, it makes it all worse. Life itself is nasty: it keeps saying 'do more, do more, try to play baseball, try to make love,' but I can't. So I give up those things I want to do, and that makes the suffering a little less because I'm not reminded of how bad I am. Sometimes I think life is cruel because it won't let me crave out and throw away those 'desires to do things' that still live in my memory. I need to cut them out of my thinking. I know suicide is the ultimate pain killer for me, but there is a

> thing in me which says that I just so much prefer to live. Suicide would cut me out of the pain. But it would also cut me out of life. I don't like that option. Help me figure this out"

Surrendering one's wants takes away much of the way we live, so in a sense it can put people into a state of non-existence. People often say they 'I cannot exist anymore the way I did before.' One poetic Latino man said that "in that sanctuary of non-existence is a refuge from the 'diabolic Satan' who endlessly weaves a web of suffering that he joyfully uses for torture."

> "So I said, ok, all the old stuff has to go....no temptation, no memory, no feelings of loss, and then maybe there will be less suffering. I see that suffering comes from comparing what I am to what I want to be. If I want to be less, then I suffer less. Still the devil makes me suffer by reminding me of what I don't have in my life anymore. The next step is to get rid of the devil."

Woven in this line of thinking is the suggestion that giving up one's will to be pain free will lessen the pain. Not everyone agrees with that line of thinking.

> "I'm not going to fight the pain anymore. I just can't win, so I'm giving in. Mr. Pain, the bastard that you are, you won. Now, can I expect to have less pain?"

What happens, and what are the ethics, of telling people to seek higher goals? Do we cause extra pain knowing that such encouragement may worsen the pain because it raises hopes of (unreachable) expectations? Is pain the product of some misguided drive to get more out of life? How do we reconcile pain and existence? If we change the parameters of our existence, then might we suffer less? Engaging in these considerations can markedly alter a person's personality. A snippy lady said "those therapists keep urging me on, saying I can do it. Hell, I know I can't. I realized that a long time ago. I failed so many times that I no longer want to feel that failure again. I'm okay now with being what I am. I'm better when I don't try to get better. That was a doozy of a thing to accept, let me tell you! The nurse, I think, probably feels she is failing me by not being my cheerleader. She's sweet, but wrong. She doesn't understand my pain and me, and what type of relationship we have."

Does this translate into 'get used to the pain, stop fighting it'? Does this mean that not working to get better will make the pain go away? Might this mean that those who suffer have to give up their 'existence' in order to 'exist'? Or does it mean that to survive, in any desired manner, the patient must develop a new-fangled approach to a new personal 'non-existence'?

This line of thinking is as rich as it is complex. It makes people think about the role of suffering in their lives. Sometimes we have to hunt for ways to live despite handicaps or injury. It is not always easy to achieve this state of mind. Emotional balance is expensive.

Perhaps medication use is justified in complex chronic pain because they reduce the psyche's boldness and willful instincts. Medications can undo the will and allow an indifference that may create a non-existence state such that 'Satan's web of suffering' can be ignored. In short, perhaps the use of medications is to take away the will that constantly compares the pain patient to the days when he did not suffer pain. Is it a calming down? Or is it a type of induced indifference? Is indifference the way to avoid uncontrollable pain? When is this the right way to think about medication use? What if such an indifference actually improves personal functioning, and it is not causing a muddling of a mental state?

In a society that wants an easy release from discomfort and pain, rather than to engage in the "noble growth potentials of suffering," can pain treatment take away the potential service that elevates its victim into an improved person? Is treating pain blocking this growth potential? This sounds backwards. It sounds like heresy!

Some argue that when the suffering is taken away, the pain loses its constructive components. Most chronic pain patients see that the pain did make them more realistic and appreciative of the good parts of life. But the construction is often matched with too much destruction as well.

> "I can tell you how much better I am. I can also tell you how much worse I am. Pain is a funny partner."

Illich says that pain becomes a "meaningless, question-less, residual horror. The sufferings for which traditional cultures have evolved endurance sometimes generated unbearable anguish, tortured imprecations, and maddening blasphemies; they were also self-limiting. The new experience that has replaced dignified suffering is artificially prolonged, opaque, depersonalized maintenance. Increasingly, pain-killing turns people into unfeeling spectators of their own decaying selves." [46] Illich still suggests that some growth is possible from being in pain. This is true insofar as it can have a maturing effect on a person's life.

Many metaphors and notions swim throughout our ethical heritage. They influence our thinking and color our judgments. When we experience profound events in life, we can learn from them, try to change from them, or try to ignore them. In any case, this process causes personality changes.

> "Many prosecutors see only liars and criminals, but the defense sees victims. The clergy sees lost souls or sinners, social workers see the underprivileged, and psychologists see the traumatized. My friends see me as a confident but my foes see me as depraved. Some doctors choose to see many as addicts while others take the time to see how even the addict suffers. Some think tough is enough and some think tough is not enough. It's all in how one sees people, as good, as trustworthy, with constructive potential, or as deceivers who are lazy, expendable and scoundrels. It is all in how someone strives towards what a person wants in life.
>
> I want different things in life. I want what most people assume. Now, I'd give up my career to have a painless night of sleep.
>
> I put my old personality in storage because it doesn't work anymore, but between you and me, if this pain goes away, I plan to bring some of that old 'me' out of storage. But I'll never be the same. Never. Some memories don't go away. My personality is the sum of my good and bad scars."

CHAPTER SEVEN

Addiction, Pseudoaddiction, and Iatraddiction

> "Not everyone has a soul of fire, and in actual human life, even in the case of the great mystic, this struggle against pain exacts a high price.
>
> Pain is always a baleful gift which reduces the subject of it, and makes him more ill than he would be without it. One must reject, then, this false conception of beneficent pain."
>
> R. Leriche, French Surgeon (1939)

Pain is commonly treated with narcotic medications. So one of the chores of living in pain is to explore the role we assign to medications. This frightens people because they envision of life of addiction.

Addiction is a real thing. But is it not necessarily dangerous. It seems more dangerous and menacing when it involves someone else's pain than when it is about our own pain. Knowledge about the real nature of addiction can be as soothing as the medications which may cause the 'addiction.' This chapter joins Chapter 20 in an effort to understand the issues of addictions.

Fears of addiction should not be the principal reason to avoid using pain killing medications. Under controlled and reasonable conditions, which include a straightforward relationship between a doctor, patient, and family, 'pain killers' do more good than harm.

Addiction is frequently referred to as being 'hooked.' Addiction is also not limited to narcotic medications. In fact, the same concepts and fears apply to the improper and uncontrolled use of all substances. For example, the National Academy of Sciences[47] noted that people who use methylphenidate (Ritalin®) for non-medical reasons may cause brain changes associated with the process of drug addiction. However, and this is so important, they also point out that hyperactive children don't usually show signs of addiction. This is because the medication is matched to a real condition. Recreational users of medications are far more likely to develop substance abuse problems.

> "This is kinda interesting, ya know. People using them ADD drugs and all.....I wonder if the reason so many people can down a beer and not be an alcoholic is 'cause they are putting out the real fires in life, not them neurotic ones. See, them neurotic fires, they never go out with beer. But a crazy day at work will be washed out of your mind with a beer or two...."

Interestingly, the phrase 'addicting pain killing medications' is misleading and unfitting. Addiction would never develop if pain was truly killed. The correct phrase is either 'pain controlling medication' or 'pain lessening medications'. They don't kill pain, though we wish they did.

When pain relief is the hunted treasure, then any resulting 'addiction' is not to the drugs but to their ability to reduce pain.

An astute person will ask if there is any connection between being addicted and the pleasure of being intoxicated. The desire for intoxication goes back to pre-historic times. Most people seek or experience some intoxication at one time or another in their lives. Intoxication can shift a state of consciousness. Such a shift follows the use of caffeine, beer, tobacco, a hard endorphin releasing hike, and so on. Most people use intoxicants without falling into addiction. Seeking intoxications is also not unique to humans; apparently elephants will seek out alcohol when stressed.

What is it that attracts living creatures to the psychoactive intoxicants? Ronald Siegel writes about a strong biological urge towards intoxication.[48] He called it the 'fourth drive' after hunger, thirst, and sex, and he refers to it as a 'holiday from reality.' The goal of intoxication is to feel pleasure and to sense that we will survive through a stress. How odd that the desire for relaxation is associated with the word *intoxication*. The presence of "*toxic*" in the word conjures up dodgy notions.

Intoxications can have utilitarian values insofar as medicating a tortured mind. The chronic pain patient, on an adjusted and proper dose of medications, almost never shows signs of intoxication. In fact, the chronic pain patient uses the 'drug assisted' state to have a holiday from his painful reality. This is a key concept – the proper use of pain medication 'assists' the user to return to a more normal life. Perhaps we ought to convert the word 'intoxication' into 'medication assisted change in mental status."

Many studies show that the incidence of addiction from narcotics use in pain patients is very low. Yet so much time is spent on this topic that we are forced to provide a discussion of addiction in the pain patient.

There is a constant flow of new research on this topic, but let's begin with some basic points. First, many pain patients have their own definition of addiction:

> "It is something I don't like, but addiction to me is a temporary remission from my handicaps. My addiction is a lifesaver. Without my addiction I would be hopelessly handicapped. My addiction, if you want to use the word, is good."

The pain patient uses drugs to escape pain's dreadful cruelty. He hopes the medications will help restore a normal life.

> I tell pain patients that the difference between the addict (in the common usage) and themselves is that they use drugs to join life while 'street' addicts use drugs to avoid life.

Some people argue that non-pain people use medications as their fountain of elixirs from which they get the courage and emotional fortitude to work or play. They are correct. This pain group uses drugs to join and go into a more normal life. A common example is of those who need antianxiety medications to control what would otherwise be a disruptive and unruly anxiety. Medication use, including narcotic use, is not always an erosion of reality. It may be a step back into it.

There are also many biological differences between people. We are able to measure only a few of these differences. Many still remain beyond our present scientific ability and dexterity to define and benchmark.

In 1984, Miller offered the idea that people with 'psychogenic pain' had a greater than normal level of neural activity.[49] He postulated that nerves regulating incoming pain signals were not inhibited in a normal fashion, making the person unusually sensitive to incoming pain. He felt the problem rested in a part of the brain known as the corticofugal inhibitory system. Simply put, he suggested that there is some inherent biophysical error, a 'biochemical inability,' to stop pain signals. This may be from a 'typographical error,' so to speak, in the way the brain is wired or in how the brain reacts to the hormones whose job it is to reduce the sensation or transmission of pain.

David Weissman[50] brought together a number of key issues about the importance of a trusting relationship between patients and treatment staff, of the problems when there is the under treating of pain (which happens in many situations), and how this flawed process often results in patients being mislabeled as addicts. He looks at the problems that arise in situations when, perhaps, a given medication dose is too low, or when the pain relief ability of the pill lasts only three hours, yet it is only given every six hours. Historically, this observation opened a strategic new line of reasoning in the evolution of the attitudes towards pain treatment:

> "The patient responds by requesting more frequent medications, often [asking for] opioids that they have recalled from the past that have been beneficial to them... most commonly meperidine (Demerol®) and Oxycodone (Percocet®, Percodan®, Vicodan®, etc). Phase 2 develops as the struggle for analgesics increases. The patient realizes that to obtain medication he must convince at least one member of the....treatment team...that the pain is both real and of sufficient severity to warrant additional medication. To achieve this goal, the patient engages in progressively escalated pain behavior, such as vocalizations, grimacing or holding affected body.parts.... As the suffering from inadequately treated pain continues, the patient may become less cooperative with ward routine, regressing to an immature level of interaction with the staff. As this point the patient is perceived as having a behavioral problem. The staff is concerned that because of the frequent requests for medication the

patient is becoming opioid dependant and therefore continues to prescribe medications on an as needed basis, at an inadequate dose and schedule, assuming that this will prevent or at least delay the onset of both opioid tolerance and dependence. The third phase occurs as the patient responds to continued, as yet unrelieved pain, by exhibiting increasingly bizarre drug seeking behavior. Emotionally, the patient will feel both angry and increasingly isolated from the staff who will in turn try to avoid contact with the patient because of the frequent complaints and requests for pain medications. This will set up a vicious cycle of anger, isolation and avoidance ultimately leading to complete distrust. Sometime during this cycle the patient will be labeled as an addict and all pretense of providing adequate analgesia will be lost because fear of contributing to the patient's addiction.

We have termed this...pseudoaddiction....an idiopathic opioid psychological dependence.... caused by the under medication of pain.... The consequences of inadequate pain relief... include loss of trust, feelings of anger, isolation and loss of self-worth....[which] may develop [into] a clinically significant depression."

Weissman's 1990 paper makes a reference to a paper published in 1973 by Marks and Sachar[51] which describes similar events. Patients are puzzled when they read these articles. So often, after reading them, they ask why their doctors failed to read the literature and treat them accordingly. "What are they afraid of?" one man asked me while he rubbed a terribly painful neuroma in the stump of his amputated knee during our discussion of his discovery of the term pseudoaddiction.

The fear of causing an addiction once existed even with the terminally ill. This has become less of problem as a result of the hospice movement. Up until the ending of such fears, there was a great risk of being under treated for pain. Other non-lethal diseases can also have extremely painful complications. Diabetes and AIDS can both cause bitingly painful leg pain. The issue in these diagnoses is treatment of pain in the living and not just in the dying.

Amenta and Bohnets' [52] chapter on the assessment of pain in the terminally ill offers some interesting notions which should be considered. They stress the importance of accepting this definition of pain:

> "Pain is whatever a person says it is, existing whenever he says it does. If the patient claims pain, believe him or her."

She makes four points about the attitudes of health professionals towards pain:

> **One**. Professionals fall easily into the belief that they, and not their patient's, are the authorities on the patient's pain. This moves the focus away from the patient's comfort and back to how the professional perceives someone else's pain.
>
> **Two**. Professionals mis-conceptualize the difference between acute and chronic pain. Acute pain is usually a warning that some damage has happened and that it will heal itself or it will respond to treatment. Chronic pain does not

resolve itself. Chronic pain may be as severe as acute pain, but chronic pain may defy treatment, which frustrates the patient.

Three. Many professionals try to get their patients to withstand their pain. But the levels of tolerance vary from person to person and from day to day. However, many professionals "overtly or covertly admire stoicism in patients. They admire those who tolerate pain and look down on those who do not seem to bear up."

Four. Too many professionals think that giving pain medications on a PRN (as needed) basis will prevent addiction.

She recommends that professionals correct these attitudes.

By the way, PRN is Latin for *Pro re nata,* which means 'according to the circumstance' or 'for the thing born.'

Amanita and Bonnet's chapter endorses the position that too many professionals still insinuate to their patients that addiction is a problem worse than the pain, that drugs to endure pain is socially 'bad', or that suffering holds a higher honor, distinction, glory, and homage than admitting that one needs medications to live comfortably.

This attitude comes in part from what doctors learned in medical school. Rarely do doctors develop clinical positions and perspectives about pain management prior to their medical trainings. This is how a major medical textbook discussed intractable pain:

"If pain accompanies a mortal disease and the life expectancy is measured in days or weeks,

> opiates in sufficient doses are best. Opiates modify reactions to pain more than perception of it and this provides the dual advantage of easing anxiety as well as pain. However, it is tragic when a patient with chronic pain and a normal life expectancy is provided opiates. Although temporary relief for both the patient and the physician may ensue, the problems of addiction inevitably complicate management and aggravate morbidity." [53]

Doctors who trained during the 1960's or 1970's were taught this approach. Doctors who trained in the 1980's were taught by the doctors from those earlier years. The attitude was passed along, and far too often this attitude towards pain lacked the sophistication needed for this area of medicine. Recent training attitudes, however, are much more in line with the real patient needs. It is, however, a slow transition.

> "The most vexing problems of intractable pain are presented by patients for whom pain fulfills an emotional need. These pain prone patients often have pain that is bizarre, defying rational explanation. The physical findings are seldom commensurate with the pain described. The physician, frustrated by repeated efforts to relieve the pain, may unwisely undertake operative exploration. This approach may be repeated many times, resulting in multiple surgical efforts to no avail. Psychiatric treatment, though quite obviously necessary, is frequently rejected by such patients.

> Intractable pain may also be perpetrated when disability may provide some gain. Pending litigation for damages resulting from injury may so magnify a patient's reaction to pain that effective treatment is impossible until the legal proceedings are concluded."

Or:

> "I never was sure about pain treatment. Medical school and residency left me certain it was needed, but not quite sure how to do it. And there was always a fear I would be hoodwinked by a clever addict. Or that I might be too soft on people's needs. I didn't know how to measure the real pathology. It was too close to psychiatry for my comfort."

Even the best doctor can be fooled by clever people with outstanding façades that hide their sinister motivations. Such dishonesty is bound to occasionally happen. Patients with complex psychiatric problems may also make it difficult to separate the physical from the psychic pain.

But these are relatively rare, and with take time and skill, many of these problems can be avoided. Fewer errors also occur whenever there is an effort to learn the *real* psychological make-up of the patient.

> "I was asked to evaluate a woman whose migraine headaches defied treatment. Partial relief was possible with Demerol® injections. Her frequent emergency room visits for Demerol® resulted in one emergency room physician

calling her an addict. They subsequently refused to treat her. During our psychotherapy sessions I learned of a history of childhood sexual abuse, her losing her children to foster care because of her ex-husband's violence, and of her current husband's terminal illness. She realized, after about 30 psychotherapy sessions, that about half of her headaches were indeed stress related. I choose not to concern myself with her narcotic use (keeping it to pain controlling levels) while I worked on the core problem.

She kept asking why I wasn't concerned with her drug use. I told her that while I was concerned, I also knew that productive psychotherapy would be impossible if she was tortured by pain. This built a trust between us "that," she said, "no other doctor gave me." Over time, and due to psychotherapy, her drug needs dropped markedly."

Many medical work-ups fail because physicians lack the skills to find the real problem. Too often these failures drop the burden of 'how to survive with the pain' onto the patient's lap. The doctor effectively washes his hands of 'impossible' tasks.

"My doctor told me he could not resolve my headaches even after an exhaustive work-up. So I asked if he would at least provide pain medications. After all, nothing curative or preventative could be done. The doctor refused, saying he could "not do *just* that." I left the office feeling that suddenly he was also beginning to doubt my pain. My husband was furious, saying the doctor could not tolerate being involved with something he could not fix. That really made me think that the doctor could really not look at my suffering. I initially thought he was sensitive to the suffering, but I lost full respect for him when he wasn't gutsy enough to stick with me and treat the pain anyway.

This is the type of experience that makes us pain patients so cynical and tough!"

This observation is from an articulate patient:

"Oh! the exhausting road and strenuous stream of hazards from the first complaint of pain to the use of continuous narcotics that patients must pass over, including the enormous hurdle of convincing the treatment givers that the existence and level of the pain is real, that the pain is not primarily a psychological or designed event, and that any addiction to a drug is better than the pain or my death."

Most people think of an addict as being someone out of control in some aspect of their life. For pain patients, 'addiction', to use the term, puts them into *better* control of their lives. Patients in pain use narcotics because they are addicted to no pain.

Much has been discussed in an effort to properly separate the 'addict' from the 'pain patient.' Some of the traditional differences that suggest a improper motive – which is put under the 'addict' label – are when there are (1) unsanctioned dose increases, (2) the altering of prescriptions, (3) going to several doctors simultaneously, (4) any unapproved use of other drugs along with the narcotics, (5) the use of the drugs for symptoms not noted by the therapy, or (6) the use of drugs during periods of no symptoms.

The haunting preoccupation of needing to keep a reliable medication supply is an understandable psychological dependence, and it should not be seen as pathological. Simple reassurance that a doctor and a pharmacy are available for emergencies ought to resolve this behavior.

Patients with obsessive compulsive traits may find that being a chronic pain patient is exceptionally difficult. The reason is obvious – their sense of comfort is dependent on an external factor. Having no controllable and reliable access to medications routinely produces survival driven changes in behavior. One common result of being in chronic pain is the development of compulsively flavored personality traits. This may appear to have the style of an addiction because of the motivational overlaps. But the compulsion is merely to insure a medication supply. It is driven by the memories of what it was like to not have adequate treatment.

Indeed, part of the definition of the word *'addiction'* is the feature or component of being *'compulsive.'* A compulsion is an act that cannot be stopped, or if it is stymied, then a tremendous amount of inner tension develops until the behavior can be carried out. Imagine if there is a monstrous uneasiness in your life. Hours and days pass being unable to do little more than to keep the irritation in check. Time is drawn away from work, family, and play just in order to quiet the aggravation and anguish. Maybe there is no quieting the pestering pain. Maybe all that can be done is to shove it back an inch or so, so that it is not the center stage in one's life. Perhaps this compulsion has the effect of stopping or slowing the endless 'stalking by the pain,' so it is not a constant menace to one's sanity.

Imagine the rush of joy when a treatment makes things better. Less energy is needed to hold off the predatory pain monster. Life gains back some freedom. Would it be any wonder if an obsession developed to insure the constant presence of this treatment? Would it be reasonable that a compulsion should evolve to keep the medication supply intact?

An escape from pain is a dose of euphoria. One patient said that because of the uncontrolled pain, "my time in life" was unusually nasty. "But the pain medications take me out of that diseased cage for a while." One of the rows against using narcotics is that they are self-reinforcing drugs because of the euphoria they produce. This suggests that more and more drug will be needed to maintain the euphoria. Wikler[54] described the euphoric effects of narcotics as a "positive reinforcer," which makes repeated intoxications more likely. Addiction, then, is allegedly to the euphoria, and any physical dependence is a secondary item attached the process of getting endless euphoria. On-going drug use is therefore arguably used to avoid the dysphorias of things like anxiety, depression, or withdrawal.

But wait. That logic implies that using narcotics always causes euphoria. This is not true. Pain patients feel relief from pain, so by comparison to their pre-medication use state, they might indeed feel 'euphoric.' This type of euphoria is spiritual, not physical. The euphoria that comes from escaping reality versus the euphoria getting pain relief are separate experiences. The transition from an unhealthy life into a normal one is quite different than that of going from a normal one into escapist euphoria.

"My doctor asked me if I got euphoric from the meds. I said not at all. But I looked up the

> word, and it means a feeling of happiness, confidence, or well-being. So I went back to the doctor and said I feel confident and not as afraid because of his medications. I like that better than euphoric."

There is no pleasure in having the typical street addiction. It is a miserable existence. Life is wasted in pursuit of the drug. It is a reality of daily fear, loneliness, façades, raw survival, physical agony, emotional anguish, hiding, and no growth. Those who have addictions well know the enormous energy they put into keeping every bit of balance in their lives. Many people who were never addicted view narcotic use as a desire for pleasure without effort, or as an lazy way to go through life and avoid responsibilities. These are not true.

Two old notions are of the 'addictive personality' or of an 'addiction proneness.' These concepts are supposed to reflect the effect of the first experience of drug use on the user, such that the user will immediately slip into a repeated, downward spiraling, pattern of drug use. Thomas de Quincey, in 1804, is often used as an example of addiction proneness, but reading the below about his pain, and how he controlled it, casts a very different flavor to his situation.

> He was suffering from facial pain when a "college acquaintance recommended opium....I took it and in an hour, Oh Heavens! What revulsion! What a resurrection, from its lowest depths, of the inner spirit.... That my pains had vanished, was not a trifle in my eyes this negative effect was swallowed up in the immensity of those positive effects which had opened before me, and in the abyss of divine enjoyment this

suddenly revealed. Here was a panacea... for all human woes here was the secret of happiness, about which philosophers had disputed for so many ages, at once discovered happiness might now be bought for a penny and carried in the waistcoat-pocket portable ecstasies might be corked up in a pint-bottle and peace of mind could be sent down by the mail." [55]

Did de Quincey's peace of mind happen because his pain disappeared? Is relief a bad product of addiction? Did the pain return when the opium wore off? These critical questions prevent the formation of any negative conclusions about his drug using motivation, other than he enjoyed the fact that his facial pain disappeared.

Different dictionaries offer insights into the attitudes that exist in our society about drug use. For example, a drug that typically dulls the senses or induces a sleep is called a *narcotic*. The state of being drugged is called *narcotism*, and a drug induced stupor is called a *narcosis*.

The word *addict* is derived from the Latin *addicere*. It is legal term that means that someone is physically turned over to the court for a sentence. An addict, therefore, 'is bound to or given over to' something. This figuratively has come to mean 'given over to a habit.' The word addict is also the outgrowth of the word 'verdict,' which means to 'declare the truth.' We can extend these implications to mean that being an addict is a sentence. Sentences are punishments, and so it implies bad behaviors that are worthy of a punishment

There is also the implication that being addicted is being stuck in something. Therefore, using the concepts from the above paragraphs, an addict is 'someone stuck in bad behaviors.'

The word addict has become associated more with a value judgment than a behavioral description. Call someone an addict and observe the reaction! A host of defensive explanations spout up! The protest may say "Okay, I may be out of control, and maybe there is an addiction problem, but I am not a bad person!"

The word addiction should be retired because it is pejorative. It should not be used in the professional literature.

It would be better to use the word 'dependence' to describe the relationship between a patient, his treatment, and a substance. *Dependent,* as a word, comes from the root word *aggravate,* which means to *upset or put a heavy strain on someone.* The Latin word *gravis* means 'heavy' or to 'put a burden on.' Its figurative use is to 'add to one's burdens or troubles,' and to annoy oneself greatly. Grief is also from the same root *gravis.* Close to this is the Latin word *pondere,* which means to 'hang or lean forward.' Dependent, therefore, means *'leaning upon or hanging from.'* So to be dependent on drugs means to lean on them for something. There is no judgmental or sneering connotation attached to the word. Hopefully the term 'dependence' won't one day become just a new vogue and slang way to say addict.

Narcotics palliate pain. A treatment which does not cure a problem but controls or swaddles the symptoms is known as palliative care. *Palliate* comes from the Latin word *pallium,* which means to *cloak.* To palliate is to disguise things that need to be hidden, hence there is the sense that the pain needs to be hidden. Early English used 'cloak' in place of palliate, and the inference was that the cloak was being drawn over an offense, so the process was 'to palliate the offense'. They needed to remove the legal flavor to the word because there is no offense.

If narcotic use does not fix the core problem but reduces suffering, then its use is palliative.

This can be extended to mean that both street addictions and medication dependencies are palliative endeavors. To many, hospice palliative innuendos have honest flavors, and addiction palliative innuendos taste foul. Interestingly, many thesauruses' offer terms like gesture, sop, pacify, bribe, panacea, excuse or placebo as synonyms for palliative.

It would be nice to see the word dependency used with a describer, such as 'dependency on morphine for control of intractable pain.' The label is cumbersome, but it is also more truthful and nonjudgmental. Initials make it into a shorter label: "DOMCIP."

If some people insist that a labeling reference to addiction must persist, then the terms pseudoaddiction and iatraddiction should be more widely used. This would force a shift from the older, traditional theories and practices into a healthier state of enlightenment.

Let's end this section with a look at hard numbers about the incidence of addiction in chronic pain patients. We being with an excellent summary in a 1990 paper by Portenoy [56] It is also important to remember just how much new research exists on these topics. The major trends are the same, that the misuse of pain medications is not the norm for the greater and vast majority of legitimate pain patients.

> - Sixteen patients with narcotic treatments for back pain were followed over 2 to 14 years, and over 75% had improvement in life styles without any evidence of opioid toxicity or drug abuse in any patient.
>
> - Patients with refractory neuropathic pain, followed for 22 months, on methadone, all had

greater than 50% pain relief. No problems with toxicity or abuse were noted.

- Nonmalignant pain patients, who failed various pain clinics, began chronic opioid use. Fifteen patients were able to return to work and they had fewer medical visits. In a second survey of 52 patients with different pains, who were also on narcotics, and were followed for an average of 12 years, it found 'adequate' pain relief in greater than 88% of patients, and partial relief in the remaining 12%. Abuse behaviors developed in 9 patients, but these are not well described, so questions exist as to why this happen, and even if they matched the characteristics of the other patients, etc.

- In the Collaborative Drug Surveillance Project, more than 10,000 patients without prior drug abuse problems were given opioids for pain control, and no cases of addiction were reported.

- A large headache clinic found narcotic abuse in only three of 2369 patients.

Pain treatment does not turn pain patients into dysfunctional addicts. Portenoy reported this same theme with two subsequent papers. [57] [58]

Many other similar papers and reports exist. [59] [60] Some did reach different conclusions, so care must be made that the subtle inferences in these reports would not sway people into too rapid a conclusion in the wrong direction. For example, one variable not often considered in these studies is this: what is the expected incidence of opiate addiction in the general population? Is this different from the addiction rate seen in opiate using pain patients? In other words, what is the overall general risk, in life, of becoming a narcotic addict even among non-pain patients? Might the risk of becoming an addict not be related to the exposure to narcotics as many believe? In short, does being an opioid using pain patient carry a higher rate, or risk, of being becoming an addict than anyone else in the general population?

This remains a controversial and technical issue. Studies are conducted and analyzed in different manners. Much of the problem lies in the nature of the tested populations. For example, a 2007 review from Yale says "substance abuse disorders are common in patients taking opioids for back pain, and aberrant medication-taking behaviors occur in up to 24% of the cases." [61] That is a higher number than in the early Portenoy papers. The 2007 article said that the analysis "did not show reduced pain with opioids", but the authors admitted that no trial was reviewed that treated the pain for more than 16 weeks. Also, what role is there that the pain was not reduced?

Fleming wrote in 2007 that "opioid use disorders were 4 times higher in (primary care) patients receiving opioid therapy compared with the general population." [62] Then Kahan wrote two articles in 2006 that concluded that "misuse and dependence on opioids can be identified and managed successfully in primary care."[63] And "Opioids are effective for managing chronic pain." [64] Another 2007 study [65] said that the benefits of opioids for chronic lower back pain "remains questionable" because of flaws in how the studies were designed. Finally, in 2007 a review of the American Pain Society's practice guideline on medications for chronic low back pain was published, [66] and it says:

- Fair evidence exists that acetaminophen, opioids, tramadol, benzodiazepines, and gabapentin are effective for pain relief.

- A mean decease in pain with opioids is at least 30%

- Trials of opioids were not designed to assess risk for abuse or addiction, and they generally excluded high-risk patients. In addition, with the exception of longer-term (16 weeks and 13 month) studies, all trials lasted fewer than three weeks.

- For very severe disabling pain, a trial of opioids in appropriately selected patients may be a reasonable option to achieve adequate pain relief and improve function, despite the potential risks for abuse, addiction, and other adverse events.

In 2008, another study looked at the incidence of addiction in chronic pain patients.[67] It is a complex paper. In one subgroup of studies with 2,507 chronic pain patients, the calculated abuse/addiction rate was 3.27%. In another subgroup of those same 2,507 patients, the calculated abuse/addiction rate was 0.19%. Another set of studies with 2,466 chronic pain patients had an abuse/addiction rate of .059%. Five studies of 1,965 patients found illicit drugs in 14.5%. They concluded that exposure to chronic opioid therapy "will lead to abuse/addiction in a small percentage of chronic pain patients." Furthermore these numbers "appear to be much less if the chronic pain patients are preselected for the absence of a current or past history of alcohol/illicit drug abuse or abuse/addiction." The question, stated again, and it cannot be answered, is how many of these same people, if they had not become pain patients, would have otherwise developed an addiction based on the rest of their psychological make-ups?

Such studies are intricate and tricky to understand. Yet three points stand out: First, experts themselves are not in agreement. Secondly, the incidence of problems with addiction in chronic pain patients is low, and that risk may be no more than the general risk of addiction in the general population. The third point is that patients enter the 'pain patient world' with all the mixtures and backgrounds common to any group of people. These are needed working foundations for anyone treating pain. [68]

It is important to remember that pain patients are mostly just the same as us, but they have pain.

Older scientific reports attest that opioid use in pain patients is quite safe, though the use must be controlled. Within that 'control team' is hopefully a viable, psychologically candid, and trusting multidisciplinary alliance between the patient and the treatment team. [69]

In 2005, I coined the term 'iatraddiction' to replace the term 'pseudoaddiction.'[70] I believe the older term pseudoaddiction does not convey the real cause of these pseudoaddictive behaviors. If patients need to locate additional medications because their doctors under treat them, then the problem is 'iatrogenic.' Iatrogenic means it is a doctor caused condition. My term re-assigns the blame to the medical profession.

Good tools for pharmacologic pain control exist. Though not perfect, and certainly embracing some risks, the risks of medication use must be measured against the most important of all tests, which is the freedom and ability to properly join in and enjoy life. A unenlightened and blinding alarm about addiction should not block the use of these tools.

...Thought...

> "...we told the Iroquois that we know all things through written documents. These savages asked us 'Before you came to the lands where we live, did you rightly know that we were here? We were obligated to say no. 'Then you don't know all things through books, and they didn't tell you everything'."
>
> Louis Hennepin (1626–1701)

The problem so many pain patients report is that they feel pre-judged. The system clumps them together rather than seeing them as unique individuals. One patient said it was as if treatment teams assume that their knowledge of pain and the pain patients' needs was complete and un-blemished. One patient said: "How different it was when the nurse really got to know me as a individual...."

Jesuit Jose de Acosta was an early explorer. He wrote:

> "I will describe what happened to me when I passed to the Indies. Having read what poets and philosophers write of the Torrid Zone, I persuaded myself that when I came to the Equator, I would not be able to endure the violent heat, but it turned out otherwise.... What could I do then but laugh at Aristotle's Meteorology and his philosophy? For in that place and that season, where everything, by his rules, should have scorched by the heat, I and my companions were cold." [71]

The sick, especially those with pain, tend to be regarded and pre-assembled into a pre-defined group rather than arduously kept as individuals. Like the early explorers, the treatment teams need to sail to the horizon to see what is really out there, and they should not rely on widespread, but not always tested, stories.

One cannot assume anything. A few bad patients should not paint another entire group as bad. This is the sin of broad brush assumptions and generalizations. Too many people lack the honesty and courage to admit to their list of overgeneralizations. Even the pain patient must accept such self acknowledgements if they are to learn to live with pain.

> "Three groups of pain patients worry me. Those with mental retardation, those who cannot speak, and the very psychologically impaired. I am not sure we can teach them much. How do we improve a life that is already so impaired? They surely need completely individualized care, but what system is prepared to support the level of needs these people need. Yet somehow, we need to reach them, and not give up. They may fear and feel they are bad people but can't say so, or they might only be able to act out instead of speaking, but we can look into their eyes and know they are feeling. What did they do to deserve the agony? God will probably attack me, but I wonder if we are doing any good in keeping them alive – oh, what a dreadful thought...."

God's will was once assumed to be the ultimate, though not always the immediate cause of illness. Disfiguring illness or epidemics were once taken as evidence of a Godly scorn and punishment. An illness was a defect.

Renaissance thinkers comfortably blamed social or cultural subgroups as the source and cause of a disease. Societies were barbaric to each other, so diseases assumed names such as the Spanish pox or the Neapolitan evil. (This "pox" disease, also known as the *morbus gallicus*, was actually syphilis brought back to Europe from America by the Spanish explorers, but its appearance was often blamed on social or politically targeted groups.) So sub-sets of groups developed that put a flavor of danger into the minds of the larger community about other subsets of groups.

Opiates, when abused, is a danger to society. Efforts to explain the abuse use patterns as a disease, infirmity, defect, or as coming from some other origin, are underway and, as expected, it is the topic of enormous debate.

The reality is that opiate abuse exists. Work is underway to make opioid medications harder to abuse. The reasons are scary: in 2005, 8,500 people died from prescription opioid overdose – this is more than from cocaine and heroin use combined. The drug companies therefore want tamper-resistant opioid medications. Coming soon is Remoxy®, which is a new tamper resistant form of Oxycontin®: Oxycodone is mixed with gelatin that forms a rubbery pill which bends when it is hit or crushed. Even if it is dissolved it will not release all the oxycodone at once. Other formulations want to make the pill so tough it cannot be crushed. This may slow the casual abuse, but the determined abuser will look for a way to beat the system. Some pills mix naltrexone in the core. If the pill is crushed, the naltrexone is released, which will block the opioid effect.

Good ideas, yes, but they do not offset the reason for abusing the drugs.

Those who 'abuse' are not the same as those who 'use.' Like the brave early explorers who discovered that the general common contention that so much of what they 'knew' was simply wrong, the closer we get to the users and abusers, the more their differences come into view. The pain group ought not to suffer for the another's unhealthy deeds. But the only relationship between these two groups is that they both consume narcotics – it's just that different reasons exist for putting the same molecules into their bodies.

Placebos

There is a sneering interest in placebos because they suggests faking. There is also a scientific infatuation with placebos because they work.

Beecher found post-surgical pain relief using placebos happens in about 35 percent of patients. Morphine relieves pain in about 75 percent of people, and some propose that half of this is from the placebo effect. This speaks to the mighty contribution of placebo to pain control. It is known that non-drug induced enkephalin releasers, such as with acupuncture, stress, or placebos, can produce significant analgesia.[72] As a result it is tricky to make a clinical diagnosis based on a 'suspected' placebo response. [73] [74] Interestingly, a recent text book on pain control made no mention of placebos.[75]

Placebo is a Latin word for '*I will please.*' It became a noun meaning 'to be a medicine given more to please than benefit the patient.' The opposite of placebo is 'nocebo,' which is Latin for '*I will harm.*' Medical procedures can be as much placebo as nocebo. 'Nocent' is a 15th century English word for 'harmful'. It stems from Latin '*nocere,*' which is 'to harm.' Medicine in the 18th century labeled as 'placebo' those inert preparations prescribed solely for a patient's mental relief when there was no physical disorder. Eventually, someone noticed that harmless preparations could also have detrimental effects on user's health. It was then that the word 'nocebo' for substances causing adverse reactions was born. Much alchemy was considered to be the exploitation of placebos. But interestingly, alchemy was looking for 'cures', and the off shoot of this search was the beginning of the basic chemistry that feed into the development of modern pharmaceuticals.

Many use 'fake' as their definition of placebo. Usually someone who responds to a placebo is downgraded to a 'faker,' which then converts to a less than real, or bogus, clinical status.

Patients get quite upset if they are asked to take a placebo in a test. If they respond, then the response might mean that their pain is not real, that the pain is imaginary, or perhaps it is an invention of the mind. In truth, however, the pain can be quite real and it can react to placebo treatment.

A placebo response is a real physical response to the 'pretend drug.' But this is a false long-term positive. Repeating the placebo use again, and again, and again, and again, will see the placebo effect fade away. So while a shot of morphine will work with reasonable consistency over time, the placebo will eventually lose its effectiveness over the same time period. (A loss of therapeutic response could also be a pseudotolerance, but this is a process not related to placebo issues).

Some people are placebo responders. Somehow the brain is 'fooled' into ignoring or not feeling the pain. How wonderful it would be to identify what is happening in this process. Maybe it is an infusion of hope, which all of us know is one of the most powerful of all remedies. A positive response to a placebo is known as the 'analgesic placebo response.' It combines all the biological and psychological aspects of pain. It also brings us directly into the complex area of mind-body interactions.[76] An understanding of these interactions is far from complete.[77] Elsewhere in this book are discussions of our body's endogenous opiate systems. Perhaps the placebo response is related, in part, to how our bodies make endorphins and opiates.

A new genetic basis may explain why some people respond to placebos and some do not. A gene has been preliminarily linked to the placebo effect. The gene in question makes the enzyme tryptophan hydroxylase-2, which makes serotonin. People with two copies of a variant of this gene were less anxious in 'fear tests.' This discovery, should it stand up to repeated study, may help explain the 'why' of pain disorders, sleep disorders, depression, or phobias, etc. Great care has to be kept not to over-generalize from these early findings. But great joy can be felt that another newly found pathway may explain an important event in our lives. [78]

The challenge of a book like this is that so much new is always appearing and therefore it can never be fully up to date. It leaves us with the feeling of falling behind rather than being ahead.

CHAPTER EIGHT

Punishment for what the doctor can't fix in patients with unfixable emotional problems

It seems that we never emphasize enough that pain patients do not germinate from defective seeds. Pain patients don't irresponsibly and feverishly grow from non-medication using into medication needing people.

The metamorphosis into 'painhood' can be rapid or slow. But the moment someone realizes that they have become a chronic pain patient is a solemn day. That day can leave grisly emotional etchings.

Problematic pre-pain life experiences may be the reason why some people need extra training in stress management skills. But the force of a chronic and ever-present pain is often no match for even the strongest of us.

It would be reassuring to know what in a person's character or chemistry could help us say "With your psychological past, chemistry, and background, if you get hurt, you stand a greater chance than not of being able to withstand the pain." If we could fully isolate that 'something,' then perhaps we could fix it before it caused problems.

One interesting concept is that some people, when under stress, want to retreat into their past as a form of avoidance from the new problems. This could be especially so if there was little hope to resolve the new problems, such as facing untreatable pains and all that falls from that.

Some people are more emotionally susceptible than others to trauma and suffering. Many say that these folks suffer more due to a personality weakness or powerlessness, or to an impediment. So let's move into a discussion of personality styles, traits, and disorders. This will include the challenges and reality of treating some patients with problematic psychological make-ups.

> Personality traits, sometimes also commonly referred to as character traits, are patterns of how a person interacts and views their the relationships to their environment and self-views. The results are exhibited in a wide range of important social and personal contexts. Only when the personality traits are inflexible and maladaptive, and when they cause either significant functional impairment or subjective distress, do they constitute a personality disorder. All of us have clusters of unique personality traits – these clusters give us our individuality. Great care must be taken before the label of a personality disorder is applied to a person.

The personality trait or disorder may hinder an ability to function effectively. Sometimes the person with a personality trait or disorder will deny or not realize that they have a syndrome.

"A personality disorder is an enduring pattern of inner experiences and behaviors that deviates markedly from the expectation of the individual's culture, is pervasive and inflexible, has an onset in adolescence or early adulthood, is stable over time, and leads to distress or impairment".[79]

Culture may influence a personality style. A culture is defined as the behavioral and thought patterns of a group of people. How people approach and trust each other is often a product of their cultures. Both doctor and patient need to be sensitive to the 'cultures' they each bring into the relationship. Sometimes a person, acting in a manner that appears to be at odds with the surrounding culture, may be mislabeled as having a peculiar personality style. But it is not pathology, per se, as much as it is the product of a cultural dissimilarity.

Time and again we are quick to forget that a treatment team member may be an insurance company. A patient's cultural make-up may not understand the cultural value system of an insurance company. For example:

> "My grandfather emigrated here from China. He is humble, quiet, simple in so many ways, and he cannot understand why the insurance company, to whom he paid premiums, won't pay for his medications now that he is sick. I have never seen a man so angry and yet so unable to express it! When he acted out, the doctor wanted him to see a counselor. We said no, that's not his real personality. Thank God we Americanized children are here to explain and fight for him."

Or:

> "My Dad is Puerto Rican. He never admits to his emotions, except when he is mad. He also never liked to be told what he could and could not do. We saw him limp for over a month before he agreed to see a doctor. Then we learned there was a small tumor between his toes. It was so painful, but he refused to take 'those pain tablets'. My aunt yelled at him, saying he has a stupid old personality that is going to kill him. "This is so like you," she said.

We kids had to find an older Spanish priest to convince him to use the meds until the surgery could be done. However, he could not understand why the insurance company had a say in which doctor he could use."

A very thorough knowledge of a person's psychological make-up is needed to correctly diagnosis a personality disorder. This should not be done slapdashedly, because the ramifications of such a diagnosis can be devastating. Personality disorder diagnoses should only be made by seasoned mental health professionals. These are some basic questions to ask before the final diagnosis is made:

> Might the person's behavior make sense given some larger cultural operating problem, about which the observer is unaware? The problem could be an unresolved trauma, an emotional embarrassment or lost, etc.

> If the at-odds behavior merely disagrees with the observer's moral code, then might the observer feel justified in applying his personal moral code onto another person's behaviors? This often happens.

> Another key question is whether or not the patient's presenting behavior is an ethical, financial or professional nuisance, or other inconvenience or threat to the observer? Applying a diagnosis in cases like this are potentially more an opinion than a fact. This type of event happens when people live in conflicting socio-ethnic cultures.

> "My former doctor believed in the culture of aggressive pain management. This current doctor believes in the culture of conservative pain management. I believe in the culture of effective pain management. I suppose some of my current doctor's patients do still get better because they are lucky enough to respond to conservative treatment. I don't, I need the unusual treatments, so I still hurt. But my insurance company won't pay for me to go elsewhere. I now live in the culture of indentured pain patients."

Might a patient's unusual behavior in fact be stemming from a survival issue, such as relentless pain or hunger? Remove the survival threat and perhaps the behaviors will 'normalize.' By the same token, perhaps the behavior in question is the outgrowth of another problem, such as a phobic, depressive, or an obsessive ailment? The list of all possibilities has to be explored.

> "My old doctor, a nice guy and he tried, but we didn't know the right diagnosis. Finally the right med finally came out, and I got better. So all those nights of calling him at 2 AM, of my endless complaining and arguing, it was because I had the disease but they did not have the fix. Once, when in a hospital, another doctor said I was a borderline personality because of how I treated my doctors. Hey, did I get myself a nasty diagnosis! It was wrong, but it was branded onto my chart. Now all the symptoms are gone. I am better. And that supposed personality disorder they said I had – gone too!"

'Bad personality' labels have both political and medical implications. For example:

> "I was nasty to the new doctor. I didn't like his 'he-knows-it-all' approach to my case. I tried to speak to him, but oh no, he didn't have the time. I've suffered too long for me to get this type of treatment. He told the nurse I had a 'personality problem.' He wrote that in the chart, so the next doctor assumed the first doctor was right. Then my worker's compensation adjustor read it. Now I'm accused being uncooperative because I disagreed with a most obnoxious doctor. He's got the personality problem, not me. But his label is now my punishment. I gotta get it erased somehow…"

Some nasty behaviors that are listed as personality disorders may actually sprout from psychological seeds and predispositions that were never seen until the person faced a relentlessly mammoth stress or fear. Personality can change as workable situations become unworkable. Patients are often embarrassed to see 'that side of me come out.'

> A 24 year old woman with a mild eating disorder and soft borderline traits suffered a hip injury. Her borderline traits did not interfere with much of her life before the accident. She was able to work, go to school, and have a lasting boyfriend. There was no insurance money for psychological intervention. She admitted she was vain, but prior to the accident she managed her weight without difficulty. She could not

understand why the pain doctors "only want me on meds that cause weight gain and block my orgasms!" So she asked only for narcotics simply because they controlled the pain without the other side effects. She didn't want the antidepressants, which, by the way, she probably did not need. They told her the antidepressants helped reduce the pain, but she felt the side effects were much greater than any benefit she obtained from them. One time, her request for narcotics without the antidepressants was labeled by a doctor as drug seeking. When she heard that this label had been applied to her, she flew out of the office, leaving behind a trail of vibrant insults. She ended up using walk in pain management clinics where she got just what she wanted.

Despite the theories and textbooks, overfilled with so many opinions and notions about how to treat human suffering, fixing seriously dysfunctional personality problems is not easy. A person with a provocative personality disorder who also has a chronic pain disorder can be quite challenging. If the personality issues soften with proper pain treatment, then the 'personality problem' may need to be reconsidered as 'not that bad, after all.' All this can complicate a clinical presentation.

Other cultural barriers, including language barriers, called 'health literacy,'[80] often impede access to a fitting treatment. The doctor and patient may simply not be able to understand each other's language, dialects, etc. Most hospitals have lists of local people who can translate, interpret, and explain on behalf of both patient and staff.

"My Mom broke her hip. She was scared and in pain. I was out of town when it happened. When she gets upset, she resorts to Yiddish. No one in the ER spoke Yiddish. She got dead silent because she couldn't commutate. As it happened, a Hassidic Rabbi walked by her room. She saw him, and despite her pain, she walked to him. He was a God send, he immediately found a congregant who spoke Yiddish, he waited with her until that lady got to the ER, and Mom – it makes me cry as I say this – my Mom calmed down so much. They cancelled the psychiatric evaluation, things got set up for surgery, the nurses finally got me on the phone, and every year my family says a special blessing for that Rabbi and that special lady."

Ethnopsychopharmacology, another important variable, is the science behind why different ethnic groups respond to medications differently than do other groups. African-Americans and Asian-Americans have genetically based differences in their metabolizing liver enzymes, so they may show different issues with plasma levels or side effects. Medicine is just beginning to include these backgrounds in deciding how medications are dosed.

Cultural competency is that set of skills which allow people to work across cultures.[81] Many critical problems may arise from such cultural and personality hurdles and issues, and therefore the diagnosis and management of clinical situations can be tricky. A web site devoted to the management of racial, cultural, ethnic, and other disparities is: www.thinkculturalhealth.org

Why is this so important, and why does it warrant so much time and consideration? First, the treatment team needs understand what is right and what is wrong in the person's life. And then, although the medical basis of a problem is known, it still may be unfixable from both a medical and psychosocial perspective. This is difficult for all involved, and it is especially so if cultural issues impede the communication.

Experiencing a failed treatment can be difficult for some people. Failures need to be couched in the patient's cultural expectations as well. The patient might assume the failure is the product of a personal failure. They need to know as much as possible why the failure occurred, and what options still remain. A wise chronic patient noted to me:

> "I spoke to a nice, but passive and frightened old man whose cultural make-up made it hard for him to feel that a doctor failed, so he took the blame for the failure on himself. He had a simple belief that medicine could not fail. It took a lot to get this out of him."

Consider this particularly troublesome scenario:

> Someone is hurt. Every reasonable effort to fix the injury fails. Narcotics are introduced and the patient feels relief. But the relief is not long lasting, and a pseudoaddiction develops. The patient and his family begin looking for a doctor who has the understanding and willingness to prescribe enough medications to keep the patient comfortable.
>
> A psychologist is consulted to test the patient for being in a `sick role,' which really suggested that the doctors wanted to see if there

were any underlying personality problems. Psychotherapy, a transfer to a different pain clinic, and treatment with relaxation and biofeedback were all then tried. Happily, the efforts produced some relief. Over a brief time, the psychologist felt the patient suffered from an immature personality with significant narcissistic qualities. The physical pain had been a terrible blow to his ego, and while his personality functioned well enough before the pain, it did not do so after the pain. Ongoing psychotherapy was recommended, but there was no money to pay for the amount of needed therapy.

The chart now carries the label of "personality disorder, narcissism." To many this translates into a "warning and beware sign!" However, this label should be descriptive and not pejorative. The psychologist did, to his credit, put a letter in the chart to explain the person's life, stresses, etc., and that the 'personality disorder' was not dangerous or malevolent.

Any candid psychotherapist knows that the first goal of taking care of a personality disordered patient in crisis is to keep things as stable as possible. With physical pain-suffering personality disordered patients, one challenge is to find out why the pain become an on-going crisis. This information may then prevent a recurrence of the crisis; doctors may call this a 'relapse prevention.' Understanding and fixing this problem may take a considerable amount of time.

"My doctor, a good enough lady, she's always in a rush. Yet we need her. My therapist, I need her too, but she's not in that much of a rush. The psychological work is happening, but slowly. So I put it this way: my doc has the watch, but my therapist has the time."

A fear is often raised that people with personality disorders are more prone to addiction. This is not necessarily true. It is true, however, that doctors question which problem is being treated with pain medications. The doctor wonders: "Am I treating the pain or the personality disorder?"

> Victims of sexual or other abuses commonly enter treatment with a variety of obstinate psychological hurdles, some of which are not easy to treat. But if the presenting problem is clear cut pain, then the process may be simple. Treat the pain. All the other problems may not be significant clinical issues. The emotional issues following emotional or physical abuse may never emerge if the pain treatment is adequate. Also, it may be prudent for the doctor to steer away from the emotional issues and work only on the pain problem. This, of course, assumes that the psychological and pain issues can be separated. Automatic psychological referrals or unskilled therapy may unnecessarily open doors to old problems. A onetime consultation with a good psychotherapist may be all that is needed.
>
> Sometimes the doctor is the one who needs a 'consultation' in order to provide 'consolation.'

Many treatment attempts become complicated or fail because the basic problems of an on-going abuse, or the residuals of abuse, enter into the pain management arena. This being so, the psychological problems now sit right next to the pain problems. This compels the use of conjoint clinical psycho-medical interventions. [82] [83] [84]

Many addicts abuse substances to quell their inner emotional and physical discomforts. Narcotics are excellent in doing so. This raises the quandary of what to do with patients who suffer both pain and certain psychiatric problems. Stopping or limiting pain medications because of, or until the social or emotional storms can be quieted, has a dangerously high chance of medical and psychiatric failure. Then, to complicate matters even more, if a failure happens, the patient is often labeled as 'psychiatric.' This leaves the ego-deflating flavor that the failure occurred because of 'my psychiatric issues', and not because of the medical ones. The label may be correct to some degree, but the repercussion for the failure should not primarily rest with the patient if the patient did honestly try to make things better.

Appropriate blame needs also to be assigned to treatment plan and related limitations, such as the lack of money for good on-going psychotherapy. That is another slap of defeat, which can only worsen the patient's self-image. It takes away opportunities for new skill development, and it may add to an increased level of hopelessness and anger at themselves and their worlds.

> A 55 year old woman suffered years of a mix of horrible, treatment resistant psychological emptiness and thought disorders. Her years of good therapy efforts gave little lasting relief. Then she accidently hurt herself, and after narcotics were started to address the new back pain, her moods calmed in ways that all the prior psychiatric medications failed to do. Her narcotic dosing needs were quite constant, so the

first pain management doctor accepted the psychiatric extra-benefits she got from the pain medications. However, when the first doctor retired, the new pain management doctor was not so accommodating. He lowered her pain med doses, which put her into a terrible psychiatric crisis. He even called her an addict. Her psychiatrist saw all this happen. No psychotropic medication would calm her as did the narcotics. Since the psychiatrist knew her for years, he called the new pain doctor with the hopes that giving him more history, that she was in regular therapy, etc., would make him feel comfortable in adjusting the narcotics back up to the older doses. He acknowledged that the patient could be demanding and quite annoying at times, which was part of her psychopathology. The psychiatrist had learned how to work with her 'style', yet the new pain doctor would not modify his position. He made no changes. The psychiatrist was struck by the indifference the new doctor had to the real history. The new pain doctor even implied the psychiatrist was soft on the reality of his patient. It was an irresolvable impasse. So a third pain doctor was found who understood the situation.

It's not uncommon for prior substance abusers to need narcotic pain medications. The treatment team may worry that treatment will re-kindle a narcotic craving. This can initially be very uncomfortable for the treatment team. Considerable debate exists about giving pain medications to a former drug abuser. It is not an dangerous impasse, however.

The situation can handled in the simple and obvious manner of getting to thoroughly know the patient. The development of a solid multilayered working relationship between doctor and patient must occur. Doctors need to simultaneously 'ignore and use' the patient's past. This requires sophisticated professional skills.

Sister Helen Prejean reminds us that: "people are more than the worst thing they have ever done in their life." [85]

> A 37 year old woman contracted AIDS from intravenous heroin use. Her pre-AIDS life has been miserably hard. In her last year of life, she developed incredibly painful neuropathy in her legs. She required higher than usual doses of narcotics to control the pain. The primary doctor prescribing the narcotics was criticized for giving the drugs to a former addict. The allegation was that her pain could not be as bad as she was reporting, so, in essence, she was lying and exaggerating. His reply was that while she was once plagued with drug addiction because of a pitiful adolescence, her current problem was pain. He didn't deny that some aspects of her former self still existed, but he could regulate them. He said "I know my patient quite well. The reason for the heroin use was altogether different than her need for the narcotics now." He commented how disappointed he was in that so many of his colleagues were so comfortable punishing such patients for their prior lives.

Doctors are terrified by hypochondria. They don't want to feel blackmailed or foolish by giving unnecessary medications. A hypochondriac implies 'fake.' Anxiety, neurosis, imagined ill-health, and morbid melancholy are some of the synonyms for hypochondria. Indeed, finding a real diagnosis for some unusual clinical symptoms can, at times, be very difficult. The doctor may have to offer treatment based only on subjective reports. This is a dreadfully problematic and intimidating situation for doctors. Yet a report exits wherein two people committed suicide after their supposed 'hypochondriac symptoms' failed to get better. The fundamental question to ask is if the pain was truly psychosomatic (in the sense of it being entirely of a psychological origin), or did the lack of a diagnosis merely reflect the current limits of the doctors' diagnostic abilities? [86]

Giving pain medications to people with co-morbid psychiatric disorders is challenging and arduous. Can we ethically deny treatment because of a lack of system's patience, energy, tools, financial commitments, skills, or courage to try to fix them? So often it's our fault that they don't get better. The fault is ours, not theirs.

When medications are used in an intensive yet controlled manner, with an aggressive psychiatric input, then a human being will very likely have less pain. Over time, any other dysfunctional emotional issues can be addressed, studied, and hopefully changed. The success of the rehabilitation program at the Mayo Clinic, mentioned earlier, shows what good resources and hard work can produce.

...Thought...

What should you do if you fall into one of the groups alluded to in his chapter? (Similar suggestions are also listed in the last chapter of this book.)

> Get the doctor to really know you. Be honest in ways that may be quite new for you. Bring clinical records. Try to understand the doctor's

world. Complicated or unusual cases usually stir up outside monitoring. Don't expect the doctor to be someone she or he is not. Don't expect to present your entire life, with all the problems, etc., at a first visit. Give the doctor a chance. Don't give up your role as part of the treatment team. But by the same token, all doctors are not equally caring, skillful, clever, dedicated, empathic, engageable, benevolent, and so on. There is no shame in needing to find a doctor whose make-up and style better matches your needs. We seek both treatments and relationships with our doctors. Almost anyone can give the treatment part of the association. Not all can give the relationship side of the association.

Let the non-psychiatrist become a better listener, but keep the psychiatry to the psychiatrist. Ask for a psychiatric or mental health referral if needed. Good psychotherapy is as productive as any medicine or device.

Allow and demand an absolutely clean paper trail. Show where and how medications are obtained and used, which other doctors are involved in your care, who controls the medication supply, etc. Don't jeopardize the doctor's reputation and legal standing if he is willing to help you. Help him help you. Secrets will poison the relationship. Learn to be candid, open-minded, and to trust one another. And that takes time!

Finally, some excellent advice for all of us from a very old source:

"Be quick to listen and slow to speak" *The New Testament*

...Thought...

Disease was once regarded as the product of internal imbalances. The four internal substances that could go out of balance were blood, bile, black bile, and phlegm. The discovery of microorganisms, cancers, and some definable chemical imbalances shoved medicine into thinking that disease was produced by invasive entities, that is, something wrong or bad invaded or injured the body. Find out what this was, measure it with a lab test, take the bad away, and the disease ought to be cured.

The riddle is what to do when something discrete and measurable could not be found. People thought that if a 'wrong or bad' couldn't be physically found, then it was an imagined malady. This imagined infirmity was considered to be the result of, or a throwback to, some form of mystical internal imbalance. It became a delicate way of saying that the person's constitution was imbalanced, which, in its own way, left the sense that the illnesses grew more from a psychological or ethical abnormality than from a biological one.

A central clinical burden is what to do with patients who don't get better with standard treatments, or if their pain origin is more vague than specific. These patients often face a real hesitancy among treatment team personnel against long term pain medication use. This may be because of the team's fear of legal ramifications for even allegedly inappropriate use of medications given the inexact cause of the pain. But what are the ethical obligations on the part of the team and doctor? And how does a team and doctor rise to those ethical requirements?

The doctor has to trust and believe in the patient. The patient has to prove his honesty and trustworthiness to the doctor. The clinical records need to almost be a novel, with as many non-scientific but critical and supported comments about the improvement in life that followed pain medication use. Typical medical charting styles may be too anemic. The entire process must join the clinical needs, legal realities, psychosocial pressures, and *the ethical commitment* into a product that offers the best treatment.

Chapman [87] gives us an interesting thought:

> "But what of the beginnings of ethical thought? It is convenient, as a first approach to this difficult topic, to note that many ancient philosophers made little distinction between legal obligation and moral, or ethical, duty. It would, however, be very misleading to assume that in our own time law and ethics are one and the same thing. For the present purposes we may view ethics, in a free society at least, as concerned with rules that are beyond the province of law, in that they summon the individual to actions that are nobler, and usually more altruistic, than those required by law. Legal requirements, in contrast, are in a sense minimal in some instances (for example, the common law of negligence), the standard of performance requires by law is by design mediocre. Ethical standards, to the contrary, require the best performance the individual can, by virtue of training and natural endowment, deliver."

CHAPTER NINE
Lying

"Oh, but you can't hurt *that* much," said the doctor.

"But I do!" said the patient.

How often do we hear this conversation?

Lying is a common and deeply rooted activity that penetrates into many people's thinking. We know this is true because we all know how to lie.

Often, when others don't themselves feel or experience something, they conclude that that the 'something' is not likely to exist. This is egocentrism. How many times do doctors, nurses, family or friends say or suggest to a pain patient that "it cannot possibly be as much pain as you complain about."

> Egocentrism means that "if something doesn't make sense to me, or I don't feel it, then it doesn't exist."

There is no doubt that some pains are exaggerations and 'embellishments with a motive.' This evokes accusations that the patient is lying. This process happens to also reek throughout the business, personal, medical, political, insurance, and legal worlds. A lawyer told his patient that she "couldn't possibly need that much medication." This effectively accused her of a fraud. At her deposition, however, he painted a portrait of how much she was suffering.

Many insurance companies limit the quantity of pain medications they will pay for. They may also refuse to pay for pain medications if their experts' feel 'the patient doesn't have real pain.'[88]

Medical records also often misrepresent the patient's clinical truth. Every chart reflects only what the writer chooses to write. Every record, therefore, contains some editorializing and bias. This can have the effect of alleging that a patient is reporting excessive pain. In such cases, the patient could be honest and the chart is lying.

These problems can be solved when people better know each other. How inopportune it is that so many doctors and patients, whose lives are intimately involved with each other, still fail to know each very well. Allegations of "lying" typically reflect the lack of a time tested and honed familiarly.

It is important to underscore and highlight this: That any malfunction in the nature of the affiliations between patient and treatment providers (including insurance authorities) will most certainly destroy, skew, or add antagonism into physician-patient relationships. That then results in less than optimum pain management. The different parties may lie to make their points, save money, or avoid battles. The battles are lessened when the parties – i.e., doctor and patient, know each other. A relationship that stands atop a lie will not withstand the real test of time.

In 1935, Henderson felt that the doctor-patient relationship had not changed in centuries, that this relationship was a mini-social system, and that the doctor "must not only appear to be, but must be really interested in what the patient says." He emphasized that the possible harm coming out of this system rests as much with the level of technical skills as with what the doctor says or fails to say. [89] That mini-social system supports and nurtures the ability to get good pain management.

A doctor's style may actually encourage patient's lying so they can get that they need. In 1987, Merril et al.,[90] examined the patient characteristics that physicians dislike:

> "Among the complaints where those patients with trivial and un-diagnosable problems, those who are not sick, those who are hypochondriacs, request medical procedures, who are substance abusers, hostile or 'dumped', and those who waste the doctor's time. An overview...reveals that physician's find it a hassle to deal with patients for whom the prognosis is not clearly positive or patients over whom they believe they have little control."

Merrill points out that if a physician changes his practice style, then what had been normal or abnormal in the past may have to be redefined to meet the new relationship style or setting. This is called *'observer shift.'* This is an important concept that can re-define the core elements of a doctor-patient relationship.

The "theory of the *observer shift* holds that the intensity of a stimulus is judged by comparing it to the mean of the most recent occurrences being weighted most heavily." What this complex sentence means is that we make conclusions based on what we see and the values of the group around us. Something that was once 'abnormal' may be re-labeled as 'normal' when new reference points are used. So if a doctor spends additional time with his pain patients, the result should be a greater familiarity with the gestalt of their lives.

The inclination to say a patient is lying should change as the *'observer shifts'* go from a theory to a fact. Basically this means that getting to better know someone can often convert distrust (theory) into trust (fact). It is also much harder to lie to those who know us well.

Hard data doesn't exist, but one must wonder which groups of doctors are more likely than others to suspect that a patient is lying to them. And by the same token, it would be interesting to know which groups of doctors are most likely to be lied to?

> This same theme applies to nursing attitudes as well. "A patient's behavior, then, does strongly influence a nurse's willingness to accept (a patient's) pain rating and to administer a higher dose of an opioid. The nurses who discussed the survey results ... appeared to be unaware that their personal biases ... could influence what they recorded in a patients chart, and what they choose to do about pain relief.... Some nurses rely more on the patient's behavior than on what he says about his pain." If a behavior is not believable to the nurse, or if the patient is difficult or unlikable, then the nurse is likely to downgrade the patient's reports of pain. In effect, how does a patient communicate in such a way that the nurse believes him. [91]

> Could this frustration or fear force a patient to lie about his symptoms in order to survive?

A suspicion of lying or exaggeration may be posted in the chart if the nurse doesn't believe that the pain intensity reports are valid. But what if another nurse believes the pain levels are valid. This introduces inconsistent assessments. Who is right? Should this happen, then the patient must then diplomatically confront these differences with the treatment team. But not every patient has these political skills. And not every treatment team is interested in discussing such inconsistencies.

> "I spoke to the good nurse last night. Wow, what a difference when she's on. The meds are on time, I sleep better, we laugh a little, and I feel like a real person. But that other nurse treats me like I would steal money from her purse. I heard her mumble to another nurse that I was lying. So I asked her why she was so uptight about my meds, and she gave me a bothered 'huff'. I asked the good nurse why the bad nurse was so stubborn; I was told "that's her way... " So just before I left the hospital, I put out pamphlets about pain for the nurses to read. Someone picked them up – maybe this will educate the bad nurse about pain a bit. But maybe she has her own problems and she is sicker than me. But damn, sick or not, I'm the patient and when she was working, I suffered from her illiteracy or attitudes. But I had to lie and put on a decent face when the bad nurse was on, because I feared I'd never get the meds at all! By the way, the good nurse was told by the bad nurse that she was weak-willed on pain and needy patients. I wanted to ring the bad nurse's neck!"

Many nurses have the misconception that postoperative pain lasts for about 3 days. Studies have shown that significant pain can endure for 4 days or longer. Some patients do have less post-operative pain. The key is to ask the patient. Pain from major surgery typically peaks on the second postoperative day. Yet, caregivers tend to consider the second postoperative day as the time to convert the analgesic administration from the parental to oral routes.[92] This misconception, the reversal of which might actually reduce the overall amount of pain, may run counter to what a patient may be actually feeling. So if the patient wants more medication, then the possible 'lying' problem is born.

Many doctors will not or greatly hesitate to prescribe narcotics. One wonders why. Do they doubt the need? Do they not trust the patient? Do they think too many patients lie about their real needs?

> "The doc says my hip is bad and yes, I should hurt, but he gave me only 30 Percocets. I tried to tell him that wouldn't cut it, but he refused to give me any more medications. It was like he was afraid and didn't trust me. I felt he thought I was lying about how much I hurt just so I could just get drugs.... that hurts, emotionally, that is, it really hurts me as much as the hip itself. I guess he can see the hip on an x-ray and prove it is bad, but he can't see the pain, so he can't prove it. I told him I wouldn't be a bother or call him all the time for medications. I don't know why he lets me suffer. Are doctors that afraid to trust people, or don't they trust their own diagnostic skills enough to know I hurt? Or maybe they don't know how to tell that I am being honest. Hell! Maybe doctor's don't know how to diagnosis 'honesty', or maybe, he don't like my level of honesty, yeah, maybe that's it....never thought of it that way before... sure makes sense, don't it? I asked him if he thought I was lying. He told me not to come back for pain meds...I was floored"

The insurance companies are often no better. No one can fault them from protecting themselves from fraud, but remember that these are profit-making or cost reduction organizations. (Much more will be said about that later.) The far too common assumption is that many people lie or exaggerate to get something they don't clinically need. Sometimes insurance companies are afraid to assume financial responsibility for problems that will not end, such as chronic pain and hard to resolve psychological conditions that need long-term and costly care.

Our society, and many of our daily interactions, are based on the notion that people would be dishonest if it would be to their advantage. We constantly have to prove our honesty. A handshake is now a meaningless contract. Cheating is everywhere, and so we too easily assume the worst. Profit, as what recently happened within the brokerage and mortgage industries, is a perfect example of this. Lying to make a profit is a very common maneuver in our society. So cynicism comes from our own experience!

> Some people do indeed lie and cheat. But that doesn't mean all people do.
>
> An old legal notion is that it is better to let ten guilty men go free than to convict an innocent man. But this is not so in medicine. The legal world for the chronic pain patient consists of a judge and jury, who are often one in the same person in the form of a doctor or the insurance adjustor. There is a paucity of opportunity for the patient to argue in front of a public judge and jury. Nonetheless, the best 'defense attorney' for the patient is the data within the clinical record, which in turn often reflects the relationship between patient and treatment

team. Remember that so often the only witness to a patient's true needs is what is written in the chart.

Ask any chronic pain patient this question: of all the doctors they have consulted, how many gave the patient a true feeling that the doctor believed the scale of their pain complaints? The list of doctors getting favorable votes would be small. Ask this same patient how many times he felt he was being accused of exaggerating or lying? The list would be much larger.

Individually or privately, doctors may believe the patient's pain level. But perhaps they are not willing to put themselves at risk. Perhaps they hold a quiet fear that they could be wrong about the patient, i.e., the patient is actually lying but they missed it. The larger task, therefore, is to ask what data can move the situation into the opposite direction and make a doctor believe the patient is honest. As one patient put it: *"How do I get honesty back onto the doctor's menu of choices about me?"*

Occasionally patients report the sentiment that treatment teams subtextually say "you must be lying about the pain because we can't successfully treat you." Patients take this to mean "that if we can't get you better, then we must protect our ego's by making the fault lie within you, the patient, by calling you a liar, for if you were real, then our methods would have fixed you." It sounds harsh. Yet it so often happens in very crafty, underhanded, and emotionally piercing ways.

> "Every time they talked to me I knew they meant well, I knew they wanted to take care of the pain, but they didn't trust me that I was really hurting that much. I can't explain it more than it's real, very real, and very sad. I know

they don't believe me, I know they don't, but I'm not lying, honestly, I'm not....

They don't understand that after time and time of pain attacks I cannot sit and be passively patient. The days of waiting are long gone. I want quick relief. I can't stand it anymore. Why would I lie about the pain? So I can get drugs? Bull! Pain is a four letter word to them, except I'm not sure which four letter word it is: fake, liar, hoax, ruse, show, fuss, trap, ploy, wile—who knows? They want me to lie and say I'm better when I'm not. They also say I'm lying if tell them how badly I hurt. I just want to say that the pain is gone. Can it be any simpler?

I was told that I can't possibly need so much medication. I say back to them they can't possibly feel how bad it is. They said I must be exaggerating. I say they are distrustful. They say I can't be in that much pain. I say they shouldn't talk about what they have never felt. They say that they do understand. I tell them I'm hungry and they tell me I was just fed. I say I'm still starving. They say that that's all the food I'll get from them. I remind them why political revolutions occur. They think I'm crazy..."

...Thought...

The doctor ended up transferring me from his hell to mine. I've got arthritis in my feet, a bad shoulder bursa, and an old hip injury that is giving me terrible sciatica.

I'm also overweight and have been this way my entire life. For years the doctors told me to lose weight, but I just can't—oh, I can lose some, and I have lost plenty over the years, but me, no, I can't lose that much. Then I watched a TV show about fat people and the reporter said that non-fat people think fat people can't control themselves, like I sit and stuff down cherry pies all day long. Then it come to me, that people in this country like to be in control, and they think that because I'm fat, that I'm not in control of myself. 'You can do it, Ronnie, all ya need to do is to really want to do it', is what one nurse told me. The key word is 'really.' I'd just about do anything to lose the weight, I would. I really would. It ain't easy living in these times being so fat. I can control what I eat—you'd be surprised how good a diet I eat! But I can't control my weight.

Then the pain. No doctor would treat me. They all said I gotta lose weight, and I did try, but even when I did lose weight, then they had another excuse— then they say I gotta learn to live with the pain. Okay, sure, I can live with some of it, no problem, that's part of life. But when the leg hurts so bad I couldn't even cook a supper for my family, when it hurts too much to stand in the shower, when I couldn't go to church cause it was too far to walk from the car, when I couldn't sleep because there weren't no position in God's earth that was comfortable— that's when I changed doctors. Went to a few of them, then I found one who believed me.

Set me up with a physical therapist, looked into someone to kill the nerve if nothing else worked, he kept looking at me and saying 'Where's the balance, Ronnie, between no life because of the pain and some life with some medications.' Even though the medications had risks, even so, I knew what they were, and I accepted them risks because I wasn't living the other way.

Well, he put on medications and it helped. It was hard, 'cause the pain didn't always go away. But I had good moments when I could get things done. You can't imagine how free I felt.

Then something happened. I heard the state said he was giving me too many medications. The same for other patients, too. They investigated him—hah, but funny, they never talked to me about it! I could have told them a thing or two — but it was hell for the doctor, sheer hell for him. He was living a hell in order to give me some freedom. And the patients in the waiting room – all good and totally not a seedy bunch. Good folks. Well, it turned out an insurance company complained about him because the meds he prescribed cost so much. It was a battle over cost, not outcome. I was alive because of him. He had no control of what dose I needed or the cost of my meds. I felt horrible for him. He was taking the hit for me. And for all of us too.

Then it broke. He stopped giving me the medications. He was honest and told me why. He was innocent but couldn't afford the added risk of treating people like me – even though he was proper, right, I was better and ok, etc. He sent me to a pain clinic. They were, oh I remember the word, astounded with the amount of medication I was taking. So the first thing they did was send me to an addictionologist. I said what for?

But, you see, I had no choice. The supply of medications was gone.

So they detoxed me, took me off the medications. And while they did that, they also had me go to groups, and meetings, and see a counselor—nice enough people, but they missed the point. It was coming back. The pain was coming back. And it hit me with a sadness deeper than I had in years, cause all that was so black in my life, when I couldn't do things, when I was a dead person living in pain, I saw it all come back. So they put me on an antidepressant. I said I don't need an antidepressant, I need no pain! But they didn't listen, but I did. I listened to them talk about me. And I knew I had been labeled. I was fat and a drug user. Someone said I couldn't control my weight (but they saw how I ate), and that I needed the narcotics to hide from my self-image problems. If my family disagreed with the counselor, then my family became 'enablers'—they too were 'denying' my problem, just like I was supposed to be doing, and they were letting me continue on with my sick ways. Which devil were they protecting me from? The devil of 'addicting' drugs, or the devil of a lousy life.

I made a stink. Finally they agreed to consider me for one of them pumps they put under your skin. My doctor had recommended it and we was working on it, but in the meantime he gave me too few pain medications. I mean, it weren't like I was just taking 'em pills for fun!

The last three days there, before I signed myself out of that clinic, 'cause I was hurting too bad, but they kept telling me how good it was that I was getting off them bad drugs. They said it was good that I was learning how to control the pain. Truth was, I was re-polishing some old lying skills and giving them a show.

I saw some people do real well in that clinic, and God be good to them, but they ain't got no idea about the pain problem like I have. But I also spoke to a lot of people, time and time again. These people just naturally drew to me, and me to them, like we had some real inside story to talk about.

As I packed my clothes they kept asking me if I needed anything. And I kept asking them, each and every one of them staff members, one at a time, straight to their faces, I kept saying 'but what about the pain? What do I do with the pain?'

And not a one of them could give me answer. Not a one. Like that's the one question they didn't want to answer. Like up until that question was posed, it was all some sort of game.

I felt real bad that my former good doctor suffered while he was trying to make me not suffer. I heard they beat up him for a while, but the dust settled and he was still there, and he was making a good stink for all us pain people. I made sure to tell one of the nurses about him. She just kinda smiled.

By the way, I heard the state dropped the claims that my good doctor was clinically bad. But it cost him a fortune, far more than he was making from the fees from us pain patients.

Anyway, I left that pain clinic and went back into hell."

CHAPTER TEN
Sleep

This chapter is as short as is a night's sleep for many pain patients.

> It's hard to sleep when you hurt.
>
> Its takes the mental posturing of a yoga master to lie in bed and try to relax when you hurt like hell.
>
> Sleep with pain is usually sleep from exhaustion. Sleep then leaves the bed once the sheer exhaustion is relieved. Sleep doesn't always stay long enough to give good, deep rest.
>
> Pain and good sleep are two notions rarely used in the same sentence when pain is inadequately treated.

In late 2007, 2,949 nurses were asked *'Yes or no – a patient may sleep despite being in pain.'* The correct answer is true, and 94% of the nurses got the right answer. "As most respondents know, patients sleep despite pain, especially those who've have been living with pain for a long time because they are exhausted. In the past, nurses typically perceived sleeping patients as being comfortable. This high proportion of correct answers is a significant advance in nurses' knowledge and attitudes." [93]

Being over-tired can make for confusion, slurry speech, sloppy movements, dozing off, and decision errors. Many drugs can produce similar looking behaviors. Pain patients who act that way are often accused of using too much medication. In truth, they often aren't using enough medication to be able to get good sleep. The separation that has to be asked is if the troublesome looking behavior is just old-fashioned fatigue and not drug induced intoxication. Good sleep often follows adequate pain relief.

Other circumstances interfere with sleep, such as depression, anxiety, anger, other diseases, excessive cold or heat, or just an uncomfortable bed. Pain patients are not immune from other life problems. Late night staring at computer screens can upset the melatonin cycles, which then adds to sleep problems for many people.[94] Perhaps new mattresses and pillows would help. Sleep hygiene needs to be discussed. This has to do what how to prepare for sleep, turning off TV, bed time snacks, when to take medications or exercise, and so on.

A sequence of trials may be needed in order to identify which balance of pain and sleep medications help the most. People also have to be willing to change their sleep habits as well. Sometimes sleep will normalize if the pain is adequately controlled.

Sometimes a sleep clinic referral is needed. Scientists are just learning about sleep. People enter into their pain phases of life with a variety of pre-existing sleep patterns. How a person slept before the pain began is a critical concern to any doctor, and it is important to tell the doctors about sleep patterns. There is also some work which may show a genetic basis for our different sleep patterns. The National Institute of Health estimates that sleep disorders are found in 50 to 70 million Americans. That is almost 20% of the population.[95]

> He suffered a back injury. He won a disability claim but the monthly payments were very low. Over the years his mattress became worn, and he at last joked that sleeping on the floor was better than sleeping on his old mattress. He

could not afford a new one, and the insurance company, following a very prolonged appeals process, eventually agreed to purchase a new mattress for him. He was delighted. His sleep improved, as did his mood and attitude towards life. His pain levels also dropped.

A patient wrote this beautiful comment: "Broken moods and spirits regularly follow lying endlessly, night after night, in bed, miserable and throbbing with afflicting swells of pain, not wanting to wake the bed partner, and the result is an agonizing, lonely, and offensive eternity."

Consider these three different comments from three patients:

1. Doctor, please, give me something to sleep. I can't stand the fatigue because the pain is bad.
2. Well no, I'm afraid to start a sleeping medication. I'll try going to sleep and maybe the pain will go away. But it if doesn't work, I'll be back.
3. Right doc! When's the last time you could just 'fall asleep' in the middle of a tormenting toothache.

...Thought...

A man wrote this. He also quoted his sister:

She said that her life had no acknowledgement from other people. "How could it, I don't spend time with other people." The only *acknowledgment* she gets in life is that of being a pain patient. Too often that acknowledgement is also full of doubt, implying that she really isn't as bad off as she says she is. She told me that "People give me the feeling they think I lie! Never, never. Why would I? I'm not like them 'cause they must think that way themselves, so they project it onto me. They lie, so they think I lie too."

There is always this unspoken, but intimidating suggestion that 'there just has to be' a less formidable way to control her symptoms other than using the narcotics. She only seeks a confirmation that people believe her suffering. She has an unwanted but genuine need for what she calls 'my disagreeable but damnedly needed medications.' That is why she knows all the radio and TV shows that talk about the problems real pain suffers have when they are not believed.

I remember how often she spoke of endless runs of sleepless nights. She cried to doctors to help her get sleep. She would prefer recognition as a teacher or wife than as an insomniac or pain patient, but those first descriptions have been taken away from her by the pain. It was a good insight.

She feels unacknowledged as a citizen. "People are supposed to have equal protection under the law, and that includes a right to freedom, choice, treatment, and protection against those who would harm me or deny those rights. Because I was hurt by someone else, I must pay the price of being the victim. Who is protecting me? Do I not have a right to medical treatment? Why do I have to not sleep anymore? Is society willing to protect the rights of some subgroups (and some do need the protection, so don't take this too far!), yet society is willing to ignore we medically needy subgroups? Is it because we medically ill subgroups cost money and may not ever be productive. I would love to pay taxes again.

Am I a victim who has lost my rights to a decent life? Is it that I am 'deemed not worth the money?' Is this some sort of eminent domain policy? I would gladly work if I could. I get stigmatized because of the racket I make when I scream that I want to be better.....what a twist of logic!!!

How does that make me feel? Use your imagination. I will never give up the fight, even if the first part of the challenge before me is the political fight to gain access to the medical tools which I need to continue this fight. Don't keep me off the playing field.

My fate, obviously, is to suffer. I guess I can live with that, maybe even learn from it, and I will find a way to put some joy in my life but I cannot live with the stigma that comes from not wanting to suffer.

But I would love a night of good sleep."

And I, and all my family, wish we could give it to her.

CHAPTER ELEVEN
Relationships

Trusting, and being trusted, are the currencies and safety nets of relationships.

Imagine if trust is gone. It feels so alone. It is so frightening when one's doctor, friends or family say "the pain can't be that bad!" or "you have to get off those meds," or 'you're always sick." Over time the bonds weaken, and there is an increasing sense of being abandoned. Abandonment is often followed by a feeling of chilling vulnerability and demoralizing uselessness. "How can they not trust my reports to them?" Or: "Why don't they want to be with me anymore?"

Pain can be amplified by these emotional stresses. What is worse, however, is when the pain becomes the only focus of one's life, and there is no counterforce or joy in life to dilute the pain. Unremitting pain can sever personal relationships. This produces enormous suffering.

A wise chronic pain patient offered these thoughts:

> Life becomes a lonely, secret world of suffering. And we, who have such pain, must learn to know our pain, much as person learns to know their lover, except that pain is not a lover. Perhaps it is more like knowing one's warden.
>
> The pain is mine, yes indeed, but despite that, I am a person and a patient. Pundits and their statistics are not the authority on me. How dare they speak from their lecterns about me. I feel they enjoy separating the person from the

patient. They do not understand the relationship I need to have with me!

I used to wonder about myself. My joint pain is so bad. It is so bad at times that I would have preferred to die. It was like an argument I had with a friend who never heard of cashew apples. I tried to say they were delicacies in the Dominican Republic, but he kept insisting that cashews do not have an eatable fruit. Only when he saw pictures did he believe me. It's like the pain, I knew it was real but he didn't believe me. And how do I show him what I felt!

Anyway, slowly I wondered who was crazy, me or everyone else. No one trusted me. They all initially meant well, I know, and they wanted me to learn to live with the pain, but I soon realized that the pain was something different to them than it was to me. Yet I had to survive using their perception of the pain, least I be ostracized. I had to lie to them or lie to myself. Only one time did a doctor inquire about my relationship to my pain.

Do you know about the *Battle of the Books* by Jonathan Swift? It's a wonderful book written in 1704. There's a line in it that I memorized: "The torture of the pain, whirled the valiant bowman round, till death, like a star of superior influence, drew him into his own vortex." That bothered me a lot. All I could think of is that the 'superior influence' he referred to could have been overpowered if people—my so-called friends and doctors—had given me their trust and belief. But when so many people began to doubt me, when 'all' they saw was my medication use, when I was measured not by my soul nor my suffering, but in terms of how much medication I needed, or how little I could contribute to social events, when their trust was gone, and then, and oh, this was a bad time for me, they let the powers of death subdue my spirit and I wanted to die. They let me to die—how can I say any more? Good old Jonathan Swift! [96]

But why? Why did those who once professed to love me, why did they leave me to die? I don't really know. It's been the topic of so much thought, though. Several times I went through thinking I should die and they were all correct – I was flawed, weak, useless, not loveable, and so on.

But one morning I was struck with the thought that maybe their positions came from their own denial. It wasn't me! Maybe they could not tolerate being so helpless with me, so they chose to wipe it out of their minds. Maybe they were afraid the pain could someday come live with them as it did to me. Would telling me to not be in so much pain reduce, in their minds, the chance of it ever happing to them? I felt like I broke some secret and feared code. That they wanted to see me make the pain go away – it meant it would work for them too, if they needed it to happen. They were responding to their own painful fears. I mean, couldn't this be why people without pain are so easy to suggest to us to "well, just don't think about it so much."

After all, if all of you, right now, as you hear me talk, if you can re-focus your mind from one subject to another, then you can forget about something bad. But if that 'something' is very big and very bad, it is nearly impossible to think it away. I have a friend with obsessions — he tells me he cannot stop himself from having the bad thoughts. I understand him so well.

The pain of my experience, as perceived by others, can go away in their minds. But the pain, as sensed by me, won't go away because that which they perceive is different from what I perceive.

One lady friend said to me: "Oh, we feel so much better that you're using less drugs." I do take less medication when I am around her, because I'm afraid since sometimes it makes a bit sleepy for a while, but what she fails to understand is that I doubly hurt without the full dose of medications. Really, when I take the medications they, on occasion, make me a little sleepy – that's a reality I've learned to work around. Yet I want her 'trust and companionship' so much that I gave up the better pain relief for those moments of time with her because those moments put some pleasure back into my bleak life. But because I pretend not to have the pain, she assumes I could mentally control it. I lie to feed a piece of my soul. It's all so circular, isn't it.

I met an older man who had a great attitude about his terrible arthritis. He said that he could sit home and hurt, having no fun, or he could go out, have fun, and yet still hurt. The pain was a constant event, so he added fun to his 'life in pain.' He told me that it took him a very long time to develop that attitude, and that lots of his friends think the pain is 'not that bad' because he can now go to restaurants with them. If they only knew.

He called his state of affairs as his 'life in pain.' I like that phrase. He used the first letters of each word to describe it as "LIP". He kept saying that pain patients end up giving 'lip' service to themselves and to others. Then he also showed me the pills he takes to make his outings tolerable. He said that "I can give them LIP service because of what passes my lips and goes into my body."

My psychiatrist pointed out an interesting thing to me. He said "that when the pain patient has a truly loving and believing spouse, then the experience of living as a pain patient is not as bad." I agree. I know someone who has an inoperable neuroma in his knee. The man visibly cries from pain. I've seen him rub his knee until it is red or his hands are exhausted. But his wife is so supportive, and they go through this all together. She seeks out doctors, reads literature on pain, lets go of her anger when she has to, is seen as pushy by a lot of people because of what she demands on behalf of her husband, and she thinks and thinks of anything she can do to help her husband. He told me that without her he would have killed himself a long time ago. He always says that when someone believes him, "it's so nice to hear".

Here is a story. Two men met in a pain clinic. They became good friends. The lingo of their relationship can be summarized like this: "Hi, do you know what I mean by pain?" says one to the other. "Yes I do," is the response. I like that.

My pain clinic had a lot of well intending staff. They tried to teach us coping skills. Okay, so the premise is basically good, and I too can always use some polishing up on coping skills, but they didn't look at us holistically. They assumed the presence of a believing environment at home. Sadly, my home was, well, how shall I put it, I had some serious home problems. I could have never learned any real coping skills if it had not been for my few friends at the clinic and for the psychiatrist I'm now seeing. I would like the general office staff to take a course in 'coping with pain when no one outside of the office believes in your pain.' Try that, will you! I must also say that I have a new girlfriend who is supportive and wonderful, and I feel blessed with her. But really, I don't know why she stays with me. She said that "love is blind" and that I make her laugh. Wow.

But back to the larger topic. I have to be fair. I was once in another pain clinic and they did begin to talk about the topic of trust, etc., but only after I insisted that it be discussed. There was a lady there, we called her Micky, with horrible migraines. We became the best of friends, and we saw each other almost daily until she moved away because her husband died. She was 30 years old and he was 35 when he died. It was so sad, so tragic. She loved him so much. It was pathetic that they found each after both of them had experienced years of misery and mistakes. That's life, I know, but don't let me get on to that part or I'll cry. Let me take a breath. Ok. I gotta tell you how we held each other's hands a lot.

Anyway, this lady was in a horrible mess. Remember that her husband was dying and she had so many appalling setbacks in her life that her ability to cope was less than it should be. She didn't have good insurance, the meds were also so expensive – it was a mess on so many levels. So the group therapist said that she needed better coping skills. She agreed but would come back with little comments like "but first teach me how to ignore the fact that my husband is dying and that I'll be broke and alone in the world. Look at the here and now. I don't, just now, have the time to discuss away my other problems!"

One day, in group, we were all talking about medication use and the leader asked Micky, who was, by the way, using a pretty hefty amount of pain medication at the moment, "what are you addicted to?" She quipped back "I'm addicted to no pain." The leader didn't like that, and later said that she was addicted to the pain so she didn't have to deal with the reality around her. Well, I thought Micky would go wild! I thought her phrase 'I'm addicted to no pain' was the best explanation I've ever heard. And I also thought that that is one therapist who needs to go back to school!

To continue. My friend then argued with the group leader, saying that professionals like her make people use more drugs. She then went on to tell us her story and everyone, including the leader, just sat there, listening to a sequence of 'logic' that all of us knew was true and that applied to more than just pain.

Let me tell you what she said, as best as I can remember it:

She described to us how, in her life, she had to, on occasion, do things and associate with certain unsavory people as a matter of survival. If the need had not been so great, and if real and other options had existed for her, then these associations would have never occurred. She used to say that people go to where they get help, and some help is better than no help.

One of the problems was the nature of her family relationships. No one believed the intensity of her headaches. Every time she'd see a doctor the only advice she got was to learn to live with life's stresses and that the pain medication use had to stop. In short, there was no useful relationship with the health care system. They would attempt a diagnosis, offer treatment to a point, and then let her be on her own. One rainy week, the migraines were so bad that she needed repeated Emergency Room visits. The ER doctor eventually refused to treat her, called her an addict, and told her not to come back. She says that it was then that she realized the nature of the relationship with the medications—that her best and worst friend was Demerol®. Demerol® relieved the pain, but it was a contract with the devil because the Demerol® rarely failed her. It believed in her pain. It soothed her, and made her not want to kill herself. But as she had to do so many times in her life, she had to consort with a nefarious world in order to survive. The world of 'regular' people failed her again. She began to think that her fate was sealed, that she was no good because her 'friends' were now either the medications or the less than savory people. This was not the way she wanted to live. She pleaded and looked for a doctor who believed that the pain was real, and who would give her enough medication to at least temper the pain. She used to tell me that the medications were her only friends because they were the only things that could lessen the pain. "People only worsened the pain, so I avoided people." Every time she saw a doctor the 'first order of business' became the task of her reducing her dose of pain medication. So relationships with many doctors didn't last very long. Finally, she met a psychiatric doctor who worked backwards—he kept her at a good medication dose while at the same time he began to teach her how to express anger, how to trust people again, and so on. Little by little her emotional condition improved and then, after a while, wouldn't you know, her medication use dropped in half. The headaches were still there, but less so.

Her doctor said that pain medication use might drop even further if the rest of their clinical work was successful. Picture the smile on her face when she told me that '...it did just that!'

Families delight when pain medication use is down because, to them, it is one basic measure they can see of possible pain reduction. It might mean to them—blind as it actually is—that the problem isn't endlessly bad and out of control, or that it might even be going away. Sometimes pain levels are denied by friends or family because it is hard for them to accept that nothing can be done for the patient. Their concerns emerge from their own frustrations as not being able to help someone they love.

Pain disrupts the family as well as the patient. It converts an active family into a dysfunctional one because the 'pain member' is not able to participate in traditional activities. Even the most loving families occasionally scream out in frustration, saying "can the pain really be that bad?" or "I can't take it anymore! Your endless complaints, and the burden it puts on all of us because of the pain – I hate admitting it, and I really still love you, but I need to get away!"

Pain's influence is often not completely understood by those who've never lived with it. The 'living with it' can mean both having it and living next to it.

Let's explore this a bit more. The shame of being a 'helpless' friend or relative might be so strong that people avoid the patient. One patient put it this way:

"My friends, one by one, all stopped calling me. I don't blame them. They all spoke of boyfriends, new clothes, jobs, etc., and all I could talk about was how much I hurt. I'm not interesting anymore....and I think they couldn't handle not being able to help me...they couldn't watch me suffer... and I'm not fun too. Who would want to be with me? I wouldn't. Then one day, my best friend just cried and said she can't look at me suffering so much, and so she had to stay away for her own ego's sake. Then she and I cried even more, and she came over to hug me, and then we together baked a big old fattening chocolate cake like we did when we were younger, but it was so good because we started to figure out ways to again do things together. I love her so much.

The stuff in my friend – we call it now her 'emotional pain.' It is the spin-off from my 'physical pain.' I have my friend again."

A common sequence of events is when friends withdraw or become hesitant to talk to a patient. The friend feels that "all she talks about is the pain." The patient is then disappointed in their friends, which transfers even greater anger at the pain. The pain is the repulsive villain. Pain can break relationships. There are two parts in this process: (a) the friends' inability to deal with the patient's needs, and (b) the patient's inability to know how to express the anger in appropriate ways to people other than friends. There is a delicate line between venting to and burdening a friend.

Her stomach pain began at age 46. For almost a year, doctors were unable to locate the cause. Many of the first group of doctors felt it was psychosomatic. Finally a new doctor did surgery that initially helped. But some of the pain returned. Then the anxiety overwhelmed the pain, and she became terrified that the rest of her life would be in pain, which added even more to the anxiety. The standard weaker medications failed to control her pain and anxiety. Her friends found reasons not to invite her out. Pain control doctors thought she might need more narcotics. She wanted to change psychiatrists. However, her psychotherapist felt she held deep insecurities in life. The fact that some held her pain to be psychosomatic insulted her. She came to believe that she would now be so endlessly sick that she would eventually lose all those who loved her. The secondary gain was to get the attention she needed to calm her chronic and pre-illness insecurities. This inner need was very heavy. It turned out her physical problem was indeed repaired by the surgery, but the trauma of waiting so long for the correct diagnosis left deep emotional scars which unleashed her acerbic psychological proclivities. She continues in extensive and productive psychotherapy. Fortunately, she had the money to afford the psychotherapy.

There is another story with a bad ending. A 25 year old man suffered a crush injury at work. The case was managed by worker's compensation insurance. Eventually he settled with the insurance company so he would have the freedom to get medical care away from the insurance companies control and limitations. However, private care was unexpectedly costly and he used up all the settlement money. His family also doubted his pain, and said his complaints were just a ploy for some 'secondary gain' (they used this label about him) because he just wanted an excuse not to work and to be felt sorry for; apparently the family had many levels of its own problems, with an alcoholic father and a passive mother; in fact, he'd been in a short period of psychotherapy to address these issues. But because there was no money to prepare a tough fight against the insurance company, and that he was used to being submissive in life rather than be strong, the case settled for as little as it did because no one thought he was in 'that much pain.' He tried to get his lawyer to re-open the case, claiming the settlement amount was realistically low, but that failed. Because of no money, his pain control drifted from very up-scale and organized clinics (which believed his pain and which gave good pain relief) to the walk-in clinics where it was just a matter of paying cash to get a script. He became desperate, and found that he could use a little less pain medications, so he sold the extra medication for much needed cash. His family went into an uproar when he was arrested for selling narcotics. During his incarceration, his pain was not treated, and his anger and desperation only grew. Once released from jail, he stole money so he could go back to the former walk-in pain clinic to try to control the pain. The staff asked where he had been for so long. He told them he was living with a cousin because he feared telling them about the legal problems. So the doctor wrote a refill of a former prescription, which was filled, which was then partially sold to get more money, and partially consumed to dampen the pain. But he took his original dose, which was now too high of an dose, and he died. We learned afterwards, from one friend he contacted after release from jail, that he felt abandoned by his family and friends, he was deeply embarrassed by the direction of his life, he had no insurance for any medical care, there was no plan in his life anymore, he felt the devil was his only companion, and he just wanted to be out of pain.

It's necessary to make a note of a major danger point in the cases just discussed. Introducing the concept of a secondary gain requires the skills and insight of a good psychotherapist. People tend to too sloppily throw this 'secondary gain' hypothesis around. It is, therefore, imperative to note just how professionally and ethically perilous it is to smear the label of a secondary gain on a patient. It is like putting malicious and indelible graffiti on the wall. The responsible way to consider a secondary gain is to proffer a sense of what the core motivation really might be for any secondary gain, and then properly test for it. Indeed, a 'secondary gainer' is an imposter, but it may be to fraud an insurance company, it may be old fashioned malingering, or it may be an insecure ego that doesn't have the strength and skills to function otherwise.

A professional using the notion of secondary gain can taint more than slipshod yellow-journalism. It can also be part of the 'hunt' that occurs when treatments fail and the treatment team needs to tender an explanation.

Too often the blame for the 'trust problems' in a relationship is centered on what people consider to be an out of control pattern of medication use. In fact, the medication use may not be out of control as much as the pain is out of control.

> "My best friend thought I was abusing the meds. She just couldn't understand how bad the pain was. She would talk to other members of my family and I knew something was up. I felt like a leper or a criminal. I tried to reduce the pain medications, but couldn't. I had to start sneaking the medications. Everyone was suddenly an expert on me. All people did was complain about how I was ruining myself, but no one did anything to help me find the right doctor. They wanted me to go into a drug detoxification center. God, if I had gone there, it would have been my death! A medieval torture, drawn out on a rack, with hot irons pushed into my groin, would have been gentler. It would have been the wrong focus.
>
> Someone even called the child welfare board to complain since I was so stubborn with my demands for medications. They questioned if I was a good enough parent!!! I would have never hurt my children! I'd die for my children! But these friends, so to speak, they didn't listen to me, they didn't believe me and they brought me so much trouble. They thought they were right, but it was their version of right, not the right version of right.
>
> The state child welfare investigator at least listened to the whole story. She closed the case

and offered me a prayer. That was so nice, and so unexpected. I asked her if it was okay for a state worker to offer prayers. She smiled and said "Shhhh. It can't hurt."

I think I trusted my friends too much. That was a mistake. I finally found the right doctor and things got better. But I'm still waiting for an apology. I lost many of those friends. I heard some of them were so surprised how quickly I got better after I started with my new doctor.

What I learned is that sometimes pain has to be a secret. That's kinda hard to do when it hurts."

It is well known that pain medications can also calm anxiety and hide worry. This is one of reasons why emergency rooms give morphine to people having a heart attack. But too many non-pain suffering people believe that this tranquilization is the real reason so many pain patients use medications. Of course, it is wrong, but it is astonishing how commonly this is thought. Yet, when a closer look is made, it may occasionally have some merit. Consider the desperation of someone in constant pain, who is losing relationships and who feels life is falling apart – the pain medications may indeed be asked to quiet the pain, soften the loneliness, and calm the anger.

The problem is complicated by the fact that many pain management or ER doctors see so much abuse of the system that they assume it to be larger than it really is. This goes back to the concept of observer shift. One has to ask how different are the professional views of those who work in the methadone clinics, in the walk-in clinics, in the jails, or in the upscale clinics. Too many experts forget that their slice of the world is not necessarily the entire world.

A classic interpretation of the narcotic addict is that the abuser has such an inordinate amount of internal anger and aggression that his ego cannot manage it. Opiates are used to dampen the hostility and counter the threat of internal psychological disorganization.

The mother of a pain patient said to me: "Yes, he was using drugs before he got into the fight and busted up his hand. The pain now makes it all worse. I don't know how to control him. He was an addict before the pain, his father used drugs, I once drank too much – and my son hates his Dad and can't figure out the world! So he uses drugs to run away. What scares me is that now because he needs the pain meds, he might use this as an excuse to hide from the rest of life too."

This may indeed be true for many everyday narcotic 'addicts,' but before applying the term addiction to the pain patient, one has to know if they were predisposed to, or actively engaging in, addictive behaviors before the pain entered their life. Unfortunately, too many people label other people based only on existing and observable current behaviors, and not at all on the why, or the how, that the person came to act in a certain way. These premature or unsubstantiated conclusions destroy relationships.

If someone uses pain medication in the same manner as someone uses an occasional shot of whiskey, then great risk exists that speculations will be born suggesting that the medications are used more for psychological than physical discomforts. This is how many people define an addict. Pain medication use is seen as "covering up" something. People worry that they can't trust the pain patient to be honest about their real reasons to use medications.

> "People don't realize that I can be using Dilaudid® to control pain and still, at the same time, suffer from depression or anxiety. So if I am just so angry, or so scared, and no one is around to help me through it, and, hell, my life has deteriorated to where there is little joy in it anyway, and all the coping skills I knew so well just don't work anymore, and all I see is misery, then sure, I'll use an extra dose of medication to give me some peace of mind. Is that so bad?
>
> I really know that I wouldn't need the medication if the pain wasn't part of my everyday life. I'd do like most people and have a drink, take a walk, make love, go shopping or something, but since I can't drink, and I hurt too much to walk around the mall or go swimming, then I do what little I can. Do you blame me? My friends do. My doctors think I'm a criminal. I try to explain it to them, that it's like an evening cocktail. I say to them that life is full of grey areas, and when we are all really honest, we all use those grey areas at times. But we pain patients, we got to be perfect and not have grey.....
>
> And that destroys even more of my relationships with the world. I have so much inside me that is scared, and wants to give to others, and so much of me needs touching. Someone listen to me! Damn, I hate this pain...."

A story of two friends warrants a close look because one's pain was resolved and the other's was not. Both women had similar reasons for their chronic pain. After they met, they developed a mutually soothing relationship, which included supportively helping each other with their agonies. It would include such things as talking each other through pain attacks. It also included 'girl-talk' about family, men, fashion, and so on.

The benefits of this two-member, mini-self help group was enormous. When and if additional medication was ever necessary, it was used with less guilt. The friends would tell each other "don't be silly, if you need it, take it!" They probably kept their medication use lower than would have otherwise occurred if they lacked the close emotional support. These two people were real checks and balances for each other. Together they polished their biofeedback skills, they acknowledged the loneliness of being in pain, they lamented over their impaired social lives, and they fortified each other with phrases to use when trying to convince others that pain is real. Everyone around them learned so much about pain and suffering from them.

And all was well and good until one got better.

In fact, as the events began to unfold that one was probably going to get better while the other was not, the first round of guilt appeared. The one getting better felt uncomfortable talking to her friend about the medical prognosis. She was embarrassed and felt God wasn't being fair to her friend. She prayed for God to also cure her friend, yet at the same time she could not deny that she was pleased that God seemed to be on her side. Yet their friendship was so deep that the 'not-going-to-get better friend' genuinely could not have been happier that the other one was probably going to be better. The one who got better wrote this:

"I could have never thought of a worse predicament. My very dearest friend was going to be left behind. I couldn't live with the guilt. I would have given anything for the good fortune to have fallen on her than me, yet, to be honest, I felt such a relief that my life would be normal again. As much as I truly loved her—and still love her as a dear, dear friend—I couldn't not go for my surgery. But I couldn't talk to her. I was so self-conscious. I thought she'd hate me. I was afraid that she'd be in a pain attack and rather than me being at home, I'd miss her phone call because I was out. How could I abandon her? I wanted so much to get away from the diabolical life of pain, but did I have to sacrifice my future to appease my guilt? I began to avoid phone calls to her. I made up excuses not to call her.

But for a while I missed her in ways that superseded the pain. And that is when it all came to me. The pain had been a central topic to much of our conversation, and I thought we were merely two battlefield buddies—that is, good friends while at war but little in common with each in peace. Then I realized just how much we did not have in common outside of the pain. It was so obvious. I'm even ashamed to acknowledge that a blind spot existed. This is not easy for me to write about...

Yes, I may not be in the same pain I was before, and yes, my limitations are now not what they were, but we were friends who were sharing life together, and life is more than just pain.

I realized that what we were giving each other was a life outside of the pain during the period when our lives were so much in pain. It allowed the pain to exist, and we helped each other have a non-pain life given the baseline pain. We both knew what we were not getting from our non-pain friends.

So now that I leave the ranks of the pain patients, I know what she needs and I am willing and wanting to give it to her. She is a friend with pain. I have to accept her with pain, and that's hard for a lot of non-pain people to realize. When she needs to talk about the pain, then we do so. When she needs to shout and cry, then I let her. When she needs to tell me how jealous she is of me, I will grit my teeth and bury my guilt and let her talk. But I also know when she is obsessing on the pain and I have to stop her. I say "Yes, damn it, you bet I believe you, but I'm not letting you overdo it. You've got ten minutes to blow off steam and tell me what idiots there are in the world, but then we're going to talk about movies, old boyfriends, crazy mother-in-laws, and so on." I make a point of telling her a bad joke or two. But mostly I make a point of telling her that I believe her. Despite how our lives have changed, she is not alone! Even if we somehow part ways, in my heart she will never be alone – that has to be a constant in her soul. And I hope that anyone reading this will put a bit of their prayers toward her. I wish I could fix her.

But I will never forget my pain."

As mentioned elsewhere, friends might distant themselves from those suffering pain. Many times people avoid pain patients because they fear the prospect that they too might someday suffer the same fate. It's similar to how people react when they hear of a sick child going into a hospice. They want to run away. "It's too painful for me to visit Douglas anymore. I can't stand to see the suffering." Seeing someone in pain can mean: *'That I fear it might happen to me. It's horrible. I'm not strong enough to look at it. That's why I could never be a nurse. I don't want to face that side of life….'*

The patient is then left alone, but not of their own doing. And the abandonment may not be seen by the patient as stemming from the friends' emotional inability to be around such ceaseless suffering.

Friends may feel helpless. It is horrible to watch someone tortured by pain. It can also be boring, though people don't always want to admit to this.

Pain also takes away any control that the friend has over the situation, and many people cannot stand losing control or being forced into a passive footing, secondary to feeding the pain's appetite. This same loss of control is repulsively familiar to the patient.

> "I'm used to being active. I like to get things done. I work hard and I play hard. 1 was never home. My friend used to be my best and most steadfast partner, but now, well, since the accident and his pain, it's so different. It drives me loose inside to think that nothing more is being done for his pain. I can't bear it… and I guess, to be honest, I don't like the pace that he has to live now. That pulls me down. That's a lousy thing to say, isn't it? But you asked me to be honest.

> I get angry at him. Jim, I say, in the name of Jesus, why the hell don't you find the right doctor? These guys are killing you. But he seems so defeated now. I know he tried, but I can't help but think that somewhere he can find help. I know this all undermines his trust in his current doctors. But I want my old friend back But maybe he's right, maybe the old Jim is not coming back. Maybe no one can fix him. This is all so uneasy for me. I feel so uncivilized. I feel shamefully selfish too. Being alone is easier than being in the pain of his presence. Am I bad for feeling that?"

Pain can destroy marriages. With the arrival of chronic pain must be an immediate and intense examination of the strengths in the marriage. Pain can take away the option of raising children, of maintaining a job, and it can destroy dreams. Psychiatric and spiritual counseling may be needed.

> "I lost my wife to the devil named pain! So we had to find things we could do together. That was not easy. She is really a super person. And our sex life – it just isn't here anymore, and I know she feels horrible about it, and I keep seeing myself looking elsewhere, but I don't want to step outside the marriage, I don't know, I just don't know....and that's a really hard feeling to admit to...."

A 34 year old woman lamented:

> "I married Peter and all was wonderful. We laughed and partied and talked of having

babies and seeing the world and all was so delicious and marvelous. We once enjoyed a rich, sensual sex life. I couldn't be happier. But after the accident things changed. I couldn't be far from my medications. My sleep patterns changed. I had to stop working so our money supply lessened. But mostly I couldn't have intercourse—it just hurt too much. I tried as best as I could to look for positions that would not put pressure on my spine—I even said we should try making love in a swimming pool, but it didn't work. I tried to satisfy him in other ways. But I knew he was frustrated. And it didn't surprise me—oh, it was about 2 years after the accident—when I was told he was having an affair. I had mixed feelings—if it was only sex then I tried to overlook it. But it wasn't. He left me. Do you believe it, that he apologized for leaving me? At first I was hurt, but then I realized that his love for me was probably never that deep—oh hell, I really don't know what he felt. The only thing I know is that the stress killed my marriage, and the accident will probably keep me from ever enjoying a normal sex life again.

One last thought: wasn't there a time in history when a man was allowed to have more than one wife if, for some reason, she couldn't bear him any children? We spoke to an adoption agency, but we were rejected because of my pain medication needs. That was a bomb bursting in my gut! I have this deep and sneaking feeling that if our society might have allowed it, given the fact that I was injured, and we did so want to have kids, then maybe I would not have had children with that man, at least he could still be part of my life and I part of his. But because we aren't allowed to do that I end up totally alone.... need I talk about I feel that my husband, religion, and society have all abandoned me? This whole situation is so complicated."

Many pain patients feel they have to believe there is some purpose to their suffering. If not, they lose all hope. One 30 year old man put it very poignantly:

"I want to believe in God. I don't think I could believe any harder. I look at my life and know my errors but I am a good person. But why won't God believe in me? And how can I expect people to believe me if God won't?

Dear God, all I want is to have children and watch them grow and learn. All I want to do is an honest day's work. I want to be able to celebrate Your holidays and add to my life. Why won't You let me do that? Why? Why do I have a pain that no surgeon can fix? Why? Am I not worth just three seconds of Your time? What is our relationship now? Please give me the answer, please...."

Friends fail them. Family fails them. Medicine fails them. Society fails them. Religion fails them. It looks so bleak.

"We don't dare speak for God. But we can speak for ourselves. The core of our lives rests within our relationships. Let those alliances grow, for from that growth come seeds which can soothe the suffering. If we cannot give those who suffer some help from God, and if we cannot give them medical cures, then at least we can give them some of our time, our trust, and extend an open invitation, along with the tools, to join us in life."

...Thought...

Why someone abuses drugs is more important than how the abuse takes place. Early psychoanalytic theory taught drug abuse would calm primitive and unmet oral needs. The focus has since been expanded to an understanding of the overall personality and extra stresses in life. Remember that as biological organisms we are not designed to live in chronic pain. The pain spills over into the psychology. Working with these concepts can build, repair, and fortify relationships.

People vulnerable to substance abuse are those who have some problem in the nature of their relationships. They:

Cannot, or have difficulties, experiencing gradations of feelings.

Cannot tolerate the anticipation of distress.

Don't how to activate or use effective defense mechanisms against stress, including knowing how to find relationships to help in such situations.

> Very often suffer from combinations of a low self-esteem with a narcissistic self-protectiveness, have a poor self-image, a weak object constancy, unstable relationships, too many rigid defenses, maybe a bad genetic predisposition, and encounter situations with a personal burden of poor coping or problem solving mechanisms.

All drug abuse starts during a crisis that cannot be resolved by the usual or available adaptive devices. Therefore, any emotional benefit resulting from drug abuse could maintain the motivation for drug use. Such benefit may be either an emotional regression back to a less stressful emotional state, or, in a non-regressive manner by reducing the pain, it may restore some contemporary normalcy by producing less stress.[97][98] A regressive response may be evidence of former psychological problems. A non-regressive response might actually be a move towards health because it relaxes situations enough such that some resolution may follow.

We speak of relationships with people. We also need to understand the motivation for any relationship with medications or drugs.

If someone:

(a) has a full range of emotions and reliable relationships,
(b) has normal life fears and can adequately express themselves (the inability to do this is called alexthymia[99]),
(c) has not turned to drugs or alcohol to calm and mellow their own inner rages or to deal with severe traumas,
(d) can fluctuate between tension and relaxation in what would be considered a normal manner,

(e) can feel they are not on the edge of emotional disintegration,
(f) can properly handle boredom, frustration, fatigue, delays, and related life-event depressions,
(g) can make and hold onto commitments and compromises,
(h) is self-sufficient enough to have a comfortable social life,
(i) can be acceptably and appropriately aggressive,
(j) does not fear honest self-introspection, and
(k) does not live in psychological denial of their own personal problems, then this person is not likely to become a drug addict. They will prefer relationships with people over drugs. Most people fit into this group.

Pain patients have different psychological underpinnings than do drug abusers. That underpinning is pain. And as said so many times, removing the pain from a pain patient removes the underpinning and the need for medications. But a pain patient with some attraction to non-pain based medication use requires a professional and deeper psychological look into the rest of their psychosocial lives. Just taking medication away from an addict does nothing more than alter the person's inner molecular environment and physiology.

Having viable relationships gives us a sense of power: "though which we obtain some future apparent good."

Thomas Hobbs, 1588–1679

CHAPTER TWELVE
Why medications work one day and not the next

> "How quaint the ways of paradox! At common sense she daily mocks!"
>
> *WSW Gilbert*

How do we explain that medications may not work the same from day to day?

Why might today be a two morphine day, but yesterday was a one Percocet day? It seems like a paradox. Can the paradox be solved? Yes. It just takes a little understanding of the nature of pain and the nature of medications.

Pain is a multifaceted and always varying experience. Arthritis, bad enough on a dry day, is worse on a rainy one. Back pain, tolerable on a low activity day, is much worse after grocery shopping. Muscle spasms, sometimes treatable with low dose muscle relaxants or a hot tub, are less treatable when they co-exist with worries and tension. Pain is a plant living in the constantly changing garden of life.

- I have TMJ. I also love to chew gum. So if I chew gum today, I pay for it tomorrow. So a 'no' gum day requires a couple of aspirin, but a 'yes' gum day requires a Percocet and a Valium.

- I have terrible migraines. I also have to work for a living. If I'm tired then the headaches are worse. My doctor wants me to relax. If I relax that much I'll lose my house and starve. I also know my headaches are much worse just before my menses. So my need for pain meds varies a lot because my pain varies a lot.

- My doctor tells me not to lift. But my doctor doesn't come over to clean my house or wash my clothes. I cannot live in a dirty house, and I cannot afford a maid. So some days, when things have to be done, I do them. It doesn't mean the pain is less; it just means I have to do them. But wow, do I make payments later. It's like the pain is jealous and wants to completely control my life, and so it retaliates the day after I do chores. The drugs? If I mostly lie in bed all day I can usually get away with a few MS Contin®, but if I've done housework, then I usually need an extra dose or two of medicine.

- I am basically bed bound because of pain and injury. I can walk with assistance to the bathroom, but I can't stand long enough to cook or clean. I can't drive, and people have to assist me now. I hate to use the word, but I am like an invalid. But! My sister was a patient in the hospital, and one day she called, crying, saying she needs me. Usually that means we spend hours on the phone, but this time her voice had a different, almost scary peculiarity, so I knew in my heart that I had to actually go to her. Nothing would stop me. I called a friend who literally carried me to the hospital. We cried and cried and cried together, but she needed me, and damn, the pain had taken enough of my life, and so what if I hurt some more, the pain of not being with her was worse than death. Emotionally that was a wonderful day because I helped her through a crisis, and I now lie in bed knowing I did the right thing. But for about a week after the trip I hurt with an intensity like I never before knew. Wait! Before you go, I have to throw in one

> juicier tidbit. My workman compensation carrier heard that I was able to visit my friend in the hospital – they didn't know it was my sister in a crisis. I'm not sure how they found it. It's one of the many fears I live with: that I will be seen but not understood. But because of my hospital visit, they now assume that I am now better and therefore I need less home care...do you believe it? I called my lawyer who re-opened my file. And when I told my doctor that I ran out meds early this month because of my time with sister, he said there could be no early refill. The guy must never have anything go off schedule in his life.... "

Patients can distinguish different types of pain. There is muscle pain, nerve pain, bone pain, soft tissue pain, and emotional pain. Accident victims, because of injury to larger areas of the body, usually have several sources of pain. They also soon learn how to separate the types of pain they feel. Eventually they also know which treatments are needed for which types of pain. The pain experience becomes interwoven into their lives. This is why mature pain patients know if it is a day to use one Percocet® or two Oxycontin®.

Many non-pain people make the mistake of clumping all pain as equal pain. This is not true. The pain of a toothache is different than the gum pain after a root canal.

> Post-surgical pain carries an emotionally bearable connotation because it is known to end. Chronic pain is known not to end. The differences are obvious.

Some people argue that though pain is fairly constant, it is the world around the pain that varies. Therefore emotionally or physically calmer days need less medication than do tense days. Too often the implication is that medication treats less of the actual pain and more of the amplified reaction to the pain. This process is called *pain amplification* (specifically, the pain feels worse because emotional reasons amplify it). No one objects to the reality of this process. However, it can be overused, and too often it tries to paint too broad an explanatory sweep – with suspicion – as to why the *amount of medication use* and *reports of pain intensity* vary so much. "The pain is more in your head than anywhere else...." is often blatantly or subtly suggested.

> "I remember a rabbi saying that life is 10% what happens to us and 90% of how we interpret it and put it into perspective. But the rabbi's lovely phrase short changed itself of the truth. Too many people use that 90% to impose their perspective without ever experiencing the other 10% incidents. So to understand the perspective, all of us need to also experience that horrible 10%. It's like when someone who has neither been married nor has children tries to be a family counselor. There is the feeling that they are close to an understanding, but it comes only via study or empathy. It misses the higher definitions and harmonic echoes that come from personal misery. Let's share the misery a bit before we give opinions on how to live with the misery."

Often those who do or pay for the treatments add to, rather than lessen, the pain. An insurance carrier refusing to provide enough home health assistance adds to the tension and fear of being alone, which worsens aspects of the pain.

People with pain are also not exempt from the normal and extraordinary stresses of everyday life. Such stresses influence the ability to tolerate the pain. But by the same token, it is naïve to preach that merely reducing or avoiding the stresses in life will always take some of the pain away since the physical baseline of the pain may not respond to the lessening of the stress.

> "I get the feeling that people use patient's with lesser degrees of pain as the standard against which my greater degree of pain is compared. So I am forced into being like them when in fact I cannot. It means I am forced to fail because my baseline if different. Also, I do biofeedback, but then after the sessions I go home to the same problems, etc. It's the ultimate comparing of apples to oranges — reducing my stress won't so easily improve my life! And even if all my money problems disappeared, the arthritis isn't less. Now, that doesn't mean that my motivation to get over this is not as great or as high as others, it's just that I have, if you look at the details, a much steeper mountain to climb."

A commonly cited study about stress and pain is by Beecher, who reports about how seriously wounded soldiers deny their pain and were able to refuse medications.[100] Extreme stress, and perhaps then the pain itself, can activate descending nerves in our pain systems. This can cause some level of analgesia. Admittedly, the level of stress needed to produce this effect is quite high, but it seems that sufficient emotional inputs, and perhaps the fear of death to oneself or others, can temporarily reduce pain. Those who do not study this carefully enough may overlook the fact that while emotions might control pain under exceptional stresses, not all stresses are exceptional.[101] And ongoing, high levels of stress, excitement, or arousal can be lethal. We are not designed to always be on such high levels of alert. Spurts of stress may obliterate pain long enough so as to let us deal with the larger tasks of immediate survival, but we don't daily live on battlefields. And even those who live in battlefields still wear out.

> "I would be able to suffer a short period of pain to save one of my children, but I honestly doubt my body or mind could withstand prolonged and serious pain before I collapsed. We cannot blame pain patients if they cannot perpetually endure pain. No one can."

Before someone comments on a person's pattern of medication use, it is critical that they understand the person's life.

> "Before you pass judgment on me, ask yourself what is the best and most productive way to interact with me. A person can select any one of my patterns to base their understanding of me. But remember that when we interact with someone, it is an interaction of the present moment. But studying only the 'now' is too narrow. Instead look at me as you read an entire book. That book will give you insights into my joys, love, pain, fears, struggles, and so on. That will make you wiser about the choices you make on how to make conclusions about me. So when I tell you I hurt a lot more today more yesterday, understand why today is different than yesterday."

Religion can also make a difference.

> "My Dad is very religious. After he fell and shattered his left arm, he could not put on the tefillin. He intellectually understood that he was exempt from using tefillin for a while. We had a rabbi speak to him, and the rabbi said it was ok, he need not worry. He said that God heard the prayers from the heart. But my father had laid tefillin for over 70 years. It was a fundamental part of each day for him.
>
> I think, sadly, that at first all our talking made little difference. From his frustration came anger at the pain. With that the pain often increased. He felt God was punishing him. I told him that was ridiculous, but I was glad to hear him talk that way because it gave him an emotional venting. When he spoke to other religious men, his pain would be less. It was because he was reassured that he wasn't endangering himself or his family by not laying tefillin.
>
> He felt that God caused him pain as a punishment, but for reasons I still can't imagine. He then feared that because he didn't lay tefillin, part of the further punishment from God would be some harm to his family. He finally told me that if he didn't find the strength to lay tefillin, despite the pain, we would suffer.
>
> When he felt less scared, his pain days were better. What lesson this has been for all of us! The pain challenged his relationship and trust with God. I can't tell you how repugnant that

was to my Dad. And though he took some pain meds, they didn't help as much as did a trip to the synagogue."

A quick introduction to the biology of pain medications

There are also biological reasons why pain medications work differently from day to day. These mechanisms may appear complex, but they can be plainly summarized:

Drugs pass through an intricate series of metabolic pathways and processes before they get to the pain receptors. It is the activity of those receptors that causes and/or inhibits the sensation of pain. Change any one of those pathways and the final amount of drug available to the receptor is changed. These steps include (a) how the drug is dissolved in the stomach or gut, (b) how it is then absorbed through the stomach or intestinal walls to get into the blood, (c) how it is filtered by the liver or kidneys, (d) how it is carried from the filters to the receptors via the carrier proteins, and (e) how much of it is passed through the blood brain barrier into the brain, into spinal cord, or to wherever the medications need to go to do its work.

Another variable is the changeable quantity and tenacity of the carrier proteins to transport the medications. Other drugs or conditions can change the stickiness of these carrier proteins – if they get too sticky, they will not release the drug as expected. Other variables are how many of these sticky proteins exist (their population varies), how long the drug remains in circulation, and how long is the receptor modified by the pain blocking drug before the receptor goes back to its original state.

The recent introduction of a narcotic fentanyl skin patch has also introduced another variable in these processes: the relative acidity of the skin. The patch is designed to work best when the skin has a pH of 5 (pH is a means by which we measure how acidic something is). If the pH changes or the skin becomes unusually dry or oily, then the rate at which the medication leaves the patch and diffuses through the skin will change. Also, thicker skin may be a more formable barrier as well.

We call the ratio of how much drug is put into the body to how much is actually available to the final receptor as the drug's *bioavailability*. Bioavailability is an important term to understand. Likewise, people can be rapid, slow, or ultra-rapid metabolizers, so the bioavailability will vary. Other medications or illnesses might interfere with metabolism as well.

Patients every so often say that their current batch of medications doesn't seem as strong as other batches. Is this possible? Yes, and it is especially possible as one switches brands. Generic medications may lead to differences in bioavailability. This is why: Assume a brand name medication is labeled at 100 mg of drug. Assume too, that they manufacture the pill to be within 2% of the labeled dose. (This is one of the reasons for the higher brand name costs.) This means the actual amount of drug can range from 98 mg to 102 mg.

The FDA allows generics to be within 20% of the labeled dose. That means the actual amount of drug in the pill can range from 80 mg to 120 mg.

Therefore, switching from a brand to generic could allow for a change from 100 mg to 80 mg, which is a 20% reduction. The chemistry is complex, but this can translate to a 50-100% reduction in the amount of active drug that gets to the receptor. Other fluctuations can also occur if the generics change or there is a return from generic back to brand. This is why doctors try to stabilize patients on a single manufacturer's product.

Here is the metabolic process in greater detail:

A pill is swallowed. It goes into the stomach. It dissolves. How it dissolves depends on at least two major factors: (a) the pH or acidity of the stomach acid (which can also vary food or other medications), and (b) how the pill is manufactured. A pill designed to dissolve at a pH between 1 and 2 may not do so because food, antacids, or other influences changed the pH in the stomach. The pill will then pass through to the gut. If the pill encounters a different pH in the stomach, it may not dissolve as wanted – different pHs might make it happen too quickly or too slowly. Likewise, if the pill is a cheaper generic, then it may not dissolve even if the pH is correct. The reason is that part of the price of a medication is associated with the cost of the vehicle. A vehicle is the inert substance that holds on to the active drug until pill is swallowed. A good vehicle will easily and predictably release the active drug. Cheaper medications often use cheaper vehicles, which is why some generics don't work as well.

Nonetheless, not all generic medications are bad; some are quite good! Finding the good ones, however, can be a challenge.

Some medications, or other influences, speed up or slow down the speed with which things pass through the intestines. So if the gut is working more rapidly today than usual, then the pill might be pushed through too fast; the effect is that it isn't around long enough to dissolve and be absorbed. Tomorrow may be a slower day in the gut. Diet and other medications may also change the transition time through the gut.

The major drug filter is the liver. The liver recognizes natural and safe molecules from those which are not. Liver enzymes try to inactivate the unsafe or unnatural molecules. A medication is not a natural molecule. The liver cannot inactivate all the unnatural molecules, but enzyme systems learn and actually become more avid inactivators as time goes on. This is one part of tolerance; more and more medication is needed to get an adequate supply of medications to pass through the liver's filters. Cigarette smoking and the concurrent use of some other drugs, including alcohol, will alter the enzymes' activity. The other major drug filtering organ is the kidney.

Sometimes the metabolite of the original drug has an activity similar to the original drug. For example, tranquilizers such as diazepam (Valium®) have tranquilizing effects from the diazepam itself as well as from their breakdown products. The liver converts the diazepam to nordiazepam; both substances have tranquilizing effects. Eventually, the liver and kidney remove both drugs.

Some new drugs are actually the metabolites of older drugs. Prestiq® is an active metabolite of Effexor®.

The kidney has a lesser, but still important role in metabolizing drugs. Some drugs are metabolized entirely in the kidney, though the liver is the primary organ for such operations in the body. Switching from liver to kidney metabolized medications requires some care if there are liver or kidney problems. Dialysis patients need extra thought when medications are given to them.

The liver removes anywhere from 50-95% of most medications. Medication given by injection will have a greater effect because the 'first run' of the medication through the body by-passes the liver. Eventually, however, all the medication is filtered by the liver and kidney.

After passing though the hepatic (liver) filter, any remaining drug is released into the general blood stream. To be safe, the body has other protective devices such protein binding. This helps block over 'over-dose' effect. These are the 'sticky' proteins mentioned above. Countless proteins float in the blood which bind to the different medications. They essentially grab the medication. That takes the medication out of circulation. Should there be an exceptionally great number of such proteins available for binding, they might 'suck' up most of the medication and leave very little around to serve for pain relief. The opposite can also occur—there may be a time of fewer binding proteins available.

Many factors alter the blinding protein levels from one day to the next. The number of available binding proteins is influenced by nutrition (usually not a major factor except in more extreme cases), other medications, infections (even a common cold), or stress. The key is that even identical medication doses, taken with solid regularity, face numerous vigorous biological systems which always change how much medication actually gets where we want it to go in the body.

Another protective system is the blood brain barrier. This is a membrane surrounding most of the brain. All medications, foods, proteins, etc., must pass through this to get into the brain. Considerable work is underway to learn what makes this barrier more or less permeable. This is an extraordinarily fascinating but complex part of the body. It is designed to keep toxic materials from getting into the brain. It is like security personnel outside a central computer. One factor in its willingness to let molecules pass the through the membrane is the ratio of different proteins on either side of it. The membrane itself is a fat, called a lipid, and we refer to the ability of drugs to dissolve through the lipid as lipid solubility. So subtle changes in the membrane's permeability is another potential reason why a medication will work differently from one dose to the next. Each medication has a unique lipid solubility, which accounts for why one medication feels different than another. It all comes to a matter of how easily the medical molecules move past the brain's security and into the central computer.

Lipid solubility also factors into how much of the drug is stored and released by the general body fat. If a drug is very lipid soluble, it will go into the general body fat. Eventually that fat is saturated, so little more can be absorbed. But if the drug is stopped, then suddenly the medication which was stored in the fat is released from the fat and into the blood. Putting on weight or losing weight can therefore have an effect on blood levels.

Other processes also metabolize medications. But these just discussed are the main ones, and they offer a useful premise of how drugs move through the body. In essence, medication controls symptoms differently from day to day because the pain, the pills, our bodies, and our lives are always changing. Every pain patient knows this.

> "We were visiting friends in South Carolina when a hurricane hit. As it got closer, and the barometric pressure dropped, I could feel my inner ear hurt more and more. I couldn't control the pain. I went to a ER doctor who, after he heard my story (and believed me!), well, he actually gave me some generic Percodan®. Real Percodan® always worked in the past, but this time the generic – well, it did nothing. So the drop in atmospheric pressure caused increased pain and those generic drugs provided less relief for the same number of pills. Oh, what a mess."

...Thought...

> *Good news that's bad news. Or bad news that's good news.*

> In 1992 Warfield[102] published a major textbook on pain management:

> "Long term maintenance with opioid drugs is the rule in the management of chronic cancer pain. Concern about addiction should never be a consideration in the management of malignant pain.
>
> Opioid maintenance of patients with chronic benign pain (non-cancer) always has been a controversial area. A recent study indicates that, in certain highly selected patients, this approach may be a humane alternative to no treatment or neurosurgical ablative procedures. Patients selected for this technique must have no prior history of substance abuse, but there seem to be no predictive features common to any one of their several psychological measurement scales for the patients who respond. In our clinic, we have managed a small number of patients with chronic nonmalignant pain of different origins...with opioid maintenance. With careful monitoring of drug intake and use of long-acting or slow release opioid preparations by time-contingent dosing schemes, these patients have done well and showed no tendency to increase their opioid intake over time. All had not responded to other approaches, and with this program, they were able to maintain some degree of functioning."

Though these are wonderful steps in the right direction, they show how too many old notions still exist despite what is written in text books. *The social problem* is that too many people use pain medications for non-pain reasons, and as has mentioned before, the confusion is complicated by the fact that the same medications are being used in different populations; indeed, the improper using groups are effectively clumped into psychiatrically impaired groups, which adds another layer of taint to the situation. There is no similar problem with antibiotics. *The professional problem* is that doctors have better skills at diagnosing and managing infections than for pain syndromes.

Understanding Side Effects to Pain Medications

There needs to be some consideration about the side effects of pain medications. The following material will look at the more common biological and psychological side effects. The most feared side effect is addiction, so extra time will be spent examining it.

Opioids are generally safe, yet reports do exist of the potential problems with its continuous use. The concept of a ratio of the good effects to the bad effects is known as the 'risk-benefit ratio.' It is intended to answer this question: what benefit over risk is derived from the treatment? Patients often accept some side effect if the larger effect is a quality of life enhancement.

Side effects are not always the standard ones of dry mouth, constipation, sleepiness, or blurry vision. Below are less common other side effects.

Opioid induced hyperalgesia is the loss of effectiveness after a period of prolonged use. The fear is that this might lead to an ever increasing dose of medications.

Hormonal and immune side effects have been associated with opioid using chronic pain patients.[103] Only a few definitive studies exist about this, so it is still more of a new concern that just needs monitoring.

Psychiatric literature has long known that relentless depression and anxiety, such as that from uncontrolled pain, can reduce the immune function. There is growing evidence of opiate induced suppression of the follicle-stimulation hormone, testosterone, estrogen, and cortisol. [104] [105] This can result in infertility, but it is unclear how these effects might present in any single patient. Choosing opiates for pain control requires an analysis of the risk to the benefit ratio of these medications. Perhaps any immune dysfunction from opiate use is offset by the many benefits that follow a better mental status

Addiction is a key concern. Can it be considered as a side effect? Is this the biggest side effect of opiate use? People become afraid of it. Needless to say, this topic pops up in many areas of this book.

Any argument over addiction, or the implication that a patient is 'addicted', can produce such an aggravation that it might lessen or disrupt the pain medication's ability to control the pain. Sometimes patients try to voluntarily reduce their pain medication doses to test the levels of their own possible 'addictions.'

> "Everyone said I was an addict. It got to the point where I doubted myself. That made me more anxious, which tensed my back muscles, and I got more pain from that, and so I used more meds, and that made me look more like I was an addict – well, you can see where this was going. So I had a long hard talk with my therapist. I slowly decreased the pain medicine. I was happy I could do it. Then as I used less, my brother complimented me and said I was okay. That made me feel better about myself, and so I was able to drop the med dose a little more. I succeeded. I felt wonderful, like I had some control again. I wasn't an addict!

> But I was a pain patient. I tried to go too low with the meds, and the pain snapped back at me! But I know I am not an addict. That is like winning the lottery for me."

The occurrence rates of addiction vary, which is, in large part, due to differences in how addiction, iatraddiction, or pseudoaddiction is defined and measured. Nagging issues also remain about addiction rates in chronic pain patients versus the expected rates in the normal general population. The overall incidence rates vary from 5% to 19%. [106] In 2006, about 22.6 million Americans were diagnosed with substance dependence or abuse.[107] But the estimates are that 60 million people suffer from chronic pain. The great and vast majority of drug abusers are not also chronic pain patients. The vast majority pain patients most likely use non-opiates for pain relief. These overlaps are so hard to measure, and we so need to really examine the life of a patient before they began to misuse drugs. (This topic is discussed many times in this book.)

A key clinical question is this: can addiction stem from a predilection that comes alive only after exposure to (even necessary) narcotic use? To answer this requires that we know how pain patients bring to their new 'pain-lives' all the strengths and weaknesses of their pre-pain lives. One has to probe into how they managed stress, used drugs or alcohol, prospered, etc., before they were in pain. This is indispensable background information.

For example, some current thinking is that some people have a diminished ability to experience pleasure. They might then seek pleasure using substances that produce pleasure via an artificial stimulation of the dopamine system. Getting pleasure like this is so reinforcing to repeated drug use because no natural stimulation can compete. Our bodies can't release as much dopamine as follows cocaine or nicotine use. So addiction is quite possible for this sub-group who may suffer from innate inabilities to feel pleasure. That is often why it is so difficult to fix them psychiatrically. Then, should they need pain medications, the panel of motivations become so complex – did they, through their unexpected need for pain control medications, suddenly find states of relaxation or pleasure the likes of which they never had before in life? The correct diagnostic focus needs to be on the 'why' they did not migrate into opiate use before the pain medication use started.

Our biological systems respond to other stress induced factors, such as corticotrophin-releasing factor (CRF), which regulates our response to stress. If we have a problem in our CRF systems, then when we look into ourselves for help, we will not find the systems to reduce the stress. So we look outside our bodies to find something to relieve the discomfort. Countless millions do this with a nightly cocktail. But the differences lie in that most people use the cocktail without it becoming a problem to the rest of their lives. The cocktail merely soothes a day's anxiety.

> "I get side effects from my work. Work is the pill I need to take in order to survive. It makes me anxious, scared, and so tired that I can't relax and cut out the worry. So I have a drink to calm down. It takes away the side effects. I never need more than one or two drinks. It's all how ya look at things..."

There is now work on the use of vaccines to treatment addictions,[108] and on how a person's genetic make-up may contribute to pain or addictions. One interesting area of study are the levels of brain-derived neurotrophic factor (BDNF).[109] BDNF, also known as a neurotrophin, is distributed widely in the brain; it promotes neuronal survival and plasticity. A number of psychiatric disorders, including depression, appear to be associated with lower BDNF levels. Depression is also commonly associated with addictions. So BDNF may be a rich area for research. If some abnormality with BDNF is the reason for the addiction, then it speaks to a very different etiology. Maybe the sloppy term of 'addiction personality' will have some association with a subtle hormonal imbalance.

It is important to introduce the concept of physiological dependence. A physiological dependence is an 'addiction' at the cellular level insofar as a sudden cessation of medication use will cause physical withdrawal. Chronic pain patients have real physiological dependences without the usual addictive behaviors.

Tolerance and pseudotolerance represent two different needs for dose increases. Tolerance is common – the body 'gets used' to a dose and therefore more medication is needed to get the same end effect. Pseudotolerance occurs when a person does more activity, thereby additionally straining the body, and so there may be a need for extra medications. If a person, because of less pain, leaves the sick bed to do more, such as cooking or shopping, then the patient may report that the medication is not working as well at the former dose; asking for more medication that is associated with more useful activity is a pseudotolerance.

> "When the doc finally got the dose right, I started walking. It felt so good. But the stain made the joint ache more, so I needed more meds. The doc initially said I was tolerant. He forgot to ask how much more I was doing. I maybe was tolerant, but I was also better. Now I say: Real better, fake tolerance. I like that phase! The extra med made me more alive 'cause I did more.

Then he told me about pseudotolerance. I like that term."

Sedation, constipation, and respiratory depressions are other medical side effects usually resolve with on-going use. These problems are often associated with quick dose changes, so a too rapid start or increase in medication dose is much more likely to have these problems. Sedation may stop after some continued use, but this may be controlled by the timing of medication use. If the pain medication is absolutely needed, and no dose reduction is possible, then other interventions may help, such as using Nuvigil®.

Constipation can often be managed with dietary changes as well as stool softeners, etc. Patients may sometimes stop their opioids because of constipation, which results in the under treatment of pain. Wirz and Klaschik proposed a stepwise scheme for the management of opioid induced constipation, beginning with polyethylene glycol 3350/electrolyte.[110] Other management approaches may be needed in different situations. Constipation and sedation management requires close consultation with one's own physician.

Let's end this chapter with an enlightening quote from C. Stratton Hill: [111]

> "The common societal definition of addiction is simply the chronic taking of narcotics. Unfortunately, regulators accept this definition without critically evaluating it... doctors who prescribe opioids... may be judged as creating drug addicts. The physician is not creating an addict. Another popular misconception about drugs is that a mere exposure to them will cause enslavement to them. Patients who must take

opioids over prolonged periods of painful medical conditions that eventually resolve do not become psychologically dependent on them. Treating patients for chronic pain with opioids is not a threat to the public interest."

It would be good if non-narcotics eventually controlled all the pain that people endure. But this is not reality. Though the door towards proper and even pain control is opening, there are days when it is more open than not, and we are still looking for ways to keep it open wide enough so that all those who need to pass through it can do so.

CHAPTER THIRTEEN
The victim becomes the perpetrator

This chronicle is from a patient:

> "I slipped and fell five years ago. My knee cap broke, my hip was fractured, and ever since then I've had worsening, horrible pain in my knee and hip. The doctors say the hip may need replacement because of arthritis. I say it now hurts too much to walk any distance at all.
>
> I have also become the local weatherman. I can tell when a rain storm is coming hours before any TV weather show. I can also give another meaning to the term 'killer storm.'
>
> Because I fell on that greasy floor at work— something that was totally 'not my fault'— I have to live under the direction of a workman's compensation board. All was well and good at the beginning, but when it appeared that I wasn't going to get a whole lot better, and that my care was going to be expensive, things became to change. I never realized how much I would have to fight for what I needed. I was the victim of someone else's obvious negligence, but ever since then I had to turn into the perpetrator just to keep myself above water with things. I was always the nonpolitical type, never really causing trouble. I was an honest man too, believing in getting paid for the real work I did, and buying only what I could afford. I knew some people cheated and lied, but I never did.

I'd be too embarrassed to do it in front of my family, and it's not the life I want to teach my children.

Yet because I fell, and because I hurt, and because I now need the insurance company to pay my bills, I've been accused of being a liar. They seem to say that I do not hurt as much as I say I do. They say I use too much medication, and they make it hard for me to see a physical therapist. I had to wait 3 months to get them to approve for me to have a walker for the really bad days—they said that because I didn't need it every day then they doubted that I needed it at all. Can you believe that I had to hire a lawyer to fight for a silly walker? Well, I know you can believe it if you're in the same boat as me.

I heard about a doctor up at the university medical school that was the best in the country on hip replacements. If I could afford him I'd happily pay for his services myself. But I can't work now because of the pain, and the insurance company wants me to see a doctor who will work for the rates they decide to pay. Now here's where we get testy. They are interested in the lowest price and I am interested in the highest quality. After all, it is my life.

What galls me is that I didn't fall down on purpose, but now me, being the victim, I have to fight for my rights. I'm not asking for a million dollars, no, no, I'm asking only for the best chance at getting better. And if I can't get better then at least treat me like a gentleman and help me find the way I really need. I noticed that many doctors just brush me off if they can't treat me. Only once did a doctor sit and shake his head, saying "I'm sorry, I don't know what to do..." The man actually sat there and went through some of the suffering with me. Most of them just basically say 'next' until they get someone they can fix. The rest of us are discarded like bad fruit.

So over the years I had to learn to fight. Lots of them doctors don't like it when I brawl with them over what I really need. Passive me now fights like a dog. I'm sure no one likes it when I call the insurance companies or the doctors with lots of questions. But most of them don't care too much about me, so why should I care if I hurt their feelings? They ain't feeling bad about hurting mine.

What bothers me the most is that I know I'm not lying. I do know how much I hurt. I know I may never be completely fixed. But I want to try to sleep at night knowing all is being tried. I believe I can be better with the right doctor. And once again, I didn't hurt myself. And all I want is the help I honestly need. My preacher gave a great sermon about "how we learn to see further by standing on the shoulders of giants". He said, however, that when we are so high up, that too many times we can see things that are different from what most people see.

I have to depend on the insurance company now. I hate it, but it's the truth. The only thing is I can see is where all their attitudes are going. They pretend not to see it; they act short sighted. I can see better than them because they are holding me up. Fools, they are fools, because I see the future and they think they are some sort of wonderful giant helping me out. Let them see the world through my eyes. No, they are anything but giants. I am forced to stand on their shoulders, but these aren't the shoulders of giants, these are the shoulders of idiots.

So I am a fighter now. I have learned how to kick the hand that feeds me without it stopping to feed me."

...Thought...

Buddha would speak of the lepers, the outcasts, the miserable poor who toil with aching limbs, and of those who live with scanty nourishment, of the battle wounded, those dying in slow agony, the orphans ill-treated by cruel guardians, and even of successful people who are haunted by the thought of failure and death. From this load of sorrow, he would say that a way of salvation must be found. For him salvation can only come through love.

Nietzsche sees things a bit differently. He would say '....good heavens, man, you must learn to be of tougher fiber. Why go about sniveling because trivial people suffer? Or, for that matter, because great men also suffer? Trivial people suffer trivially, great men suffer greatly, and great sufferings are not to be regretted, because they are noble.... For the sake of such men, any misery is worthwhile.'

These conflicting philosophies are not merely academic amusements. Nietzsche's position on suffering is still prevalent in today's society: those who suffer through a pain can become a better breed of people. Pain offers definition. Nietzsche gave pain a purpose: it made things grow. To conquer pain is to succeed. To succumb or even give in to it is failure. Pain is the fire that forges potency, and it gives a conviction to the goals of truth and honor.

But not everyone has Nietzsche's commitments and infatuations.

...*Thought*...

This excerpt is from a 2001 *New York Times* article titled *Pain, the Disease:*

> "But pain can be the opposite. It is a world of struggling metaphors to describe the experience. It defines a life in a negative way. Pain can destroy and shift the shape of a person's life. It can be a world to which the "modern chronicler of hell might look to the lives of chronic pain patients for inspiration. Theirs is a special suffering, a separate chamber…it is pain whose presence predominates."
>
> It continues with: "chronic pain resembles a disease…that often outlives its original causes… that is harmful to the body…there are no spokesmen for under treating pain – no one advocates not treating pain." The author further asks "And what make a doctor sympathetic to pain?" Her answer is a quote from Pennsylvania

> physician James Mickle: "Someone who has pain himself, or has an intellectual interest...who isn't interested in immediate results, doesn't want to make money, and has a lot of degrees. There's one in a lot of communities, but then they get all the pain patients sent to them and eventually they burn out and quit." [112]

Pain forces people to change. Perhaps those who lack the ability to change are those who find delight in the narcosis, and avoid the socially awakening, aspects of narcotic use.

> "I hate that this medication has the side of effect of sometimes making me sleepy. I like that it takes the pain away, however. I met a two patients in the clinic – they are so different than me. They aren't fighters. They like the sleepy part of the meds."

Elaine Scarry [113] wrote that pain throws the afflicted into "the world of cries and whispers." Pain patients struggle like aphasic poets looking to put the pain into words. They hope that the correct words will eloquently convey and demystify their pain so others will understand it.

Pain can turn the quiet meek into the vibrant vocalist.

> A pain patient often described her pain like 'hot rods being shoved up into my groin!' She spent so much time fighting her insurance company for a myriad of benefits. By chance she met another pain patient. They compared problems and symptoms, and then they both felt a spiritual emancipation in being mutually

understood. From that joint emancipation came a hearty and shared backing that enabled both of them to more uncompromisingly fight for their needs.

A 73 year old quiet and compassionate gentleman, who worked for years helping military veterans, developed pain in his lower back. The first pain doctor did an injection, but it made things worse. The doctor then removed himself from the case. The patient believed the doctor was afraid of a lawsuit. But the patient was also dismayed that he had to fight for more care. He found another doctor who agreed to work with him, but the insurance delayed the authorization. "I became a politician! I wrote letters, I made noise, I did things I never did before! I was always there to help others, and then I saw how few of those 'others' were there to help me. But I was also scared I would anger the insurance company such that they would become even more mulish and head-strong in their position." A second doctor was eventually authorized, and over many months of different injections, medications, and exercises, the patient got much better. But the experience of becoming the aggressor was "like boot camp for me – and I am better for it."

CHAPTER FOURTEEN
What is pain? A medical perspective

Pain is actually the brain code responding to the neuron code.

This book is less about the science of pain and more about the reaction to and attitudes towards pain. Nevertheless, a discussion of pain itself is needed.

This next section is no more than a sketchy introduction into science of pain and its treatments. This clinical playing field far too large and ever so rapidly changing that it cannot be condensed into a single chapter. Treatments are also so individualized that, at best, only the most general overviews can be safely given. Nonetheless, a brief overview of the nervous system will help decipher the types, the causes, the problems, and the reasons supporting why a particular treatment form is chosen. Some of this information overlaps with information elsewhere in this book.

The nervous system exists to monitor and control many of life's activities. Pain and pleasure are both nervous system activities. The ability to taste, hear, touch, balance, remember, love, cry, hate, see, feel temperatures, or sense an injury, are all nervous system events. The nerves are our body's wires whose job is to connect the body to the brain or to other control centers. That is how we get the information from which we will make decisions. The nervous system is the most amazing computer.

A nociceptor is a sensory cell sensitive to situations that are potentially damaging to tissues. The term 'nociceptive' relates to nerve signals that produce the sensation of pain. *Noci* is the Latin indicator of harm or injury.

Pain is "an unpleasant sensory and emotional experience associated with actual or potential tissue damage." [114]

Pain is actually the intricate processing and interpretation of signals. Some processing is physiologic while some is psychologic. Pain signals from peripheral nerves produce interactions in the dorsal horn of the spinal cord that trigger circuits. These circuits ascend (go up) or descend (come down) through the spinal cord and then go into and out of the brain. The result of all this is that certain signal patterns are perceived as pain.

Pain signals that continue over time have a neuroplastic effect which could enhance pain. This is known as a pronociceptive positive feedback loop. It means untreated pain can make things worse. Neuroplastic means that the neurological system is 'plastic', which means it can be changed (or to be literal, to be re-molded). It is critical to control pain before the neuroplastic effect takes place. [115]

Pain has traditionally been divided into that from either neuropathic or inflammatory origins. These will be discussed in greater detail below. Recently a new theory of pain origin is emerging. Called central sensitization, it is pain caused by neither an inflammatory or neuropathic origin.[116][117] It is thought to be a major process in the pain of fibromyalgia. The central sensitization process is defined by the unusual excitability of the neuron in the spinal cord. An impulse from a peripheral nerve sends a message to the spinal cord. The spinal cord, in the section known as a dorsal horn, ordinarily relays the pain message to the brain. In fibromyalgia, the dorsal horn neurons become hypersensitive to stimulation, so a relatively little input to these cells is required to make them send up a full pain signal. In other words, the over reactivity of the dorsal horn causes the dorsal horn to amplify or give spurious pain signals to the brain. The reason for the hypersensitivity is uncertain. It may be related to excessive amounts of excitatory amino acids, such as a glutamate, or to the activity of substance P.

> Fibromyalgia is eight times as more likely to occur in someone if a first-degree relative also has it. Genetic variations may predispose to the condition, and it is commonly co-morbid (that is the medical term for co-existing) with other disorders. The term itself is a descendent of the 1904 term 'fibrositis'.[118] Environmental stresses can also trigger its onset. Fibromyalgia affects between 2 to 5% of adults, so it is the most chronic and common pain condition in the United States. [119]
>
> Fibromyalgia's cardinal feature is 'chronic widespread pain' (CWP). From 73% to 99% of fibromyalgia patients also report some sleep disturbance. A night of poor sleep is followed by a day of more pain. Depression and anxiety are associated with poor sleep as well, but the restoration of good sleep could lower the levels of daytime angst, pain and/or depression. [120]

Many physicians believe fibromyalgia is real. Some don't. The overlap with psychiatric illnesses is very high. It is a bit confusing because many of the medications used for depressions are also used for fibromyalgia. Might the disorders actually be two discrete conditions that manifest with common symptoms? Research is looking into this.

This book has many references to the overlaps between the presence of pain and psychiatric disorders. Some psychiatric disorders actually present not only with complaints of sadness or anxiety, but rather with joint pain, headaches, or other somatic disturbances. People with psychiatric disorders may even process pain signals differently; some people may be more or less sensitive to pain thresholds. [121] A Swedish study of 45,000 patients found depression, anxiety, and eating disorders in people with chronic fatigue and fibromyalgia, and they said that a "genetic susceptibility to emotional instability may...play an etiological role in the links among psychiatric disorders, CWP (chronic widespread pain), and chronic fatigue." [122] Similar diagnostic and treatment concerns co-exist with conditions such as reflex sympathetic dystrophy or the complex regional pain syndrome.

We are now about to enter the world of biochemistry. Sometimes these concepts seem to be too simple, as if they can explain so much more than they actually can. These concepts offer targets for treatment, but these are often not the true targets. The targets often seem too obvious and reachable. These 'targets' live in a world far more complex that meets the eye. The more one studies these targets and the bullets we shoot at them, the more one is humbled by how little we really know. Sometimes it feels like we know in which direction to shoot, but hitting the right target requires a dose of luck as well. Some biochemical targets and some bullets make so much sense on paper that we overly expect them to solve many problems. They frequently fail.

We must be very careful not to give these targets and bullets more jurisdiction than they rightly deserve. Many see pain as a complex, but straightforward biochemical event. It is not that simple. Furthermore, a failure to respond to a series of biochemical interventions doesn't mean the source has to be psychological. Treatment failures may issue from an inadequate science, or from many other and powerful political, economic, psychologic, or philosophic choices or constraints.

Pain Chemistry

Pain is the psychological response to certain patterns of information relayed through the nervous system. The brain then interprets these signals as an unpleasant sensation known as pain. Pain treatments, by and large, merely modify or reduce these signals and/or the response to the patterns.

Neurons do not touch each other. The gap between neurons is the synapse, and hormones flood out of one neuron, cross the synapse, and then sit on the receptors of receiving neurons. The transmitting cell is called the pre-synaptic nerve, and the receiving cell is called the post-synaptic cell. Blocking the transmission of pain is often done by blocking or increasing (it depends on the situation) the final activity of these hormones. These hormones are known as neurotransmitters.

Disease, drugs of all types, including alcohol, can change these hormone levels or how they act.

The neurohormones wash over specialized receptors that sit on the outside surface of receiving cells. When the right hormone finds the right receptor, the receiving cell is triggered into firing, and a message is passed along until the receiving nerve encounters another nerve or cell. The 'rules' about how neurons communicate with each other is the 'neuron code.' The psychological meanings we give the neuron code pattern is the 'brain code.'[123] *Pain is actually the brain code responding to the neuron code.* Medications change the brain code by changing the neuron code.

Receptors on the neurons are fascinating items. Molecules protrude into the synapse from the surface of the cell. These molecules are similar to antennas. After the antenna is stimulated by the hormone, a series of cellular chemical reactions follow which cause the post-synaptic cell to do something. Usually it causes another set of hormones to be released, causing, in turn, yet another set of neurons to do something. The end result of thousands and thousands of these cells, all firing in certain patterns, cumulates into something that we can feel, do, or think. That's the brain code.

Some receptors also exist on the pre-synaptic cells. These control self-feedback mechanisms about the cell's own activity.

Many steps are involved in this process, and problems with any one of them could distort the system. An excellent analogy is a radio. Visualize the number of steps needed between speaking into a microphone and the sound coming out of a loudspeaker. We have a pretty good idea of what happens in a radio, but much remains unknown about the transmission and reception of pain signals.

Over the past decade or so, an interest has grown into the fascinating role that glial cells play in pain and depression. Glia cells wrap around and support the neurons. They provide glucose to neurons and protect the cells from glutamate. As a result they actively participate in neurohormone activity. Glia also helps with neuronal repair and survival because they make and release neurotrophic factors, which essentially help to keep the neurons healthy. Stress will decrease the availability of these protective factors. So perhaps pain is felt because the glia are not working as they should. This is interesting because the 'pain,' per se, may be bad because of problems in the glial cells, and not with the neurons. It is like a car that pulls to one side. An alignment may not be the problem. The problem may be tires that have different tread patterns. But if we don't think of the tread patterns, a lot of money may be wasted on repeated alignments. The same concern applies to pain treatment. The good doctor must think of both neuronal as well as glial causes of pain control.

Antidepressants appear to help the glia. This raises the question of the impact of stress that comes from pain. Such stress, if unchecked, can damage neurons because the neurons lack the protection by the glia. Antidepressants may do more than just undoing depressions. With less stress, the glia can go about their work of maintaining the integrity of the neurons.

It also appears that glial activation can amplify pain, and studies have shown that they contribute to the development of arthritic pain. [124] Watkins [125], in 2003, wrote: "Until now, all research aimed at understanding how pain amplification occurs in the spinal cord and all drug therapies aimed at causing exaggerated pain have focused exclusively on neurons." He concludes that the spinal cord glia cells are critically important because when they are activated, they release substances that amplify the pain message. Medications like Lyrica® may calm down these circuits. These are keenly interesting new areas of future pain management possibilities to watch.

We know of five types of sensory receptors:

- *Thermoreceptors* – these detect changes in temperature
- *Electromagnetic receptors* — these detect light (vision)
- *Nociceptors* — these detect injury and damage to tissues
- *Mechanoreceptors* — these detect deformations of the receptor cells
- *Chemoreceptors* — these detect chemical changes, such as taste, smell, oxygen level changes, blood sugar levels, hormonal levels, etc.

Receptors are selective. They respond to the sensory inputs for which they are designed. They may be totally non-responsive to other stimuli, e.g., a tickle is not felt as warmth. They are like microphones that respond only to a specific frequency. But there is no division in the different types of signal – the vision signal is electrophysiologically the same as a hearing signal. The differences lie in where it starts and where it goes. So the neuron code is the same. But it is the brain code which gives us a perception, an understanding, or some emotional feeling about the pattern of the raw signal. There are, therefore, two areas of treating the pain – to reduce or modify the areas triggering the neuron code, and to reduce or modify the patterns triggering the brain code.

One could say that pain lives in the neuron code and suffering lives in the brain code.

Nerves end in specific areas of the brain or spinal cord. These areas – because of the brain code – recognize the input as a particular pattern. However, sometimes the nerves also cross stimulates the pain monitoring centers in ways that resemble another experience, such as anxiety. So we get both anxiety and pain. Remember that a pain signal wants us to do something about the pain. It wants us to remove the trigger. Pain is not supposed to be constant. The pain is a danger to our well-being. Anxiety also tells us that some danger is looming against our well-being. Anxiety is our colleague because it draws us to the need to focus on removing the pain. Reducing just the anxiety might make us indifferent to the pain. If the pain is unfixable, then at least no anxiety means less discomfort about an unwanted visitor that won't go away. If the anxiety can't be reduced, then it may turn from an ally to an foe.

All receptors adapt (fully or partially) to on-going stimulation. This means they may lose their normal ability to react to an on-going stimulation. This allows us not to feel the pressure of sitting. Until a leg goes to sleep or is bent in a funny way, we lose the conscious perception of sitting. The adaptation is not permanent – that is why one reason we shift positions when asleep or we shift and wiggle in a chair. It brings the receptors back into action. Many times when we sit for a long time the blood is reduced, and the need to get food and oxygen to the tissues will also make us move.

But some receptors, such as those for pain, may never adapt. In fact, pain nociceptors may fire more rapidly with continued, or even with less, stimulation. The pain pathways then become hypersensitive. [126] This is one argument for the rapid use of pain controlling interventions.

Deeper tissues are less plentifully innervated than the skin. However, there are some highly innervated tissues, such as arterial walls, joint surfaces, and certain intracranial (inside the skull) tissues. Widespread damage to the deeper tissues can cause an aching type of pain.

Certain chemicals cause pain. These work through chemo-sensitive nociceptors. The chemicals are many, but some of the most common ones are bradykinin, prostaglandin, potassium ions, acids, histamine, and serotonin.

When a tissue is irritated or injured, certain substances break out of cells and cause an inflammation. These substances cause the nociceptors to be stimulated, and we thereafter perceive pain. If the body suspects organ damage, then the blood vessels may be triggered to dilate, perhaps using nitrous oxide to do so, as the inflammatory response cascade begins. [127] Sometimes massive organ damage will constrict the blood vessels so blood is not lost.

The process can then go either way. The nociceptors can enhance the pain, which causes hyperalgesia. Or the opposite can happen: the endogenous (meaning made in our own bodies) opiate like materials could reduce the pain signal before it gets to the central nervous system. Not everyone has the same level of endogenous opiates, so this may explain why some people are more sensitive to pain than others. Some people also have different psychological approaches to the pain, which will greatly alter the responses to pain (They have different brain codes). Having a good psychological foundation, along with the good fortune of also having a strong army of endogenous opiates, is a lucky combination.

Some drugs reduce or prevent inflammation by inhibiting the production of prostaglandin. These anti-inflammatory drugs include aspirin, acetaminophen, steroids, and the non-steroidal anti-inflammatory drugs (commonly known by the initials NSAID). Common NSAIDs are ibuprofen, Vioxx®, Celebrex®, Embrel®, and others.

Antihistamines block histamine release. Benadryl® and Vistaril® are two antihistamines are often combined with other pain medications to augment the anti-pain effect. They also offer some anti-anxiety effect.

Each time a certain sequence of messages passes through the nerves, the synapses 'learn' the pattern, and so the next time the pattern passes through the same nerves, the signal becomes 'facilitated.' After many repeated sequences of similar signals, the pattern may be experienced by the person as strong, even if the current signal is really weak.[128] Far too often pain patients are accused of experiencing exaggerated pain; this may one reason why this is so.

There are about 35 known neurotransmitters involved in the transmission of messages. The operations are complex, and often the desired effect can be an indirect one. For example, one substance stimulates a system that, in turn, inhibits another system. Pain reduction may then result from the second system's inhibition. It is a spaghetti bowl of feedback circuits.

Morphine is a neurotransmitter. Morphine is a truly great pain reliever. Traditionally, it is the one against which all others are compared.

N-methyl-d-aspartate receptors (NMDA) are thought to be involved with chronic pain. The NMDA receptor may also be involved in the development of opioid tolerance. Memantine (Namenda®) is a NMDA blocker (antagonist) used for Alzheimer's disease. It blocks the stimulatory effect of the amino acid glutamate. Much work is being done to explore the role of memantine in the treatment of chronic pain and addiction.[129] The vital notions to consider are that non-opiate systems are being explored that may account for some of the different clinical situations seen in chronic pain. For example, some people can be weaned off their narcotics with no reduction in pain. Does this mean that the pain may be coming from a non-opiate based system? Perhaps the cause of the pain is from a NDMA rather than an opiate based system problem? This is discussed in greater detail elsewhere in the book. Failure to respond to an opiate doesn't mean the pain is false. It means it is a pain being transmitted with a different code.

Descending nerve tracts from the brain use serotonin to dampen pain signals. In the spinal cord, at the same site where the pain message comes into the spinal cord, this descending nerve releases serotonin with the intention of diminishing the intensity of the pain signal that is about to be transmitted to the brain. This is a case of one neurotransmitter inhibiting the activity of another neurotransmitter.

Many antidepressants augment serotonin, and so are used in chronic pain patients. This is one of the reasons why Elavil® and Cymbalta® are widely used. Theoretically, many other antidepressants ought to be equally effective.

When an antidepressant modifies pain signal transmission in the spinal code, it is working on the neuron code. When it works on the person's mood, it is working on the brain code. It's clear, however, that the antidepressants affect the brain code by modifying the neuron code. Our bodies are incredibly complex and intertwined.

It has been said that chronic pain uses serotonin like a speeding train engine uses fuel. Eventually the fuel (serotonin) runs out, and the pain goes up while the mood goes down. Volumes of literature exist about this. Recently the press reported that when serotonin goes down, behavioral reactions can be more impulsive. Indeed one article in *Science* is titled: *Serotonin Modulates Behavioral Reactions to Unfairness*.[130] How intriguing it is that the authors chose to use the term 'unfairness' since many pain patients feel the system is 'unfair' to their needs.

> Might it be that one reason pain patients are often antagonistic or impulsive is that the pain is consuming their serotonin? This subsequent impulsivity may lead to interpersonal problems with people, including their doctors. While moods may soften somewhat with antidepressant use, the pain may not be sufficiently lowered to allow the improved mood to show itself. The patient might ask for a higher pain medication dose. Some doctors are comfortable doing this and some are not. The intricate link of pain to mood in the context of a social contract may be as complex as the brain itself. Pain needs to be evaluated using many different ideas and tools.

Sometimes the failure or success in manipulating the biochemistry of pain is related to how much medication is being used.

Sophisticated psychopharmacolgists quite often take patients to unusually high medication doses. High antidepressant doses may be 'out of the box' to many doctors, but 'in the box' for many psychiatrists. The result is that a patient may not be getting enough medications as a result of their doctor's political-professional-personal choices rather than because of any scientific rationale. The *Science* article writes: "Our results suggest that 5-HT (serotonin) plays a critical role in regulating emotions during social decision-making." Too low a level of serotonin, for whatever reason, handicaps the patient. The biochemical aspects of pain control may face greater challenges from human foibles and eccentricities than from our biological knowledge database.

In 2006, a protein called 'p11' was discovered. Mice deficient in this protein acted as if they were depressed. Sufficient additional quantities of p11 resulted in behaviors changing as if the mice were being treated with antidepressants, which, of course, increased the serotonin. This may someday play a role in pain control.

There is great excitement about the neurotransmitters known as endogenous opiates. These molecules, also called endorphins, are made in the central nervous system. They work via the same receptors as many drugs, such as morphine. Endorphins are 'endogenous' because they are made by the body. The drug store opiates are 'exogenous' because they are made outside the body. Endogenous endorphins are the basis of the 'runner's high,' and some believe that endorphins are involved in laugher.

Endorphins have the exact activity as morphine. A tolerance and dependence can develop, and the effects of an endorphin can be reversed by a drug called naloxone (Narcan®). Naloxone is given in opiate overdoses to reverse the narcotic effect. Naloxone is also combined with some pain medications to reduce the chance of overdose and euphoria. Suboxone® is a combination of buprenorphine and naloxone.

Endorphins are actually small chains of amino acids called peptides. Peptides are released by the body under certain stresses.

Sometimes large peptides are released which later are divided into smaller, active molecules. One product of such a process are the beta-endorphins. These are further broken into shorter chains called met-enkephalins. Leu-enkephalins are produced from the division of other precursors. Enkephalins may be even more potent than beta-endorphins. Though somewhat complex, here are the basic definitions of some of these incredible molecules, all of which play such critical roles in pain transmission.

> **Beta-lipotropin -** *This 91 amino acid chain may be a fragment of the hormone ACTH. Beta lipotropin has no opiate activity.*
>
> **Beta-endorphin -** *A molecule with 30 amino acids, it has opiate activity and it consists of a fragment of the beta lipotropin chain.*
>
> **Enkephalins -** *Chains of 5 amino acids, they have potent opiate activity. They are fragments of longer chains.*
>
> **Substance P -** *A chain with 11 amino acids, it is the opposite of an opiate, and is a pain neurotransmitter.*

Dynorphins - *A 17 unit chain with mixed affinities.*

Opioids are primarily made in the brain and spinal cord, but some come from the adrenal medulla, where they are released with epinephrine into the blood. There are suggestions that endorphins in the limbic system are involved with learning, emotion, and memory.

Considerable pain control can be managed by either increasing the endorphin/enkephalin levels or reducing the Substance P levels. Exogenous narcotics aid and mimic the endorphins and enkephalins. One substance, capsaicin, which is made from peppers, reduces Substance P. Capsaicin is currently available for external use only. Its practical potential does not yet match its theoretical one.

As noted above, about thirty-five nervous system hormonal transmitters are known. They are also called neurotransmitters. The following is a list of the more common and well known ones. Other chemical or neurologic systems may still be unknown to us. The literature about hormones is vast, so these are tiny summaries:

Acetylcholine. It is widely found throughout the brain and in the peripheral systems. It is excitatory in most areas, but can be inhibitory in some areas. Many drugs effect acetylcholine. Many of the side effects to drugs stem from how they interfere with the normal action of acetylcholine. The term 'anticholinergic' means that something is blocking the action of acetylcholine. Too little acetylcholine is thought to cause one aspect of dementia. Medications with anticholingeric properties might cause dry mouth, blurry vision, problems with constipation and voiding, etc.

Norepinephrine. Commonly called adrenaline, it is found widely in the brain and is generally inhibitory, although it can be stimulatory in some areas. Epinephrine is metabolically related to norepinephrine. Many stimulants alter this hormone's activity, such as caffeine, nicotine, antidepressants, blood pressure medications, etc. Moods can be affected by norepinephrine levels. Some antidepressants modify norepinephrine levels or activity.

Dopamine. This is a fascinating hormone. When deficient, it is responsible for Parkinson's disease. Too much of it can cause psychosis. It can produce emotional pleasure or pain. It is important in maintaining blood pressure. Sinemet® increases dopamine, while antipsychotics reduce its effect. It is the chemical precursor of norepinephrine. Opiates have the ability to block the re-uptake of dopamine. That is, they keep it in the synaptic circulation longer so it can work longer. This could be one of the ways opiates make us feel better. [131] In mice, the more morphine used by the animal, the greater is the increase in the dopamine and norepinephrine levels.[132]

The presence of extra dopamine leads to pleasure. Lower levels of dopamine can cause some types of depressions. But dopamine may itself be converted, that is, be synthesized, into morphine by human white blood cells. [133] The white blood cells have low, but significant amounts of endogenous morphine that are released following trauma or stress. Human neuroblastoma cells can synthesize endogenous morphine as well.[134] Perhaps within these mechanisms lie the reasons why some people need more, or some need less, medication to achieve pain relief. There are suggestions that cocaine, alcohol, and nicotine also enhance endogenous morphine. This speaks even more so to the converging of biological mechanisms that explain why some of these substances are so addicting. [135] This is one of many fascinating research threads that need careful monitoring.

GABA (gamma-aminobutyric acid). It causes inhibition of a cells activity. GABA is the hormone through which tranquilizers like Valium® and Xanax® work. GABA can modulate and inhibit dopamine.[136] Perhaps people needing benzodiazepines have too little GABA or have a problem in the GABA system, and therefore they suffer the over stimulating ill-effects of too much dopamine.

Cannabinoids. A preparation from the cannabis sativa plant, it is also known as coming from marijuana or the Indian hemp plant. The plant was indigenous to India, but it is now grown worldwide. Delta-9-tetrahydrocannabinol (THC) is the major psychoactive component. Cannabis has been used for centuries to alleviate disease.[137] It was called a panacea, and for many years it was sold as a pain medication. It has been illegal in the United States since 1937. By the early 1990's, the endogenous cannabinoid system has been discovered, which created great interest in how a system that naturally existed in our bodies might be involved in pain control. [138] [139]

In 1964, oral dronabinol was developed; it was approved in 1985 as Marinol® to treat chemotherapy induced nausea. In 1992, it earned an indication for appetite stimulation for HIV patients. In January 2006, the US FDA approved advanced clinical studies for its possible use in cancer pain. In June 2005, Canada approved Sativex® for neuropathic pain in multiple sclerosis. Later, in August 2007, Canada further approved it for pain that was nonresponsive to opioids. Sativex® is an oral spray.

These marijuana based medications work via receptors located throughout the brain.[140] Its medicinal use remains a topic of considerable debate, in large part related both to the cultural and legal status of marijuana, and the fact that the substance has psychoactive properties. Nonetheless, THC as been associated with antiemetic, analgesic, muscle relaxation, appetite stimulation qualities, and with the reduction of ocular pressure in glaucoma. The cannabinoid system is one of the main modulators of the central nervous system.[141] Recent work suggests that cannabis may down-regulate neuroinflammation, and it may reduce both neuropathic pain and the pain associated with multiple sclerosis.[142,143] It has further been suggested that cannabinoid analgesia is via endocannabinboids, which work in tandem with endogenous opioids.[144] Much remains to be learned.

In January 2010, New Jersey Governor Jon Corzine signed the New Jersey Compassionate Use Medical Marijuana Act. This bill allows patients with serious debilitating illnesses to use marijuana with their doctors' recommendations. It will also create regulated compassion centers at which patients and caregivers can obtain their medical marijuana. New Jersey is the 14th state to endorse the use of marijuana in pain as useful in debilitating medical conditions. The bill also addresses the thorny problem of how to supply medical marijuana to appropriate patients. However, the bill does not allow marijuana to be used for chronic pain; perhaps the chronic pain label is too broad. It does allow marijuana to be used for multiple sclerosis, cancer, glaucoma, epilepsy, Crohn's disease, AIDS, muscular dystrophy, and Lou Gehrig's disease. Clearly, pain is part of many of these diseases. The fear seems to be that if access to medical marijuana is too open, the policy and its effects cannot be "measured." The issue will be revisited in two years when other ailments could be added, such as neuropathic pain conditions. Questions of how to dose it, to be sure it is being used in appropriate clinical situations, and that dispensaries will be controlled, are central concerns. In January 2010, Los Angles was considering an move to limit the number of marijuana dispensaries.

As with all similar legislature events, the details may change without a moment's notice, so on-going monitoring is needed. What is perhaps the oldest medical text, *Shen-nung Pen-tshao Ching*, suggests that cannabis be used to reduce the pain of rheumatism and some digestive disorders.

Without question, the use and role of cannabinoids and its derivatives in chronic pain needs a very careful and a very objective scientific inquiry.

> The problem is not with those who use marijuana correctly. The problem is with those who abuse the intent of the law to make it more accessible to the sick.

Attitudes towards the use of medical marijuana have varied with the differing political situations. In October 2009, the Obama administration refocused the police efforts away from prosecuting medical marijuana users. The DEA posted this on October 22, 2009:

> "DEA (www.dea.gov) welcomes the issuance of these clarifying guidelines pertaining to the use of federal investigative and prosecutorial resources in states that have enacted laws authorizing the use of marijuana for medical purposes.
>
> "These guidelines do not legalize marijuana. It is not the practice or policy of DEA to target individuals with serious medical conditions who comply with state laws authorizing the use of marijuana for medical purposes. Consistent with the DOJ guidelines, we will continue to identify and investigate any criminal organization or individual who unlawfully grows, markets, or distributes marijuana or other dangerous drugs. Those who unlawfully possess firearms, commit

acts of violence, provide drugs to minors, or have ties to other criminal organizations may also be subject to arrest.

Prior administrations took different positions. This is an example of an on-going medical-political evolution. One of the key questions is if the many medical marijuana dispensaries are indeed supplying marijuana to other than legitimate medical patients. The other key question is for medical science to extract the therapeutic aspects of marijuana, and to find the where's, if's and how's of its use as a medication.

Glycine. An amino acid, it causes inhibition. There are yet no available medications that directly alter glycine functions.

Glutamic acid. Found in the sensory pathways, it causes excitation. High concentrations are associated with cell death. NMDA antagonists block or slow down the receptor response to glutamic acid. Memantine can do just this. Despite the theory, its use in pain has not yet been established. However some patients can reduce their opioid dose without loss of pain control when memantine is added. Memantine, approved for dementia, is marketed in the US as Namenda®. Elsewhere it is known as Ebixa® or Axura®. A poster at the 11th World Congress on Pain[145] reported with memantine: "Migraine frequency fell to an average of 4.1 migraines per month, or almost 56% less than at baseline, in 14 of 20 patients. Remaining migraines were rated as less severe and easier to treat. Acute migraine and rescue medication use dropped by two-thirds." Another study supports findings that memantine may be useful in the prevention of refractory migraines.[146] Its use in painful neuropathy has shown poor or mixed results.[147]

It has also been suggested that memantine reduces the development of tolerance to morphine[148], and that it reduces central sensitization.¹⁴⁹ Memantine itself may not ultimately play a huge role in pain management, but the research into its mechanisms may produce a rich harvest.

Glutamate (the other name for glutamic acid) is found in virtually all brain neurons. Its role was discovered only about 25 years ago. Research is beginning to appear that links glutamate levels to pain processing pathways and how pain is being maintained.¹⁵⁰ It has been suggested that the anticonvulsant medications gabapentin, lamotrigine, and riluzole reduce the development of hyperalgesia (increased pain sensitivity) in rats by reducing the release of glutamate in spinal cord.¹⁵¹ Changes in glutamate levels in parts of the brain (the insula) are associated with changes in fibromyalgia pain.¹⁵² This rapidly expanding area warrants careful monitoring.

Substance P. It causes excitation of the pain transmitting fibers. Capsaicin, an over the counter pain medication, is thought to deplete and prevent re-accumulation of Substance P in peripheral nerves. This is a peptide.

Nitrous Oxide. It is a regulator of vascular and inflammatory activities. It has even been associated with glutamate (NMDA) neurotoxicity. One theory suggests that NO (nitrous oxide) can un-do the body's alerting systems in the midst of pain. NO dampens the excitatory pathways and promotes relaxation. ¹⁵³ ¹⁵⁴ Medications which enhance the normal release of NO are used for erectile dysfunction disorders.

Serotonin. Commonly found throughout the brain, it inhibits pain and greatly effects moods and sleep. Many medications influence its activity. Serotonin, also called 5-HT, is made from the amino acid tryptophan. Antihistamines and antidepressants alter the functions and availability of 5-HT. 5-HT receptors are also found in the spinal cord and can inhibit pain transmission. Serotonin levels can go up during periods of relaxation. The amount of on-going scientific work done to understand 5-HT is enormous. This is one of the central substances involved the regulation of so many body and psychiatric systems. Efforts to increase 5-HT with dietary supplements are of questionable use.

Vasoactive Intestinal Peptide (VIP), Thyrotropin Releasing Hormone (TRH), Galanin, Cytokines, Calcitonin Gene-Related Peptide (CGRP), and Cholecystokinin (CCK). These are other neuropeptides that have been shown to have roles in pain transmission. Much work remains to be done.

Brain derived neurotrophic factor (BDNF) – This is a fascinating new area of possible pain control. The brain is made up of neurons and non-neuronal glial cells. Glial cells support, protect, remove dead neurons, offer nutrition, form myelin (an insulator between neurons), and participate in signal transmission in the nervous system. Glial cells outnumber neurons by about 10 to 1. They are also known as the "glue" of the nervous system. When glial cells activate to protect the neurons, they may employ BDNF and other growth factors.[155] These factors can potentiate pain.[156] The research into this process is rich, complex and compelling.

Morphine, Heroin, and Codeine – A bit of history

In 1803, Fredrich Sertüner tested different fractions of crude opium. He found a fraction that caused cerebral depression and spasms of the extremities, and yet it also relieved toothaches. He called the fraction morphine after *Morpheus*, the Greek God of sleep.

Opium appears to have been used to control pain since pre-historic times. Third century Arabian physicians used it. In the Orient it was used for dysentery.

Opium is obtained by drying poppy seed juice. Before Sertüner, only crude opium was used in medicine. Opium is rarely used any more, although tinctures (laudanum) do exist to control diarrhea. The word "opioid" comes from the word 'opos', which is Greek for juice. Opium is the juice of the *papaver somniferum*, the opium poppy.

Morphine is made from the amino acid tyrosine. This is a complex, but the sequence is this: tyrosine → norlaudanosoline → reticuline → salutaridine → salutaridinol-I → thebaine → codeine → morphine. [157] Notice that codeine, a widely used medication, is converted within our bodies into morphine. So, our bodies convert the codeine in a Tylenol #3® into morphine. The pain relief comes from morphine, not codeine. By the way, eating extra tyrosine does not make our bodies make more morphine. But eating a correct diet will keep our systems in an appropriate biochemical balance.

Morphine can both stimulate and depress the central nervous system. The depressive aspect can cause analgesia or respiratory problems (mainly an issue with patients who are new to morphine or when there is a large and sudden dose increase). Morphine can depress the cough reflex, and cause sleep. The stimulating aspects of the drug can cause vomiting, miosis (which is a contraction of the pupil), some hyperactive reflexes, and very rarely, convulsions. It can change the mood either into euphoria or dysphoria, and it might cause smooth muscle spasms in the biliary (sphincter of Oddi), bladder sphincter, or gastrointestinal tracts. This can lead to constipation or urinary retention because the muscles are in a state of tonic (continuous) contraction. Some other side effects are a possible blood pressure drop, sweating, and pruritus (itching). The usual duration of pain relief from immediate release formulations is from 4-6 hours. The long acting formulations last longer because they dissolve slower, (like a slow continuous infusion of medication), but the morphine they release is the same molecule, and it lasts the expected 4-6 hours.

It was once thought that morphine had no addictive potential. In 1874, heroin was first produced from morphine by CR Wright, an English pharmacist at St. Mary's Hospital in London. The name 'heroin' is from the German word *heroisch*, (heroic), because of its apparent 'heroic' effects. About 25 years later, the pharmaceutical company Bayer put heroin into cough medicines because it too was thought not to have addicting properties. So from 1898 through 1910, heroin was marketed as a non-addictive morphine substitute and cough suppressant. Bayer also marketed heroin as a cure for morphine addiction before it was discovered that it rapidly metabolizes into morphine. However, it proved to be more addicting than morphine. Therefore, morphine remains a mainstay pain medication.

Some discussion remains claiming that heroin should, at times, be used because the medical literature suggests that heroin might be better than morphine for some types and levels of pain. Renamed diamorphine, heroin has been used as strong analgesic in the United Kingdom.[158]

Heroin, whose chemical name is diacetylmorphine, is a semi-synthetic product made from morphine. Interestingly, it is hydrolyzed by the body back into morphine; that is, heroin turns into morphine, and it is the morphine that addresses the pain! (Morphine goes into diacetylmorphine, then it is changed into 6-monoacetylmorphine (6-MAM), which is then, in turn, changed back to morphine.) Heroin is more lipid soluble than morphine, so it will more readily pass into the brain than morphine, and that is why it is so dangerous and so abused. Though in 1898 it began to be used to treat cough and to treat morphine addictions, it was soon seen to be very problematic, and in 1924 heroin was banned in the United States. It is now illegal throughout the world. Yet, it still has use in England. Some say it has no good use at all: "It does not, and this misconception should be dispelled permanently." [159] These issues are still being debated. [160]

> "I found an article that British doctors use diamorphine – that's heroin – as a pain killer for the terminally ill and after serious operations. Then I read that Kabul doesn't have much of a opium abuse problem because most of it is exported to Europe. Then I read that the idea of cultivating Afghan opium for medicine use was stopped because it is too difficult to keep safeguards going and to keep the opium standard high enough. So I see it this way: Maybe in the world of diamorphine there is something to help those who need it, but as a layman, are the problems more medical or political....I'm not sure...but the automatic notion that heroin is 'so, so very bad' now has a question mark rather than an explanation mark. I don't know."

The natural opiates are opium, morphine, and codeine. Semi-synthetic opiates are heroin, hydromorphone, and oxycodone. The completely synthetic medications are propoxyphene (Darvon®), hydrocodone, and meperidine (Demerol®). In early 2009, the FDA recommended that propoxyphene no longer be marketed because of its addiction potential. Also, many patients felt it was not that effective of a medication.

Codeine was discovered by Robiquet in 1832. It is about 60% as strong as morphine. It becomes effective only after it is converted to morphine in the body. Again, it's interesting that codeine, like heroin, is converted by our bodies into morphine. That is why morphine is considered the standard against which we compare other pain medications.

Before the turn of the last century opium was commonly mixed in many over-the-counter preparations. It was used to treat food poisoning, parasites, other stomach disorders, and anxiety. Opium seed pods were found in Spanish burial plots, which suggest that it was used in 4200 BC. A long and colorful history of opium trade between Britain, China and India resulted in the Opium Wars. Thomas Jefferson grew opium at Monticello, and medical groups praised the virtues of opiates. In the mid-1800's, Chinese immigrants brought opium smoking to this country as they built the American railroads. Opium use and addiction was often too quickly associated with this entire group of immigrants.

> *Papaver somniferum* existed in the ancient civilizations of Persia, Egypt and Mesopotamia. Archaeological evidence suggests that Neanderthal man may have used the opium poppy over thirty thousand years ago. Perhaps the first written reference to *Papaver somniferum* (opium poppies) was in a Sumerian text dated around 4,000 BC. The poppy flower is also known as the plant of joy, and it has been called the Sacred Anchor of Life, the Milk of Paradise, the Hand of God, and the Destroyer of Grief.
>
> Its use had spread from its mid-Eastern origin throughout Europe by 2000 B.C. By the 8th century it was cultivated in India, China, and throughout mid-Asia. Opium poppy flower pods form a lettuce-like base, atop a single tall stalk. The beautiful flowers grace gardens

world-wide. The poppy seeds are commonly used in baking.

Opioids work by sitting on opioid receptors. The major receptors involved in pain transmission are the *mu* (μ) receptors, *delta* (Δ) receptors, and *kappa* (κ) receptors. These different receptors are found in different ratios in different places throughout the body, and they also respond to different medications or opioids.[161] The μ receptor activation primarily results in the analgesia, euphoria, the other common side effects, and is linked to addiction. The κ receptor also produces analgesia, but is associated with dysphoria rather than euphoria.[162] The mesolimbic pathway appears to be the brain circuit that, when stimulated by opiates, is responsible for addictive behaviors.

Re-introducing dopamine – a return visit

Though μ opiate receptors are associated with addiction, there is bit more biochemistry to discuss. The opiates themselves are not the sole cause of the addiction. Opiates themselves cause a dopamine release. Dopamine is the award hormone. It makes us feel good. What is clear is that unnaturally high levels of dopamine – such as from taking cocaine or tobacco – is related to the onset of many addictions. Evidence suggests that opiate addiction is not just to the opiate, but it is also to the lack of 'higher than normal' levels of drug induced dopamine levels. In short, addiction to pain medications may really be an addiction to dopamine.[163] [164] There still may be other and yet unknown biochemical mechanisms that explain addiction. One excellent source of new data is the National Institute on Drug Abuse at www.nida.nih.gov. This information is constantly changing and growing.

Legitimate pain patients rarely report euphoria from opiates. It is as if they respond to the pain reducing aspects of the opiates, but not to dopamine induced euphoria.

> "I've been on these narcotics for years. And so many times when I see a new doc or nurse, they keep staring at me like I live a life of drug highs! If they only knew! And it's a secret between me and my Mom, but I tell her that I'd kinda one day want to know what that euphoria is all about...I never had it.....maybe just a small dose of it every now and then would be a great break from this life...."

The lack of euphoria makes it easier for a legitimate patient to psychologically remove themselves from opiates once the medical need has disappeared. It gets complex if, during the course of narcotic treatment, some psychological problem is also reduced by the sensations caused by the dopamine release. An old expression says pain medications go to the pain and not other places. A healthy person has no other places for the medication to go. But a troubled person may have other places for the medication to go. Perhaps the different responses to the dopamine release reflect the wisdom of the old expression.

Impaired dopamine release is involved in the physiology of depression.[165] Dopamine in a pain patient may be depleted from the prolonged stress of under treated pain, so introducing an opiate may reduce the pain and improve the mood.

> About twenty different medications activate opiate receptors. Why a medication works in one person and not another may be due to tiny molecular differences in the receptor conformations. Medications have to sit like keys in

a lock. Not every key fits every lock. And nature doesn't guarantee that all of us have exactly the same shaped lock, or that our bodies can make the right shaped keys. This may be why a response to a medication varies so much.

In 1914, the Harrison Narcotic Tax Act was passed.[166] But a closer look at the law reveals that only untaxed and unregulated opium and narcotic use was prohibited:

> This bill was not a prohibition law at all. Its official title was "An act to provide for the registration of, with collectors of internal revenue, and to impose a special tax upon all persons who produce, import, manufacture, compound, deal in, dispense, sell, distribute, or give away opium or cocoa leaves, their salts, derivatives, or preparations, and for other purposes." The bill also required those physicians or manufactures of narcotics to pay a small fee in order to be licensed. The Harrison Narcotic Act was merely a law for the orderly marketing of narcotics. It did not stop physicians from prescribing narcotics. The bill did not prohibit narcotics as many thought it would. And it did not rise to the level that many Americans hoped it would insofar as having an ability to rid the country of the 'evils of addiction.'

> The Geneva Opium Convention of 1925 was sponsored by The League of Nations to regulate the growing international drug trade. The Geneva Convention to Limit the Manufacture and Regulate the Distribution of Narcotic Drugs of 1931 placed a limit on every country's ability

to manufacture narcotic drugs. The production had to match international medical needs, and as a result, many opiate factories were closed. However, the act caused drug traffickers to establish their own laboratories within the United States. The Conference for the Suppression of the Illegal Traffic in Dangerous Drugs of 1936 produced a treaty in which member nations agreed to cooperate in stopping narcotics trafficking. Harry Anslinger was the Commissioner of the then new Federal Bureau of Narcotics in the United States, and he pushed through Congress the Marihuana Tax Act of 1937; that made trafficking in marijuana illegal, but it did so by applying a transaction tax.

Morphine's popularity grew in the middle to late 1800's because of its ability to control pain. But many began to use it for euphoria. It found widespread use during the American Civil War, which caused a huge upsurge of addiction in the second half of that century.[167] Of note, and an often unanswered question, is why there was not equal surges of narcotic addiction among soldiers after earlier wars when opium was used for pain. It may also speak to what questions were then being asked about addictions, pain control, how carefully were records kept, was the surge related to the onset of the hypodermic needle for opium administration during the war, were there other variables in how available opium was to soldiers after a war, etc. There are many questions.

A similar conundrum lies on the horizon today. A USA Today article from October 2008[168] reports a rise of monthly narcotic prescriptions to US troops from 30,000 to 50,000 because "doctors rely too heavily on narcotics..." By 2005, two years into the war, narcotics were the most abused drug in the military. Pain is the most common complaint from Iraq and Afghanistan era veterans. In this same piece, Robert Kerns, the National Director for Pain Management in the VA system, reported that about half of the 350,000 veterans suffer chronic pain, and about 30% suffer so badly that it limits their daily living. The VA's problem was highlighted after six suicides and seven drug-related deaths in the Army's special treatment units. The government is making an 'aggressive effort to manage prescriptions drugs.'

These aggressive efforts should also focus on items like post-traumatic stress disorders and the other nasty financial and sociological problems facing these veterans. This could then properly re-assign the narcotic use patterns to multiple etiologies.

Two patterns of morphine use were common at the turn of the last century: (a) physicians used it relatively without fear, and (b) many of the early patent medicine manufacturers, because they were unregulated, caused a burst of narcotic use in Americans; this was especially so in the late 1800's. As a point of interest, the soft drink Coca Cola contained cocaine until 1903. They now use caffeine. (Cocaine is not a narcotic, but is listed here as an example of how freely drug and other vendors added psychoactive substances to their products. These were the sorts of practices that eventually lead to the creation of the Food and Drug Administration in 1906.)

As touched upon above, the introduction of the hypodermic needle in 1853 enlarged the drug abuse problem.

The immediate physiologic effects of injected narcotics is so much greater that the number of subsequent addiction problems rose proportionally. At the same time many patent medication manufacturers hid the ingredients in their products because the atmosphere against morphine would have hurt sales. By 1900, it was estimated that at roughly 250,000 Americans were addicted to narcotics. (The US Census reports the 1900 population at 76,094,000, which calculates to be that 1 in 304 Americans were addicted. Of course we do not know the precision of these numbers, nor which definition of addiction was used.) The problem was shifting from a medical to a large societal concern. Lay reformers then took on two problems: first, they attacked the corporations whose interest in profits ignored the public welfare. They then also attacked issues of the individual's 'immorality' that lead a person to drug addiction. The Southerner's fear of the African-American, and the Westerner's fear of the Chinese, affected the focus and quality of the laws wanted by the anti-drug movement. There was a fear that the Chinese would introduce opium smoking to so many Americans that the American society would be undermined. Many feared that cocaine using people would, because of the drug's effects, cause them to be heedless of their social boundaries, and they would then attack and ruin decent society. Morphine was associated with the underworld and lower classes of people, who in many ways, were also felt to be dangerous to the continuation of American society.

The laws at the turn of the last century (1800 into 1900) "had one great loophole: the patent medicine manufacturers repeatedly obtained exemptions for certain quantities of narcotics in proprietary medicines. These loopholes permitted the narcotized patent medicines to be sold. The public was lulled into believing that the new laws would bring the abuse of narcotics under control. "[169]

For years, the Federal Bureau of Narcotics insisted that all, or substantially all, narcotic addicts were criminals who supported themselves by preying on society. But President Kennedy's 1962 Ad Hoc Panel on Narcotic and Drug Abuse indicated that many addicts are from the middle class, and that indeed many of them are even in the higher socioeconomic classes. They often receive narcotics without detection or apprehension by law enforcement agencies. Only after a 1960 audit of the Federal Bureau of Narcotic's files was the data in those files shown to be contrary to the earlier claim that "all, or substantially all, narcotics addicts are criminals." Indeed, testimony in 1969 before the House Select Committee on Crime disclosed that approximately 30% of all 'drug abusers' are in fact legitimate users who had jobs.

> The history of drug use is a huge and fascinating topic. Only a tiny bit is presented here. Perhaps this quick overview will tantalize the reader into larger study of how and why some of these attitudes came to be. But clearly the use of these very same molecules – abused by addicts but critical to those in chronic pain – compounded and sullied so many of the social and professional attitudes towards the legitimate patients needs, backgrounds and actions, that the residues of those problems still remain.

Other non-narcotic treatment choices and notions

Pain follows tissue injury. The injury often induces inflammation, and so the inflammation has to be controlled. The inflammatory response is actually an immune response, and it can be controlled with aspirin or with steroidal and non-steroidal anti-inflammatory medications.

Acetaminophen, known widely as Tylenol®, reduces pain but does not reduce inflammation. It can augment pain relief when combined with other medications. Percocet® combines oxycodone and acetaminophen. Percodan® combines oxycodone with aspirin. Other opioids are combined with other non-steroidal anti-inflammatory drugs (NSAIDs), such as Vicoprofin®. Steroids, such as cortisol, will rapidly reduce inflammation. Sometimes people will need one of these medications on a chronic basis for such ailments as arthritis, although the long term risks of on-going steroid use needs to be considered.

Inflammation is characterized by redness, swelling, tenderness (hyperalgesia), and pain. There are three phases to inflammation: the acute phase when blood vessels dilate, the delayed subacute phase when white blood cells and phagocyte cells infiltrate the injured area, and the chronic phase in which tissue degeneration and fibrosis occur. An inflammatory response is a natural means to deal with an injury or pathogens (such a bacteria or viruses) in the body. Sometimes the inflammatory response is exaggerated or does not have any survival benefit, as in some arthritic conditions.

NSAIDs, steroids, and aspirin inhibit an inflammatory response. One of the enzymes needed in the inflammatory response is a prostaglandin known as cyclooxygenase. There are two forms of cyclooxygenase, known as COX-1 and COX-2. COX-2 produces inflammation and is not found in the stomach, so the gastric upset common to many NSAIDs and aspirin are not issues. Interestingly, steroids inhibit COX-2, so this may one of the ways cortisol inhibits inflammation. Aspirin, acetaminophen, ibuprofen, naproxen, and indomethacin all inhibit both the COX-1 and COX-2, so the stomach's side effects to these older medications are greater than with the use of new exclusive and selective COX-2 inhibitors. This is why there was such excitement when the COX-2 medications appeared.

Acetaminophen (also known by the initials APAP) lacks many of the side effects of aspirin. APAP will not interfere with blood clotting. It is important to remember that APAP is largely devoid of anti-inflammatory effects. The reason is that APAP inhibits cyclooxygenase mostly in the brain and not in the periphery – that is, it works inside the central nervous system. Excessive APAP use can be toxic to the liver. It was first introduced into medicine around 1886 to reduce fevers. It is the rather safe active metabolite of phenacetin, which was known as the coal tar analgesic. The current convention is that no more than 2000 mg of APAP per day should be used, though just a few years ago higher doses were considered safe. APAP is preferred for those who cannot take aspirin or a NSAID. Liver toxicity must always be kept in mind in cases of chronic or higher dose use. But on the whole it is a safe analgesic when properly used. Two famous APAP combinations are Tylenol #3®, which is 500 mg of APAP and 30 mg of codeine, and Percocet®, which is oxycodone 5 mg and 325 mg of APAP. Preparations exist with other ratios of opiates to APAP.

Aspirin comes from the bark of the willow tree. The active ingredient is salicin, from which the name salicylates evolved. In 1875, a chemist named Hoffman, who worked for a company named Bayer, prepared a formulation that was eventually introduced to medicine in 1899 under the name aspirin. Aspirin is actually the original brand name for acetylsalicylic acid. It wasn't until 1971 that aspirin was found to inhibit the production of prostaglandins. Interestingly, aspirin's popularity declined after the introduction of APAP in 1956 and ibuprofen in 1962. Long term aspirin use does not result in tolerance. Its use is primarily for fevers (antipyresis) and pain control. It also blocks platelets from clotting, and which is why many people take the 71 mg, low dose formulations. The history of aspirin is quite interesting.

Elemental gold has been used for many years to treat itching pain. Currently it is used to treat rheumatoid arthritis for those who fail to respond to other treatments. Gold does not have anti-inflammatory effects, but may impair the maturation of the cells which cause the immune response and inflammation.

Ibuprofen, with common names such as Motrin® or Advil® are also NSAIDs. Naproxen® (Naprosyn) is in the same group of medication. All NSAID's are arylpropionic acid derivatives that inhibit cyclooxygenase (COX-2). It is usually impossible to tell in advance which of the NSAIDs will work best for any one person. Choosing one these medications is usually a function of weighing the possible side effects (such as gastric effects) and price. Rofecoxib (Vioxx®), introduced in 1999, and celecoxib (Celebrex®), introduced in 1998, are selective COX-2 inhibitors. Rofecoxib does not interfere with blood clotting, which gives it a somewhat broader use potential. Interestingly it was first approved for osteoarthritis, acute pain and dysmenorrhea. Initially there were concerns about its safety insofar as the cardiac system and aspirin hypersensitivity were concerned. Celecoxib has a similar side effect profile to refecoxib. The data regarding these medications, as effective as they are, is a developing story, so using them requires the most recent safety data available at the time that the prescription is being considered. The COX-2 inhibitors, except for celecoxib (Celebrex®) were withdrawn from the markets because of a risk of heart attacks and stroke. Celebrex® is still used but with more caution.

Diclofenac has been available in an oral form for years. It is now available as a patch (Flector Patch®)[170] or a gel (Voltaren Gel ®).[171] Like the lidocaine patch (Lidoderm®), these formulations provide alternative methods of medication delivery. Using creams, ointments, patches, or sprays to control pain is known as topical analgesia.

An injury to a nerve requires that the nerve itself needs to be quieted. Over-firing nerves issue pain signals. By and large, nerves cannot be quieted with opioids or NSAIDs. The NSAIDs will help if the nerve is inflamed. Anticonvulsants are used to settle down the nerves. Pregabalin (Lyrica®) is indicated for fibromyalgia, diabetic peripheral neuropathy, postherpetic neuralgia, and adult partial onset seizures. Lamotrigine (Lamictal®), valproic acid (Depakote®), carbamazepine (Tegretol®) and others can slow down a nerve's firing rate and the sensitivity to being stimulated. These medications work basically on the neurons themselves and not directly on the neurotransmitters in the synapse, although the release of neurotransmitters may be effected because of changes in the neuron's behavior. Injured nerves are the basis of neuropathic pain. ('Neuro' meaning nerve, 'pathic' meaning illness, so it is an illness in the nerve.) Neuropathic pain is defined by the International Association for the Study of Pain as "pain initiated or caused by a primary lesion or dysfunction in the nervous system."[172] These pain signals come from within the nervous system itself and without the usual stimulation from a peripheral pain sensing nerve ending. Neuropathy can be hard to treat.

Recently duloxetine (Cymbalta®) was approved for use in certain types of pain, including fibromyalgia, though many other antidepressants have been used in similar manners for years. The fact that the anticonvulsant Lyrica® and the antidepressant Cymbalta® both work in fibromyalgia opens a huge territory of study about why two different medications both work on the same condition. Are these two medications somehow more similar than not? Or might there be different forms of fibromyalgia, etc. ?

Another source of pain is muscle spasticity. In these situations antispasmodic medications are indicated. These work by blocking the feedback mechanisms which instruct the muscle to tighten up. The classic anti-spasmodic is diazepam (Valium®). Clonazepam (Klonopin®) is another effective benzodiazepine antispasmodic. Metaxalone (Skelaxin®), baclofen (Lioresal®) are other antispasmodics. Other medications also work if they help to relax the muscle.

It is interesting that riluzole (Rilutek®) helps to control the spasticity, and it also extends the survival or time to tracheostomy in amyotrophic lateral sclerosis (Lou Gehrig's Disease). It does this is by inhibiting glutamate release and blocking NMDA receptors.

Clonidine is an alpha-adrenergic receptor and can block the transmission of pain signals to the brain. It is used with epidural opioids to enhance relief not obtained by opioids alone. It is useful in only certain parts of the body, it does not compete with opioids, and it is thought to mimic the action of norepinephrine in the dorsal horn of the spinal cord. This is an excellent use of an older medication that takes advantage of new knowledge of how pain messages are transmitted.[173] Clonidine is sometimes used for opiate detoxification. Lofexidine is quite similar to clonidine, and may expose the patients to fewer side effects.

There is concern that morphine reduces immune system function.[174] Morphine has been called immunosuppressive in that it can inhibit cellular and humoral activity. Yet it has been suggested that endogenous morphine helps keep the immune system in check. Lowering immune system activity may increase the chance of infection. Addicts using non-sterile needles clearly increase their vulnerability for infections, but it may be more from the concentrated force of an injected infection than from a weakened immune system. Recently the National Institute on Drug Abuse pinpointed the trigger that sets off the inhibition of the immune response:[175] Morphine suppresses the activity of three white cells: the T lymphocytes, the B lymphocytes, and the natural killer cells (NK cells). The NK cells are a natural force against viral infections and cancer. So dirty needles plus morphine induced changes raise the risk.

Of course, using morphine is a matter of weighing the risk to the benefits of its use. Certainly most people who use opiates do not suffer from infections. Immunologically healthy people do just fine, and have a better life because of the opiates.

> When considering morphine use, one is compelled to look at its potential for improper use, which raises problems for the legitimate pain patient. A fivefold increase in the number of prescriptions which allegedly were for nonmedical purposes has been reported.[176] Part of the evidence comes from the Drug Abuse Warning Network (DAWN) which showed an increase of oxycodone related emergency room visits from 1996 through 2000 of 239%.[177] Smaller but significant rises exist for other medications as well. "One area of concern highlighted by the survey was the growing role of misuse of prescription drugs. For example, nonmedical use of prescription drugs among young adults increased from 5.4 percent in 2002 to 6.4 percent in 2006, largely due to an increase in the nonmedical use of pain relievers." [178] The role of the biochemical manipulations in this non-legitimate use group is aimed more at the brain code than at the neuron code. But the other aspect of this problem lies in the nature of the patient-doctor relationships, how the doctor controls the treatment, etc. It is so important to keep in mind that these abuse/mis-use

problems occur when the use of these treatments are improper. No one really counts the frequency of proper use.

It also speaks to the size of, and attraction to, drug misuse in the community.

Opiates will continue to play a major role in the treatment of pain. But many other medications, plus new interventional or surgical techniques, are keys parts of the overall armamentarium. One part of any clinicians' armamentarium must be methods to limit medication use only to the groups of people who properly need and use them.

Ziconotide (Prialt®) – A new tool for pain treatment

Ziconotide is indicated for severe chronic pain in patients who are refractory or intolerant to other treatments. A study suggested that it can reduce pain in patients whose pain is no longer controlled by opiates. The medication interferes with a complex biochemical process known as calcium channel blockade. This mechanism is essential for the nervous system to transmit a painful event. Blocking the calcium channels decreases the release of neurotransmitters important to pain perception. Ziconotide is a synthetic peptide based on a snail toxin, the *Conus Magus*. Currently, ziconotide can only be administered with a pump that delivers it directly into the spinal cord. Ziconotide differs from opiates in other, but equally complex ways. It does not involve a system known as the G-protein (which plays a role in opioid tolerance), and it does not interact with opioid receptors. So it works on a different mechanism that reduces pain using non-opiate pathways. However, it is like opiates in that both medications reduce the influx of calcium into the cells, which makes it harder for the cells to fire, and which in turn reduces the pain signal.[179] This medication opens fascinating areas for research to explore.

Psychiatric side effects have been reported with ziconotide use, including confusion. It should not be used with patients with a history of psychosis. This medication allows for pain relief using different biological mechanisms, but choosing to use it requires a careful consideration that may well be worth the effort.

Gene therapy for pain

Investigators are using the herpes simplex virus to deliver a gene that makes enkephalin (an opioid) in the pain transmitting sites in the spinal cord.[180][181] One challenge is getting the gene only to needed areas in the body. If this proves to be safe and effective, then another intriguing means of treating chronic pain will exist.

Pain Pathways

The physical layout of the nervous system is known as neuroanatomy. It is complicated. It is hard to visualize the systems. But it is an incredible arrangement.

Pain signals travel via the peripheral nerves to the dorsal (dorsal means back) horn of the spinal cord, where there they are modified before being sent up to the brain. Once in the brain, they travel to different areas. Some signals go to the thalamus, which then projects the signal (that it, it sends the signal) to the primary and secondary somatosensory cortices. The thalamus is the primary relay station for sensory signals. Some of the signals are also sent to the limbic system, which is important in the emotional aspects of pain.

A part of the brain known as the *insula cortex* is important to the experience of pain. It is thought that this cortex associates the physical (visceral) states with the emotional experience. The unraveling of the interplay between the emotional and the physical aspects of pain is an exciting and ever changing area.

The combined spinal cord and brain is known as the central nervous system (often referred to as the CNS). All other nerves, outside of the central nervous system, are known as the peripheral nervous systems, or the PNS. The peripheral systems bring information to the central nervous system where the data is evaluated, recognized, and acted upon.

Nerves fibers are classified (a) by size, location and function, and (b) whether or not they are wrapped in a substance called myelin. Myelin is basically an insulator. Some nerves are myelinated and some are not.

Delta fibers are small, thinly myelinated nerve fibers that transmit sharp or prickling sensations from the mucous membranes and skin. In contrast, the type C fibers, as noted below, are small unmyelinated fibers that transmit pain messages from the body's inner organs (often called the viscera), and from other tissues.

Type A Delta fibers transmit information at speeds that range from 6 to 30 meters a second. This is very fast. The slowest delta fibers can carry a message from toe to head in about one-half second. These fibers give the prickling type of sensation. People usually say "ouch" to delta fibers.

Type C fibers are slower. They carry messages at velocities between 0.5 and 2 meters per second. These fibers give the burning, aching, deeper pain sensations. People 'moan and groan' from Type C fibers. A fast, prickling pain will often be followed by a slower, burning pain. The rapid pain is a signal of 'quick' damage, which often goes away. But the slower, duller, burning pain can become more painful over time, and it can become the basis of much severe chronic pain. Blocking C fibers removes the burning and aching types of pain.

A very important point to understand about pain transmission is that messages conveyed by delta and C fibers can be dampened if nearby, and larger, sensory (i.e., touch, vibration or temperature) nerves are stimulated. This is why people rub the site over or near the injury! It is a natural way towards some pain relief. It is as if the stimulation of the surrounding sensory fibers acts as a gate through which the pain messages are reduced or cannot pass. This is known as the gate theory,[182][183] and it is the rational for the TENS unit (transcutaneous electrical nerve stimulation). Specifically, a TENS unit stimulates fibers in the larger sensory nerves, which, in turn, inhibits pain transmission. It is widely used, but questions exist about its range of effectiveness. [184]

Blocking a transmission – also known as a 'nerve block' - works by injecting alcohol or a medication directly onto the particular nerve that is transmitting the pain. The problem with this method is one of specificity, or, in other words, how precisely the injection can be placed. If the doctor's aim is perfect, then a very specific area could be blocked and few side effects would occur. But sometimes blocking one nerve segment will unavoidably or accidentally block another nerve as well. It is the 'what else might be blocked' question that determines the 'if, how, where, and when' of nerve blocks. Nerve blocks usually need to be done as a series, and sometimes the series need to be periodically repeated. Experienced clinicians can be very accurate with the placement of nerve blocks.

If a nerve is permanently blocked, then the procedure is called a rhizotomy. Rhizotomies can be done mechanically (by cutting or scaring), with chemicals, or with radio waves. The last two procedures may also be referred to as neurolysis. Sometimes a chemical or radio wave block will require repeated treatments.

Once a peripheral nerve brings the pain message into the spinal cord, the message is transmitted via a hormone called Substance P. However, at the same time the nervous system may try to offset the intensity of the message by using another hormone called serotonin.

Pain signals pass to the brain primarily via the lateral spinothalamic tract. It is important to understand that the spinal cord carries messages about the right side of the body in the left side of the spinal cord. So events in the left leg are transmitted by the right spinothalamic tract. Spinal tract names indicate where tracts start and end. For example, the 'spinothalamic' tract starts in the spine and ends in the thalamus.

Given the name of a spinothalamic tract, it is not surprising that the thalamus has a role in pain perception. If the thalamus is damaged, perhaps from a stroke or tumor, then thalamic pain might develop. This is when horrible pain is felt without a peripheral source. The concept is of a damaged computer chip which is sending false, but still painful, signals. This is known as phantom pain.

In some severe pain cases, a part of the spinal cord will be cut so pain signals are stopped. This is a cordotomy. It is like cutting a wire. However, more than just the area of pain may be affected, and the person may lose sensation or motor functions below the level of the cut. The choice to do this intervention demands a very through consideration by the patient and the doctors. Increasingly sophisticated surgical techniques make it easier to cut only the needed nerves.

Dorsal column stimulators place electrodes directly into the dorsal (back) side of the spinal column. It is the equivalent in many ways to the TENS unit. It is effective for about 50% of the patients. It is interesting, and it therefore shows the intricate interplay between hormones and pain, that pain relief from dorsal column stimulator can be reversed with naloxone. (Naloxone [Narcan®] is a drug which reverses the activity of opiates.)

Brain Volume and Pain

Data is accumulating that chronic pain may change the brain matter volume, suggesting that the pain, as a disease, may change the brain morphology (i.e., the form and structure of the brain itself) in chronic pain patients. These fascinating and important findings remain preliminary, though they emphasize the speed at which initial pain management interventions should occur to prevent such structural changes. Some recent findings are that older adults with chronic low back pain have structural changes in the corpus callosum as well as within the gray and white matter.[185] One study speculates that gray matter density might increase in young patients with chronic vulvar pain over shorter periods of time of being in pain, but the volume may decrease in older women with longer periods of standing disease.[186] A study of brain changes in people with a chronic complex regional pain syndrome found regions of atrophy and a reorganization of white matter connections; these areas also encompass the emotional and pain perception regions, which suggests a strong interconnectiveness.[187] The complexity is considerable, but the theme of this evolving area of medicine is fascinating and hopeful because in all of this, new treatments may be found.

A 2004 report that compared the brain morphology of 26 chronic back 'pain to non-pain' control patients (a control group is the comparison group), found that those with chronic pain showed 5-11% less grey matter volume than the control subjects. "The magnitude of this decrease is equivalent to the gray matter volume lost in 10-20 years of normal aging." [188]

Interestingly, if alternations of neuronal connections occur in pain syndromes, then a 2003 study by Flor becomes very interesting.[189] He notes that physical change (known in medicine as plasticity) in the somatosensory cortex is possible, which is contrary to early thinking that such plasticity was modifiable *only during early life experiences*. In other words, the nervous system can physically change even after we are grown up. This helps understand the effects of chronic pain. In patients 'with chronic low back pain and fibromyalgia,' the amount of reorganization of the brain increases with the length of time of being in pain. (This is referred to as the pain's chronicity.) "In phantom pain and other neuropathic pain syndromes, cortical reorganization is correlated with the amount of pain." The suggestion is that the negative (negative now meaning unwanted) plasticity induced by the pain can be modified by behavioral interventions or with medications that prevent or reverse maladaptive memory. This intriguing area needs careful study. Once again, this speaks to the importance of rapidly getting adequate pain relief.

Acupuncture

Acupuncture may be better than placebo in chronic neck[190] and back pain.[191] How acupuncture provides lasting relief is unknown. Studies suggest that acupuncture treatment enhances the resting *default mode network* (DMN) within different brain areas. The theory is that these changes alter the 'memory or perception' of the pain. But no conclusive understanding of its mechanism yet exists.

Acupuncture is the practice of piercing specific areas of the body with fine needles. These points are known as acupoints, and they are along the peripheral nerves. This process can reduce pain or even induce anesthesia. Acupoints can also be stimulated with electricity or lasers. Korean hand acupuncture assumes the hand represents the entire body, so stimulation of different areas on the hand will cause effects elsewhere on the body. Traditional Chinese acupuncture uses manual manipulation of the needles. Modern acupuncturists may choose to use electrical stimulation.

* * *

Anatomy, politics, sociology, and chemistry blend in the most complex ways when we have pain. These interactions are not fully understood. A patient who fails to respond to ordinary treatment often means that the 'science' of medicine needs to marry the 'art' of medicine in order to reduce the product of pain, which is suffering.

...*Thought*...

> "Hey doc, stick with me. Let me get this right.... you say my own body makes morphine just like the poppy plant?"
>
> "Yep."
>
> "Okay, so maybe you make more than me. And so when you hurt, you got more morphine in you to start with, so you may need fewer pills? Is that logical so far?"
>
> "Yep."
>
> "And no one measures the blood for that, what do you call it, endogenous morphine."
>
> "Yep."
>
> "So we may be on to something here. Maybe someday this whole concept will explain why I need more medication than others. Or maybe it will explain why some people are so much calmer than others. It's really interesting, isn't it? Maybe it'll give us a whole new set of eyeglasses to use when we look at pain folks."
>
> "Yep."

CHAPTER FIFTEEN
I had a friend who got better

"We went through three years of pain together. We met in a doctor's office. Different accidents but equal pain. Only now he is better and I am not.

I shouldn't be jealous. Any maybe I'm not. I love him, and he loves me. But the love is from the war we fought together; we were partners in adversity. Only he escaped and I'm detained.

I can't measure the joy there is in me as I watch him walk away from pain. But I also have sorrow and grief. I'm scared to think that my joy is not as deep as I would like it to be because his joy may be a return to my loneliness. I'm afraid of my own selfishness.

We used to make love, holding our limbs up, or cushioning my back with pillows, so some little normal joy and intimacy wouldn't be gashed open by pain. We laughed at our acrobatics, and giggled when it hurt too much to have an orgasm. Our joy was in the sharing and in trying. We laughed when it didn't work! Funny how God didn't fix the pain but He was in bed with us.

He doesn't need pillows anymore. Will he soon not need me too? Friendship and love should be all we need. My heart is happy and pleased but I am not relieved. I'm scared."

CHAPTER SIXTEEN
Doctor shopping: it looks like an addict, but it's just looking for help

A patient told me this story:

"Oh, I know there's going to be flack over this! Are you sure you want me to say this? Are you sure you won't kick me out? I hope not.

There are two reasons why I use two doctors. One is the simplest and most obvious reason: I need to guarantee a predictable supply of medications. Several years ago my regular doctor, basically a good guy, went on vacation and the guy covering him would not renew my pain medications. That's before I got to know my doctor's away times. The covering doctor said he didn't know me well enough to give so much medication. I had to then find my regular doc in California and make arrangements for him to call my local drug store. I also learned to manage my inventory better.

It took a long time to find my two current docs. I must have interviewed or tried out dozens.

The second reason I need two docs is because it is nice to know that two doctors believe me. And these aren't walk-in clinic guys!

I'm like General Motors who needs to have two reliable supply sources. An Army quartermaster would understand perfectly.

I know how some people will look at this. They think I am double-dipping. That maybe I'm taking twice the amount of medication, or something like that. NO! My use of medications is consistent. Look closely at the prescriptions I've filled and you can be relieved—there's no hanky panky at all. My dose is 100% consistent and unchanging.

Neither doctor knows about the other. Reason? I'm not that sure I can trust them to understand why I need the 'secret' backup systems. It's like a hidden bank account or extra food in a closet for times after a bad snow storm. I get a regular supply from one doc, and a bit of an extra from the other. The first doc won't go above a set upper limit. I really need only about 10-15% more for my life to be really good. I pay for the second, smaller scripts myself. But I have the meds supply that make me work better. I just wish my primary doc would give me that little bit more, and then the second doctor would be really for back up only. I so want one doctor to do it all.

My dishonesty gives me great peace of mind and nervousness at the same time. Yet it's such a shame. I mean really, isn't that a shame! Damn, look what pain and the system makes me do. And you know what, I can't really recommend that others do as I do, but I think a lot of pain patients will understand my reasoning."

Finding the right doctor is a difficult, expensive, and time consuming task. This is hard because doctors may be afraid to treat a chronic pain patient, or they limit the range of their treatments too much (i.e., they under treat), or they won't accept insurance assignment as payment and so they are too expensive for many patients, or they fear being drawn into litigation in injury or malpractice cases, or they don't know how to treat the complexity of some patients, or they don't want relationships with patients who chronically suffer in such a massive, endless, and emotionally draining way.

Patients often feel embarrassed admitting how many doctors they've used. But in their embarrassment is an anger that comes from how hard it is find the right or best doctor. Many times the notion of the best doctor is abandoned in favor of the 'affordable' doctor. This process raises the question of if any long term relationship with a single doctor can ever be developed. Are the doctor-patient bonds too transient or too shaky?

Other concepts apply to the world of the chronically-in-pain:

> **Jiggery-pokery** is a wonderful old term referring to a dishonest or underhanded manipulation of a situation to make it work the way one wants it to work. It comes from the sense of dodging and moving away from the truth in a sly, shrewd, or artful way. Many traditionally motivated doctor shoppers are assumed to be masters of jiggery-pokery.
>
> **Velleity** is another word which can apply to this topic. It means to say one will do something, but in fact the intent is to do the opposite. Many pain management programs work on the assumption that pain patients will say whatever is needed to get the prescription, but they have

no intention of actually following through with a treatment plan. Many patients feel doctors do the same thing. They promise a strong defense against the pain, but in fact they don't follow though – they do what they can just to engage the person into becoming a paying patient.

Doctor shoppers are often considered addicts. This is not necessarily so. Let's take a look. In 1998, Albert Ellis wrote:

> "Other addict's, such as some gamblers and potheads, seem to be mainly neurotic, and have abysmally low frustration tolerance. Because they like some substance or activity very much, they childishly insist that they absolutely must indulge in it, even when they 'know' how harmful – to themselves and their loved ones – this indulgence is. Addiction, then, comes in many shapes and sizes, and has multiple 'causes,' several of which tend to overlap and interact with each other...." [192]

Ellis further asks what drives addicts to their "almost certain destruction." He believes many of "these inveterate addicts" have severe personality disorders. He believes people with personality disorders are more prone to addiction.

He did, however, make the point that a pain patient looking for relief is not the same as a typical 'addict.' Indeed, there is a real discomfort in applying the word 'addict' to this pain-relief seeking group. The pain patient wants to stop the destruction of their lives. They are 'addicted' – if we use the word to mean 'attached' – to an end product which will undo the decline in their lives, will let them return to work, enable them re-join friends and family, and un-do the feelings of worthlessness and hopelessness. To do this often requires looking for the right medical mechanic who understands and practices according to the patient's reality. So like any good consumer, one has to go shopping for the best fit, the best product, and the best buy.

What results from doctor shopping? New doctors are less likely to go out of their way for a patient if they suspect that the patient will be with them for only a short period of time. It is important to allow time for a doctor-patient relationship to deepen. The better one gets to know a patient, the greater will be the comfort in taking risks for the patient. This is because the 'logic of the risk' is substantiated by the documented history leading up to it. Too many doctors become alarmed that a relatively new, insistent patient might actually be a dreadfully clever person who is inappropriately seeking only medications. Only when the patient knows the doctor and the doctor knows the patient will both feel safer with each other.

> "I am a physician who will be more aggressive in pain management treatment. I try to get to know my patients, and most of the time the effort pays off. Sure, I'm occasionally been lied to by a few – and the key word here is 'few' – patients. But when there is anything that breaks the trust, like them changing a prescription, I have to cease treating them. I know they live in a funny and precarious world, much of which is forced upon them by my profession, but I have no choice. It gets to be so full of difficult ethical decisions at times. I tell patients to value and think carefully about the trust with any doctor

they use. I also tell my physician colleagues about the same trust needs they have to offer to their patients."

Bates observes that:

"Because many Anglo Americans have accepted the legitimacy and effectiveness of biomedicine, if such treatment proved ineffective, members of this group often become extremely angry at individual providers when they were unable to effectively repair the body and free it of pain. However, this anger did not for the most part lead to abandoning biomedicine in general, but rather to continuing the quest for the one biomedical physician who would finally find and fix the mechanical problems the patient believed must be causing his or her pain." [193]

Patients often change doctors with hope of getting relief. For example:

"Wow, I can't wait to see the new neurologist in town, I hear he's great.... maybe he can fix me"

However, one might just as easily hear this:

"Hell, I've seen them all, and nothing new has yet come from any of them..."

Patients who have seen many doctors – with little therapeutic success – may present themselves to a new doctor in a suspicious, oddly subdued, or doubting fashion.

That does little to foster a good relationship with the new doctor. Patients tire of re-telling their stories. This especially comes across if telling the history contains hints or doubts that the new doctor may not be able to any more than all those who have failed before. Patients grow tired of empty promises and of doctors who have nothing new to give.

> "The new doc and I spoke and spoke. Then he said he could offer me nothing. I still had to pay the bill. Yeah, he did spend time, I know, and maybe I'm too cold about all this now, but I don't need to pay to be told what I already know."

Most doctor shopping has a spin-off: honest patients become quite self-educated about the full scope of their own problems. They need to do this as they face the need to explain themselves. Real patients know their histories and conditions and can enter real dialogues. Addicts looking just for pain meds tend not to know their conditions and avoid dialogues. These are key differences.

> "I finally found a great doctor. He can't fix the pain, but he understands my plight. And he actually knew about the implant that's in me. We even talked about some pain management legislation in Congress. I'll stick with him. Maybe he'll help me find a surgeon who can fix my hip."

Occasionally doctors force a patient into awful emotional states. These may be triggered by a legitimate concern in the doctor about a patient's treatment needs. The patient must take it upon themselves to take an honest (and occasionally agonizing) look at their contribution to the tensions in the doctor-patient relationship. An example is if a doctor sees that a patient is not addressing important issues that are part of the pain treatment plan.

> "(Pain behaviors are) misdirected activities that are superficially linked to pain, but are often unconsciously directed at ends other than pain relief. Such activities include exaggerating symptoms to get narcotics to which the patient is addicted, doctor shopping because of a phobia of cancer or the AIDS, remaining disabled to retain a spouse's attention, or malingering to get compensation." [194]

Hyman's entire article, from which this above quote is taken, is interesting because this quote is actually the fifth paragraph in the article about pain. There are some troubling allegations in that comment. The patient and the doctor need to mutually resolve itchy 'hunches' about each other before the 'hunches' are given the status of fact.

Another subtle suggestion is made in the Hyman article.

> "When pain does not respond to treatment of the presumed injury or illness, it may lead to chronic disability, fear, and depression. As successive diagnostic tests fail to reveal an adequate pathophysiologic explanation for the severity of the pain, mounting frustration on the part of the physician and desperation on the part of the patient can lead to a premature end to their cooperation."

The question is therefore asked: who is actually ending the cooperation? Is the doctor no longer cooperating in efforts to control the pain? Or is the patient is no longer cooperating because the doctor is saying "hey, I can't find anything wrong, and therefore I can't treat you anymore." Will this force the patient to look for another doctor? Subtle innuendos are made very early in the article to "be careful with pain patients. They can be difficult; they might deceive and not be honest with their motivations". This tenor is chilling. The dilemma is that while this concern can be correct some of the time, those few times should not be over generalized into a sticky set of inaccurate labels.

Boodman wrote an article in 2008 saying how an alliance with a doctor is not an easy one. She spoke of her own illness: "I tried being the good patient. Becoming difficult," which she called empowered, was her "natural reaction to doctors who were 'incompetent, rude or domineering.' This is a careful dance for patients. You can't make doctors too angry, because you need them." The article also quotes Robert Arnold at the University of Pittsburg: "My worry is that it locates all the problems with the patient, when the question for the doctors is why the relationship is not going well...A lot of doctors, including me, have a problem with control." The article goes on to quote Nathaniel Beers from the American Academy of Pediatrics that "patients who seem difficult may just really be advocating for high quality care for themselves or a relative." The article also copies a statement by Tony Miksanek, a family doctor, who says the worst thing a doctor can do is to terminate the relationship by saying "there is nothing more I can do for you."[195]

This same theme appeared in the New York *Times*. Friedman said "when all else fails, blaming the patient often comes next." He notes that "chronically ill, treatment resistant patients can challenge the confidence of therapists themselves, who may be reluctant to question their treatment; it's easier – and less painful – to view the patient as intentionally or unconsciously resistant." He further writes "To be sure, some patients really do want to be sick....but a vast majority of patients want to feel better, and for them the burden of illness is painful enough. Let's keep the blame on the disease, not the patient." [196]

This skirmish often swells out of the clout of the first impression: tell someone that a patient is nice, honest, and good, and he'll be treated as such. Tell someone that a patient is designing, dishonest, and insincere, and he will be so treated. This identical problem warranted a 1992 article in the Reader's Digest. Pekkanen talked of people whose illnesses initially eluded an accurate diagnosis by many doctors.[197] The first story noted "After routine tests, a physician told her that her problems were all in her head." Ultimately she was properly diagnosed and treated, but there was such a great "anger towards the physicians who dealt with her so off-handedly."

It's so simple in so many ways: People who know something is wrong with them are simply going from doctor to doctor in search of an answer.

> Believe nothing, no matter where you read it, or who said it, even if I have said it, unless it agrees with your own reason and your own common sense. *Gautama Buddha*

CHAPTER SEVENTEEN
Under-treatment and mistreatment

Many treatment teams either insufficiently or improperly treat pain. Too often patients report that doctors treat according to what the doctors expect the pain to be, and not what it actually is. Physicians often dole out too limited a supply of medications because they doubt or underestimate what are the patient's real needs, or they are concerned about a patient's inability to properly self-regulate their own narcotic use.

Many honest pain patients get washed into the group of dishonest pain patients. Perhaps the exploding number of pain clinics reflects the extent to which honest pain is not being treated. But perhaps this same explosion of pain clinics reflects the degree of substance abuse in our communities. As with so many things in life, the truth lies somewhere in the middle.

> A comment in a 2008 text on psychiatric medicine reads: "Greater than half of all the patients do NOT receive adequate pain control." [198]

One widespread question is what to do for the pain from the time it starts until the real cause is found. Will blocking the pain will make it harder to find its origin? Some medical rationale exists to this: after all, a surgeon will need to see where it hurts when he pushes on the belly. But what happens during the search time period between pain onset and some 'fixing intervention' is a epoch full of horror stories. Weeks may pass before there is an appointment with a specialist. Should the patient be denied treatment with medications during the waiting period? The same logic applies to the period after the deciding the evaluation and the start of treatment. "The pain is real bad, but I gotta wait 3 weeks until the surgery. What do I do in the mean time? If I can't take a pain med because it'll not mix with the other meds I need, than I can kinda understand. But if I'm not on other meds, well, doc, what ya goina do 'bout the pain while I wait?"

> "I hurt my toe on Saturday. The emergency room doctor suggested I see an orthopedist as soon as possible. The earliest appointment was in five days, on Wednesday. The toe hurt a great deal, so I followed the emergency room doctor's suggestions and took the Percocet through Tuesday night. Believe me, it was hurtin' plenty by Wednesday morning, and I had no trouble wincing when the doc touched the trouble spot.
>
> He wanted to do some surgery, which was okay, but it couldn't be done until Friday. So I asked him for a few more Percocet and I promised to stop them Thursday night. He said no! I don't see why he did that because he knew what problem I had, and that I would merely be taking them to make the waiting less arduous. He seemed annoyed by my pain medication requests. I thought it a might archaic and felt like he was making me spend the night in the arctic cold—old fashioned, untrusting and nearly a punishment. Later I heard another orthopedic doc had no problem giving out small supplies of meds while people waited for surgery. Isn't there some standard here that applies to all doctors?"

Fortunately, if a treatment plan exists, and the doctor knows his patient, then more and more doctors are comfortable treating this type of time-limited pain. But of course, this plan has an outcome that hopefully will remove the need for continuing pain medication use.

It can never be forgotten that the medical environment has become so litigious that doctors fear being sued or of being pulled into a regulatory challenges. Patients may forget how this often under-recognized, but tremendous problem, colors the way many doctors approach their patients. This is even true with the most honest cases if there is some unusual aspect to the clinical situation. Patients may suffer as a result of these external influences. Tort and legal reforms have reduced some of the concerns. But these demons and fears remain.

Different 'sets of attitudes' towards treatment exist. Hippocratic medicine says that medicine should not 'treat those who are overmastered by their diseases, realizing that in such cases medicine is powerless."[199] Disease alters the natural state of health, so medicine must focus primarily on the 'fixable' changes that take us 'away from health.' Therefore, the traditional doctor, who strictly follows this thinking, accepts the fact that medicine should not be used if a disease is incurable. Offering treatment to incurable conditions has, as a result, been called madness and ignorance, as if the doctor was foolish to even attempt to reverse the illness. This, of course, leaves the patient to suffer. This can be circumvented if the suffering itself is considered to be a disease. Much of modern medicine has moved away from this way of thinking.

Plato added to this philosophy. Plato says "medicine (is) for those who were healthy in their nature...but were suffering from a specific disease. (But) for those, however, whose bodies were always in a state of inner sickness, he (the doctor) did not attempt to prescribe a regimen or to make their life a prolonged misery. Medicine was not intended for them and they should not be treated" [200] The 'slip' in Plato's comments is his reference to a 'specific disease.' This can mean that once something is understood it becomes specific and will then warrant a treatment. But the 'not understood' conditions too easily fall into the classes of 'non-diseases' that are not (yet) legitimate, and so they do not (yet) warrant treatment. As above, if suffering is considered a disease, then treatment should follow.

History records countless situations before specific diseases were understood. Countless stories exist of overpowering medical conditions for which all medicine was powerless. People suffered until science or attitudes changed. The more enlightened and munificent doctors tried to use whatever existed as a means to reduce the pain, suffering and misery.

> "I'm guess I'm waiting for science to catch up to my disease."

A spin off these philosophical incantations was that it was once wrong to treat the unknown. Greek physicians thought of medicine as a *techne,* which means 'doing'. In order to do something, one has to be limited to the realistic boundaries of the act. Doctors were expected to act only within the natural limits of their treatments—for example, they might be able to set a broken bone but could not treat a skin cancer. Even trying to treat skin cancer was 'foolishness' and outside of the accepted technique. To try to treat outside of the usual technique was considered an error, a *hubris,* which was scoffed at by Greek doctors as a sin of excessive confidence. Interestingly, this approach gave doctors a broad type of permission to walk away from patients suffering from certain unexplainable conditions. As it turned out, we now know that some conditions once considered as inexplicable now have very explicable medical explanations.

Trephination, as an ancient surgical opening of the skull performed with primitive tools and techniques, is one of the most fascinating surgical practices in human history. Some people still believe in it. It probably started at least 7000 years ago, and is still performed in parts of Africa, South America, and Melanesia. Evidence of its use has been found in many other parts of the world. *Trepanation*, derived from Greek, means an auger or borer, or to make an opening with a circular saw of any type.

The motives for trephination are unknown, but the speculation is that it was performed to allow for spirits to escape or enter the head. It was done for therapeutic reasons, such as for headaches, fractures, infections, insanity, convulsions, or for religious reasons. It has also been suggested that the motive was to make charms, amulets, or talismans from the disks of bone obtained from the cutting of circular holes in the skulls.

Another old fear was that some diseases were actually the products of witchcraft, possessions, moral weaknesses, and so on. Treatment of these had to be careful so not to give these conditions the status of a 'real disease.' It was a time when non-medical political-like pressures tried to define the origin of a disease. It might have been blasphemy to say someone was, in truth, not possessed, but that they actually had a seizure disorder. The trend was to convert the explanation in ways that that the seizures became the products of witchcraft. So, choosing to treat one of these disorders was viewed as an effort to convert the peccadillo into a real disease that was not anchored in alleged moral or ethical improprieties.

Hippocratic doctors are not supposed to work against, or in defiance, of nature. Doctors have the task of restoring to normal the imbalance of natural elements in the body. Therefore, a Hippocratic doctor might not put a patient on a respirator, start tube feedings, prescribe insulin or cardiac medications, insert a dorsal stimulator or cardiac pacemaker, or use chronic pain medications if these therapies were seen as an effort that would not restore the natural balance in the body. Doctors did not try to bend nature into their patient's needs. Doctors were the servants of nature. It was from within these prospects of how much of a balance could be restored that the decision to treat or not emerged. These definitions were often ambiguous at best. What should a doctor do if the normal course of nature is to let a patient die? It also raises the question of what part of a disease is to be treated. Maybe treating a cold is permissible because we expect colds to resolve, but treating a nasty cancer is not acceptable because the normal course of it will be death. Yet treating arthritis itself may be impossible, but the product of the arthritis, that is, the pain, is part of the disease process and therefore it should be treated. As medicine progresses, so too do the number of lethal diseases drop because of knowledge and new interventions. The playing field is changing.

So what about the chronic pain patient for whom no correction of the basic problem is likely? Would this patient, under the old schema, fall under the umbrella of not being treated?

Every modern physician swears to follow the Hippocratic Oath. But the oath is often made without studying the words of the affirmation. The oath says that only if 'I understand the disease and am not fighting the normal course of nature', will the doctor prescribe a treatment. Here again is the sense that it is not okay to go against nature if the effort might produce little or no benefit. The issue is that the lack of understanding may be equally the fault of either limited science or of an under skilled diagnostician. The Hippocratic Oath has no sense of what modern day medicine is like.

Many years ago medication prescribed beyond the 'powers of the art' are were seen as wrong. Giving narcotics to a chronic pain patient was once seen as bad medicine since the core problem is not being fixed. Part of that attitude was often the notion in the sense that the 'real' core problem was more psychological than physical. But as is often the case, the 'powers of the art of medicine' are actually often restricted not by the limits of the art, but more by the limits of the artist.

Occasionally ethics, decency, and clinical reality require a treatment to go beyond the standard interpretations of the art. Herein lives creativity. To practice at the edge of an existing art is sanctioned only if the both the doctor's and patient's expectations believe such actions will offer relief to the patient's body, mind, and soul. But such intervention may not be sanctioned by colleagues and insurance companies. The problem is further complicated when outside people do not know and 'feel the process' that lead to the choice of an unusual intervention; if they did, then perhaps they too would have arrived at the same decision to pursue an unusual intervention. The criticism of the plan by others may simply come from the fact that these critics are neither compassionate or true scientists.

> "Wait…I'm reading this book. This in interesting background stuff. My doctor took the Hippocratic Oath. Hey, no wonder he is afraid to treat my 'can't-find-what's-causing-it' pain."

Any judgment about the extent of a therapy's effectiveness must come from the patient or family. If no *improvement* is possible, there still may be *stability*. The patient can still be alive and emotionally active, though less than what was in the pre-disease era.

One patient put it this way:

> "I ain't no better, but I ain't no worse. While the hip gets worse, and they ain't goina be able to fix it, so I take the morphine, and at least it balances me out a little. I can sit through a TV show and get some sleep."

This is the treatment style that softens the misery and suffering until the problem can be solved.

What needs to be repeated, and repeated, and repeated, is that the vast majority of treatments for chronic pain, including nerve blocks, TENS units, medications, and biofeedback, are all bandages. They do not correct the basic problem. Take away the treatments and the pain returns. The treatments do not restore the natural balance of things in the body. Hence, by strict Hippocratic thinking, they ought not to be done. But if suffering is a disease state, then they ought to be treated. I believe suffering is every bit as much a disease as cancer or asthma. Suffering is, however, a disease of the psyche and the soul. Perhaps 'pain treatment' clinics need to be renamed as 'suffering treatment' clinics.

> "I told the doctor that I don't expect any balance in my body anymore, but I sure would want him to balance out my mind again. Make me be able to ignore the body for a while. That would be great."

Francis Bacon (1561–1626) had a different opinion about medicine. Unlike Hippocrates, Bacon would not stop at nature's limits. He wanted to bend nature to our needs and our wills. He did not revere nature, and he thought we should 'conquer and subdue her.' He thought it noble to extend our power over the universe. He said that 'nature to be commanded must be obeyed,' but the doctor does his 'obeying' by plundering, hounding, exploring, and uncloaking her laws and secrets. Bacon would put a patient on a respirator; he would perform cardiopulmonary resuscitation. Bacon wants science to master nature! So many people agreed with him that he is called the father of modern medicine and the major prophet of the Scientific Revolution.

The reason Bacon and others are discussed in a book about pain is because the pain patient needs to be familiar with the history of the many attitudes that they face. These pieces of knowledge are very illuminating and powerful tools. A patient or family simply has to know as much as possible about the politics and history of the factors that can sway the way in which a condition is treated. This is a huge topic, and what is offered here is the briefest of outlines, but hopefully it will inspire some to look further into the history of medical approaches and attitudes.

> Bacon would be more likely to consider suffering as real a disease as an obvious tumor. He would seek aggressive tools to reduce suffering in the same manner as he would find a surgeon to remove the tumor. He would look at the whole of a patient, and then build a series of axioms to understand the patient's complaints, and if the complaints could not follow a known axiom, it did not eliminate the possibility that the complaint was real but the science

was limited. Given enough time, the science would evolve such that the condition could be explained or corrected. The patient remained worthy of treatment until that scientific evolution occurred.

Over time the focus of medicine has changed from the Hippocratic notions (correcting the body's imbalance) to the disease concept. The disease concept is focused on the process of isolating and destroying foreign organisms or repairing injuries. By the mid 1800's, much disease finally was seen as the result of germs invading the body. By the mid-1900's, antibiotics were performing miracles. Once surgeons learned of aseptic technique and began to use anesthesia during surgery, their techniques made them appear as if they had almost magical skills. Medicine's new tools propelled its image upwards like a glossy new ad campaign. After all, people were getting better who, just a few decades before, would have had no opportunity for health. But people also began to see medicine as increasingly mechanical, such that it was referred to in this way: "If you can't see it, give a pill, or cut it out, then it doesn't exist." Medicine, cloaked in its own success and science, had returned to exorcism. The place, role, respect and concern for human suffering began to slip away.

It seems that even parts of psychiatry have drifted into exorcism. Many mental illnesses do come from chemical imbalances. This pleases many people; medications rather than a personal responsibility is expected to remove the imbalances and problems from their lives. Good fortune rests, however, in the fact that the better mental health practitioners adhere to the mixture of *biochemistry and life's situations* as the cause of many conditions. Many psychiatrists mix the important social factors into their diagnostic trees.

But in truth, many ailments still defy clear any etiology, or they remain outside the corral of possible or successful treatment. Most mature patients accept these limitations.

> "I hear my doc say to the nurse that some things they just don't know. They don't know what to do for me. Why doesn't he say that to me? I can take it...but they gotta keep the pain meds even if it ain't fixing nothing for sure. Well, it is fixing the pain a bit, that's for sure. I can live with reality more than thin promises."

Many chronic pain patients see themselves as having no prospect for improvement. They have medically futile conditions, with unyielding expectations of on-going suffering, and a downgraded life style that goes into the state of being a slave to the hardness of pain. Hippocrates would say that it is madness to treat them. We say it is madness not to treat them.

Many patients have asked me the enticing question about how different might a treating team might approach chronic pain if the team members themselves suffered from a similar pain. I suspect the tone would be quietly but genuinely different.

An elderly man told me this after his doctor said it was bad and unethical medicine to prescribe narcotics:

> "Ethics are problems that apply to others. Practical is when ethics apply to myself.
>
> Ya know, Doc, I'm an old, old country farmer, and in my day I've seen many a person and had many an idea. Been keeping my own tally, if ya know what I mean, and now that I'm old and festerin' with ailments like old men have,

I've come to realize how much this world I'm leaving for ya has gone astray. When I's a kid, the doc's were treating us people and they didn't have the fancy tools ya'll got, so yes, many a disease or two killed us. But they knew how to treat the sufferin'. Ya'll now got mighty good tools to knock away the diseases and ya'll should be thanked for that, but a sick person got's more than the disease, he's got sufferin'. And when they ain't got the cure for something, ya'll move away, like the sufferin' ain't just as real as the disease. Son, ya gotta treat the sufferin'. Mighty strong medicine is God's glory when it's aimed towards the sufferin'. Why, I'd seen an old lady who'd had cancer live longer than ought to 'cause her old country doctor treated her sufferin'. But ya can't down grade the sufferin' like it ain't as high powered as the main disease. Being a doc means ya gotta pay attention to both them pieces of life, or you'd might just as well be just fixin' old automobiles.

See here, now doctoring use'd to be a joyful service, done as a service, done with heart and trustin' and real carin'. Now a days I mostly get the feelin' ya doc's work more out a fear, like you's too scared to be brave. Gotta have a disease. Is that how you got all A's in school? Findin' the diseases? We ain't machines. You be good to us and we'd be good to ya. Yeh, don't hold me to it, I know it ain't quite that simple, I know, but maybe we ought to try to make it so. So now, how 'bout you and me talk of this sufferin' that comes from my nasty old knee..."

...Thought...

Growing and learning from challenges could make us larger than giants. Such challenges drive us to perfect our minds and bodies. We learn to prorate dreams into impossible or possible ones. Some challenges allow growth. Some just keep the focus on survival. We would like to have options to change things for the better. We want the freedom of choices. Does the adversity of pain made us stronger? Does pain give or take free will from us?

The process of making good and well grounded choices requires both intellectual and emotional components. The emotional component is sometimes called the will. Let's take a closer look at this important, albeit knotty notion, so we can better appreciate how it impacts those whose live with chronic pain.

> A chronic pain patient, who is also a philosopher, said that pain patients need to understand some about free will because that is part of their challenges. "Being in pain means I have to be a thinking patient. I have to know the history of my condition and how people look at it. I have to campaign for my care. I do have enemies out there whose actions can take away my life-lines. The will is the part of the process which helps me chose from among a set of non-emotional options. So when you get a chance to teach about pain, you have to be teach about life too...you have to...the patient's need to learn to survive....and a grounded and informed attitude is one of our best allies.... I know its convoluted and hard to think all this through and through, but it is worth the effort. I ask pain patients to please try to read this

material carefully and slowly. And wouldn't it be incredible if they had a therapist or minister to help them learn about this."

Free will is an important concept. Free will is often seen as having two ingredients: first is having the 'ability' to choose from options, and second is having the 'right' to act upon the choice. This is somewhat complex, but understanding one's own will can help adjust to living with chronic pain.

Free will is also when the "absolute freedom of the mind assumes that man is able to reach decisions while being completely independent of either natural or metaphysical controlling forces." [201]

Existentialism is a philosophy of existence. It maintains a hefty concern for the whole person, and not just of the intellect. It focuses on how a person both experiences and takes responsibility for their world. This is a self-deterministic approach to life, as opposed to an external cultural or biologically determined one. Existentialism gives choices which have the power to change things. If choices cannot change some things, then our wills offer us the power to modify what we can change in order to live with the unchangeables. Pain patients often struggle with existentialistic problems when they try to 'figure out the logic and strategy of how to live my life!'

Some existentialists argue that religion is a cowardly way to explain away problems in life. Religion is labeled by some as a crutch against one's personal weaknesses; its embracement is more likely to be found in those who prefer safety and security over less risk. Some existentialists (e.g., Soren Kierkegaard) encourage a restoration of religious faith while others (i.e., Friedrich Nietzsche) encourage the opposite.

Other existentialists use the concept of phenomenology. It may appear complex but it says that we have to work through a sequence of tasks before we understand our lives. It says that we must *understand* the essential structures of an experience 'before' we can *comprehend* our human consciousness. The task, simply put, is to find out what to do with oneself in the world in which we live. This will then hopefully help us discover what is vital. Only then we can use our experiences and perceptions to foster decisions which better define ourselves. That developed definition will plot the course of our lives. Being in chronic pain has to become part of a personal definition, so pain characterizes, and tints, colors, and gives a unique flair to a pain patient's signature and existence.

John Paul Sartre felt that humans are free to choose. But we are not free from not choosing. We have to make choices. In those choices is the ability to cancel or deny certain aspects of the world in which we live. Sartre felt people have both the freedom of, and a personal responsibility, for their own choices.

Will and reason are two separate activities of the mind. Will comes from decision and choice. "I have decided that I will live!" Reason comes from argument and calculation. "I have found a way to live!"

Choices are often based on the assessment of a perceived reality at the decision moment. The choice says: "Here's the current facts, make your decision now!" We understand why a person makes a particular decision when we understand their background of experiences, prior choices, and how they process information. That understanding of others is empathy.

Assemble pain patients so they might share their experiences and listen to the walls echo with empathetic comments like "hey, yes, that's how I feel too!" Or "I really understand why you refused that surgery." They understand each other because so many of the choices they each made relate to the same problems. So many of them have the same set of options. These similarities may not have existed in their lives before the pain started.

Too often patient's are not allowed to have an existence or will that is different from others. This is especially so if the 'others', such as treatment teams or insurance adjustors, have positions of power over the person's life. This situation may become what Harry Stack Sullivan calls a *parataxic distortion*.[202]

Parataxic means there is a lack of harmony between ideas, attitudes, and other aspects of a relationship. It's a useful term. Pain patients often have parataxic distortions imposed on them. The below quote will highlight it in everyday terms. But let's first try to take a look at it in more technical terms: a 'parataxic distortion' is a term for the inaccuracies in judgment and perception that occur when a viewer needs to perceive subjects and only have relationships that are in harmony with his own set of prior attitudes or experiences. In other words, how I act today is based on what made me the most comfortable when I was in similar, past situation, so the doctor may speak: "I need you to see it my way, and if you want my treatment, we will follow that way only." This parataxis produces a disharmony between the patient and doctor. The patient will feel his free will is being denied.

> "The doc was used to dealing with drug addicts. His view of me was distorted because I used the same drugs but without the addiction. I don't think he had many real trusty patients like me. That's a sad thing to say. Me, well, I'm different. I haven't been dishonest a day in my life, except the time I cheated on a girlfriend 29

years ago. Been in a great marriage since. So my life experiences have been trust and honesty. The doctor's life seems to have been of mistrust and lying. He used 'his' past to explain 'me'. That is not fair. And like I said, he distorted me by his own past. He defined me according to his past. That was wrong. This type of thinking is like we did in role playing in a psych class I took in college. I never realized that having this bad awful back pain would make me think about that psychology stuff again."

Sullivan viewed these distortions as defenses against one's own anxiety. Doctors and patients can both suffer from parataxic distortions. The distortion might build into untrusting interactions which effectively keep relationships too narrowly focused, unrealistically stilted, unilateral, or too simplistic.

"I think the doctor was nervous when he treated me, like I symbolized something out of synch with his background. I was fine. He was neurotic! He kept thinking I was something I ain't!"

Might the complaints of pain fall on deaf ears and become the victims of parataxic distortions, to the extent that the suffering and understandable requests for empathy are also overlooked or downplayed? The distortions mute away the pain complaints. Patients may feel that "the doctor doesn't seem to want to listen to me!"

Maybe these distortions protect the emotions of the non-pain people who must deal with pain people. This then puts the pain patient in a subtle but real bind. Assume that 'you' are accused of being in more than pain than you 'ought to be', and the assumption is based mostly on the accuser's own emotional needs and make-up. To survive 'you' have to make choices that act more in the flavor of a capitulation than a genuine free choice quality, especially if insurance or other forces limit your choices. Free will does not exist for many pain patients unless they limit their choices to either less than needed or no treatment. The style, form and manner of treatment options may be limited to the menu offered by the treating doctor. And that menu may be based on the doctor's parataxic distortions of you.

> If all life is predetermined before birth, then we merely act according to fate. Then there is no free will. No one can apply blame or argue on any account. But does pre-determination include suffering? Might a person adjust his fate?
>
> Judaism believes that "human behavior and actions are not either free or determined; rather they are both free and determined. Judaism acknowledges the ability of freedom of the mind. According to the Talmud and its main interpreters, the engagement in a medical practice is permissible, disclaiming the notion that by doing so one is abrogating G-d's deeds."[203] The assumption, therefore, is that perhaps it was predetermined that a person would go into medicine to beneficially alter another person's life. But is this all like the Star Trek theme, that Captain Picard cannot alter the history of another civilization. To fix someone who's fate was to be sick leads the thinking person into circular logic. Perhaps the real fate is to be sick for

> a while, and then to be lucky enough to find a repair person. Then perhaps some wisdom accrued from the time of being sick.
>
> Yet consider the agony of those who cannot be fixed: will they think that their fate is to suffer and not to be lucky enough to find a repair person.

Religious convictions hold that we are asked to keep ourselves in good shape and not to harm or destroy our bodies. Introducing medications in a prudent and studied manner might be the "doing good" wanted by religion because we are not letting the disease destroy the body and spirit. Some people feel differently. They feel that pain relieving medications lead to harm, destruction, and are violations of the value of life. But the outcome of good pain control is often the opposite, leading to improved qualities in life. This leads to some interesting discussions.

An ill person ought to self-determine their care, provided they have the presence of mind to understand their condition or fate. Protecting a patient's right to do so is an act of ultimate respect. This has been beautifully dealt with in various euphemisms:

Put yourself in their shoes.

Do not do unto others what is hated upon yourself [204]

Respect your fellowman as you would have them respect you [205]

Love your neighbor as thyself [206]

> It is critical to encourage and measure emotional growth, especially if under the weight of a chronic problem, as a way to know how we

come to our decisions. This is a challenge for all: the patient, the professional, the family and friend, the regulator and the judge. We have the skills to do it; the tools to this reside in the nature of our conversations and dialogues. It is hard to understand oneself or others. But it worth every bead of emotional sweat, for everyone grows and reaps a splendid bounty from the process.

Let's end this chapter with a chillingly focused 2006 quote by Ballantyne [207] as she wrote about opioid use for chronic non-terminal pain.

> "The general finding is that patients attain satisfactory analgesia using moderate non-escalating doses, often accompanied by an improvement in function, and minimal risk of addiction. It must be remembered, though, that these studies are anecdotal, comprising reports written by experts who likely carried out the treatment with unusual care. This inherent bias is particularly relevant to chronic opioid therapy, which requires considerable dedication, patience and caution to be successful."

She refers to works by Portenoy and Foley, both of whom are pioneers in pain management.[208] The success or failure of a pain treatment relationship may indeed rest more so with the nature of the doctor than the nature of the patient. Ballantyne's reference to "unusual care" is touching. The message explains itself.

CHAPTER EIGHTEEN
Suffering

It is extremely difficult today to recognize the capacity that suffering is a possible symptom of health. [209]

So, as this statement suggests, if the ailment from which the suffering emerges is under enough control so as to not kill our bodies, then, in some ironic extension of being physically stabilized, should the sufferer be grateful to have the opportunity to be alive so they can suffer? In other words, should someone be happy to suffer given that the alternative would be death or even a greater disability?

This is one of the difficult conundrums of logic that face all who suffer. Suffering is one of the most complex emotional experiences in life. It is all about the quality of life. What is suffering, how should we measure it, how should someone live with it, and how do the rest of us empathize with it? These challenges ripple through the arts and science of all our lives.

Clinical pain descriptions use a scientific language. Suffering uses a poetic tongue. Patients want doctors who are both scientists and poets.

Artists delight and excel in words, but words are relatively worthless when compared to the world of facial expressions.[210] Physician's who overlook the art gallery of a patient's facial vocabulary miss the purest clues into their patient's worlds and dreams. A face can speak to suffering more than words.

Though great advances in medicine have improved life, the over reliance on technical advances to fix everything is still much too strong. It is also a young and naïve position. Medicine has become too much of a purely technical venture. Using the better mechanical interventions are medicine's technical obligations, but its first moral obligation should be to reduce human suffering. Yet the fear of failure, or of unknowingly maintaining an undesirable pathology (e.g., addiction), or of the incredible time and money needed to deal with suffering, move many doctors away from the 'the obligation of managing suffering.' They may accept the need to 'treat the suffering', but they rationalize the relocation of this process to someone else by saying it requires a different skill set to treat then they have. That is fine in many ways, but the doctor himself, with just a little personal interest, time, and effort, can add immeasurably to the control of suffering. Patients don't expect their doctors to be psychotherapists or clergy, but they do expect human kindness.

"Science without a conscience is the ruin of the soul," wrote the French monk and physician François Rabelais.

> "I know my doctor is better with needles and pills than he is with words. And when I said I need the name of a psychotherapist, he said fine. But he did it like he fixed my car. Without emotion, he then directed me to someone else like I was going to change the car's oil. I don't know, it was ok, but it was cold. Like it lacked that sense of real concern with the consequences of my treatment; I wanted him to give me just a tiny bit of his soul. I kinda like him as a doctor, but I wish he'd be a little warmer and talk a little more 'to me about me,' and not so much about trigger points. If does have a deep conscience, then I just need to feel that every once in a while. It feeds my soul and softens the suffering."

The rivalry to become the best medical technician is far more robust than it is to become the preeminent medical moralist. Too often, any physician who works on moralistic grounds, usually doing so when all else has failed, is chided, damned, or has to go to horrendous extremes to justify their 'less than scientific' work. Interestingly, many physicians and their teams quietly and privately endorse the need to take the moral stand of treating suffering, but this covenant seems to weaken when they are in the public eye or when in groups of other professions. Physicians have to be brave enough to announce that once all technical interventions have failed, that only compassionate care treatment courses remain, and that the reduction of suffering may need to use any technology, evidence based or not, to achieve that goal. This is medically-legally risky for doctors to do on many levels, despite being the proper ethical and moral road to travel. Doing such requires a very tight doctor-patient relationship, with consultations, extensive documentation, consents, etc. The treatment of suffering may end up producing a paper trail larger than the original efforts to control the pain.

> A doctor said: "I began to treat a 'difficult to control the pain' patient about 10 years ago. We got his pain under fairly good control, but it was not as controlled as I would have liked it to be. However, in our visits we started to talk a lot about his life, his interests, etc. My pain prescriptions did not vary that much, but our discussions grew deeper and more honest. I then realized that I was actually treating his suffering, and the good outcome of his care from us was from the treatment of the suffering. It was as important, if not more so, than all the narcotic prescriptions and trigger points and so on."

'Pain' and 'suffering' do not mean the same thing. Pain is a physical sensation. Suffering is an emotion. Pain does not destroy life. Suffering does.

What is suffering?

Suffering involves a sense that there is no future. To suffer is to feel a potential loss of wholeness and self-identity. What used to be may be no more. Suffering anticipates that "I will not continue into the future. I will never again be what I was. I am crumbling."

> The Jewish holiday of Sukkot is called *zman simchateinu,* which means the time of our joy. Joy is different from happiness. Happiness is getting pleasure from what one currently has. Joy is the pleasure of anticipating a good future. Suffering reflects the lack of joy.

Suffering is the dreading of psychological disintegration and permanent disappointment. An aspect of suffering is dependent on what the patient was before the suffering began. Patients measure this change by comparing their present life to the life and station they had before the injury or disease. This comparison then becomes the yardstick from which they project – and fear – additional and unwanted changes in the future.

> "Ya know what suffering is. It's the lost of 'me' and that queasy sense it'll never come back."

Suffering grows increasingly foul as life passes by and things which should have happened do not come to pass.

> "I've already spent 10 years in a wheelchair. I would love to get married and have a child, but I cannot have sex. I can't move, and when I tried it, it hurt so much. People seem to think that people in wheelchairs don't get the urge. The accident cut my spinal cord but not my spirit or sex drive.
>
> The older I get, the angrier I get that there is less and less future for me, that no cure has yet been found, and that I am watching so much of life go by. The real suffering for me is what I am missing. My friends are great and family wonderful, my psychotherapy insightful, and I can be mature about this whole mess, but deep down inside I want to be the one playing football and not just cheering on my friends."

Pain may stop, but suffering might continue.

> "When I allowed the doctors to operate I knew I might lose the feeling in my arm. So now I am without pain but I look like a stroke victim—I traded the pain for numbness. Both are bad, but the days of the pain were worse than the suffering I now have. Yet it's embarrassing to be at dinner and not know my hand is sitting in a cup of hot coffee—then there's always a long story to follow—and I know it's not so bad and I'm lucky when compared to some of the other patients I knew in the pain clinic, but there is still suffering. There is still a price...."

Suffering is the inability to do what was previously easy and important. Goode called this 'role strain.' [211] Simply put, role strain is the feeling that someone is having difficulty meeting the obligations of a role. For example:

> A 35 year old woman underwent surgery. Unfortunately the surgery failed and she became a pain patient requiring a great deal of medication. Little by little her ability to take care of her children eroded because she could not sleep at night, drive, or even sit still long enough to read a bed time story to her 5 year old. She had to leave her job. She could barely socialize. Her sex life with her husband disappeared. She grew angry and depressed. The delightful obligations of being a wife and mother were too much for her, and the strain she put herself under to meet those role obligations of motherhood and spouse hood eventually exhausted her. She felt she would never get better, that her children would hate and not know her, that her husband would look for a 'healthier' woman, that her doctors and friends didn't understand her need for medications, and that her life, as she had known and wanted it, was over.

> "There has to be a hope that I can find a normalcy again, to wear pretty clothes, to have dinner out with my husband and friends, to enjoy wearing make-up, to feel part of being a full woman in this world... let's be real honest, that hope just doesn't exist much anymore...."

Suffering begins not as much when the illness begins, but rather when a person realizes what little prospect for improvement that the future holds for them. In this feeling is the horrible sense that nothing can modify the downward progression. Suffering converts the central interest in life (that is, how someone would like to live his life) from what was wanted to what is being dictated. It is the lost of free will.

Here is another story:

> "I handled my injury and its pain for years. But I began to feel uneasy inside my own head. So I entered psychotherapy, and then I began to think about where my life was going. Then, for 'no' known reason, the pain got a lot worse and, then, for a clearly known reason, I also I got older. I saw my doctor again, who referred me to two different specialists, who in turn each told me that no cure existed. My wrath exploded! This nice, cooperative patient—me!, was now a demanding and impatient one. I realized how much I'd tried to keep my old self alive. I fought to keep my usual self. I did everything to defend my self-identity. I wanted to live as a normal woman! But it couldn't be so, and then one day I put it into the simplest, most prophetic and frank statements of my last 15 years: the pain has prevailed.
>
> I went home and cried with my best friend. From here on out it became a matter of finding a new attitude based on no hope. Think about that – I had to assemble an attitude built on 'no hope' that I could ever to be what I wanted to be. Usually we build towards something that we hope will come to be. So I had

to redefine so much of my life. Thank goodness my pain doctor kept the pain under reasonable control, but I knew it was still there, like a splinter in the foot – it's tiny, but my gait is off. I know it's there……

I need my friends now. I need them to help me stabilize my life, to hold me, to laugh with and include me, and to make love to me. I remember reading about how pain patients need stable emotional environments to keep their own integrity. I never understood how true that is. I cannot explain why this is my destiny and so I need these wonderful people to keep me whole. I can't imagine not being touched by them. They are my harmony. I've seen pain patients lose their friends and drift off away from a social life. I could not tolerate suffering so many loses. My life has become a spooky metaphysical quandary. Dear God, help….and it's funny, even after all this, I still kinda hope He'll come visit me for a while….but I couldn't get it out of my mind that God was no longer interested in me."

Reducing suffering can be relatively easy. Those who suffer don't expect miracles, but their lives will be less isolated and richer if others warmly touch, engage, listen, and make an effort to understand them. The ultimate and most unbeatable balm is to help them find a purpose in life.

The below ...**Thought**... is about counter transference. This is because suffering is often a disease of broken and clogged-up relationships.

... *Thought*...

Countertransference is defined as the feelings a therapist has towards a patient. Countertransference can also easily occur outside of a patient-therapist relationship. There are positive and negative aspects of countertransference. It is usually an unconscious event that is understood after the fact. In short, we have to look for it. One definition is that it is the 'therapists total response to the patient, both conscious and unconscious." If we have a negative countertransference feeling for someone, we may act out in a negative manner towards the other person. If we have a positive countertransference, we may be too positive, kind or forgiving. We all experience bits and pieces of it across the fields of our normal lives.

By strict definition, transference is the feelings a patient has for the therapist. When people help each other, and the roles change back and forth from the helper to the helped, these feelings can also shift back and forth.

> "I idealized my lover. I could find nothing wrong. But then he made some comments that destroyed me. I spoke to my therapist about my disillusionment with him. She showed me how I idealized him much too much. It was almost a fantasy. At times I was his unofficial therapist, and at times, he was mine. She said I had lots of positive countertransference that had been broken. Then she told me not to take the term too literally, since a lot of it was transference and not countertransference. I said 'wait, this is getting complicated.' And she said yes, it was complex, and so we let it rest with the idea that we often have many unconscious feelings in us about others, and those feelings can produce

lots of feelings about ourselves, about them, about situations, and so on."

Countertransference can add to suffering. It is probably more common than is reported. Patients feel it's presence as 'something uncomfortable coming out of the liaison with the doctor or a friend who is suppose to help me." The question is always: why did the countertransference develop? For example:

> "...Yet despite the need for establishment of rapport and positive transference, the physician too frequently, even in the best institutions, displayed cynical, unrealistic and hostile attitudes towards the addict. He is indifferent to the latter's genuine complaints, assumes in advance that he is a liar, and maintains that it is a waste of effort and money to attempt a cure." [212]

Selzer [213] felt that when hostility enters the therapist's attitude against the patient, "the establishment of a positive therapeutic relationship is markedly diminished." This negative countertransference distances the therapist from the patient. Virtually every pain patient has felt it. It feeds into greater suffering. And again, what element in the patient triggered the response in the doctor or others?

> "So when I was in several of the regular 'proper' pain clinics, I actually tried to spend real time with the staff, I got their vibes. I wanted to transfer trust to them, but it hit a wall. I didn't want any competition with them. But things happened because they made some comments about me that were wrong. How'd I know they were wrong? I think they are uncomfortable with me

> because I've got a PhD in human physiology and I asked tons of questions. When I went in, we didn't talk as much as I wanted to. I really didn't want to be more than a nice patient, yet I was taken aback by their lack of new knowledge. I tried to zip up my mouth. So it grew into the cold shoulder approach. Now I go to one of those quickie-fix walk in pain clinics. I hardly talk to them, but they give me my pills. The pain is gone, and so too is the attitude I got from the 'proper' doctor. My therapist said the first doctor was having negative countertransference to me because he was afraid of my knowledge."

Patients quickly learn that medical science understands more than it can influence. They see how neuropathy might be explained, but it cannot be removed. Over time those patients who work to learn about their conditions may accumulate a more realistic knowledge of their condition than do their doctors. This is time and again reflected when patients say that the 'new doctor in the clinic wants to do surgery – he's a cowboy. He implied I wasn't trusting. Why does he think he can fix what no one else can?'

Many other reports capture what is in this quote: "How might treatment providers feel about dealing with a group of patients who are thought to dwarf the skills of experienced clinicians?" [214][215]

> "The longer I suffered this pain, and the greater the number became of doctor's I'd seen, the more I realized that my survival job was to question the doctors, and some of them were ok with it, and some of them took offense."

It would be nice if treatment teams positioned themselves to feel their patient's isolation, to remember that patients suffer both from physical ailments and a loss of self-identity, and that many patients are more experienced in the particulars of their conditions than are their doctors. If the doctor is annoyed by this, or feels threatened by this, then he may emit a negative countertransference. This feeling of a negative ambiance coming from a health care provider can seriously shatter any remaining ego strength or hope that a patient may have. That too adds to the patient's suffering.

Some patients are afraid to ask their doctors for even short moments of needed sympathy and consoling. They 'wonder if' the doctor prefers not do this because the doctor may see such a request as a need for sympathy. More often it is actually a need for empathy. Doctor's too often feel that their key obligation is to 'mechanically fix' the problem, and so they shy away from the simple act of being emotionally supportive. Yet short, kind, comforting words from doctors and nurses can be inconceivably rich and spiritually eloquent connections for patients. Patients who see professionals put up an armor against 'tender moments' take these shields as rejections or dismissals. And once again, this also adds to the suffering.

Why do some treatment providers balk at such patients? The answer is that health care providers are not all equally emotionally mature or sophisticated. A professional license does not exempt them from irritating personally styles or unresolved psychological needs, fears, or problematic attitudes. They too may suffer from parataxic distortions or from any number of other psychological quirks. There is an understandable tendency and hope that all health care providers are stable, educated, unprejudiced, responsible, predictable, trustworthy, and so on. This is not so.

Consequently, the problem that patients may have with a doctor may lie more with the doctor than with the patient.

> "With patients the problems of countertransference are especially difficult because of the aggression they include. Because patients are very demanding, expressing insatiable, endless oral fantasies, the analyst, [or health care provider] has to deal with their [own] fears of being devoured or destroyed, and often becomes concerned with giving too much to them." [71]

Correcting this problem would require that the doctors, nurses, and all other people involved in the care of the chronic pain patients should enter into some type of personal psychotherapy or sensitivity training. When more than one patient reports these types of problems with a medical team, then it strongly suggests that these problems exist within the team.

What interesting changes would follow if professionals saw reflections of their own lives in the lives of their patients?

> "I wonder what the doctor would feel if he lived in my shoes? I once went to a doctor's who wife just lost her breast from cancer. He was so gentle with me, and I knew he was busy, but he took the time to talk about my fears. He felt my fears. Then he actually spoke a little about his fears. I think we both got a little better that day.
>
> I've wondered if some doctors treat me as they do because they are afraid of how real a chance it is that they too could be injured as I

am. The randomness of my accident is proof of that possibility. I remember reading about defense mechanisms that turn on when we need to try to turn away or bury what we don't want to see...."

CHAPTER NINETEEN
What the psychologists see

In 1959, George Engel wrote a paper entitled "Psychogenic Pain and the Pain Prone Patient."[216] The paper found wide acceptance in the pain treatment community. It is still widely referred to in many pain management textbooks. Pain patients need to be acquainted with some of these ideas.

Right from the start Engel says:

> "Perhaps familiarity breeds contempt. Every physician has his own personal experience with pain and it began long before he ever became a physician. This is in contrast to other complaints which we learn about only while studying medicine....the student hence 'knows' what pain is. (But he is taught) the concept of pain (that) becomes scientific and...a relatively simple concept of pain is constructed. This leads to the...formulation that pain has two components: the original sensation, and the reaction to the sensation."

No one can argue against this basic formulation. And indeed, the basic starting point that "Every physician has his own personal experience with pain" is fascinating, but it is too narrow. For most physicians, any serious pain they may have known in life has resolved! How different might this reference be if the doctor's personal pain had not ended? Interestingly, Engel touches on the same topics as we did in the above chapter when parataxic distortion was mentioned. Clearly the doctor's own psychological make-up is a key element in the treatment style.

Engel writes that the "practical clinical problem really has to do with how the individual experience's pain." This is such a true and critical point. The patient's report is decisive. Some pain might be eliminated or modified without any change in the physical lesion, such as what happens with acupuncture. When this happens, it cannot be suggested that because the pain responded to acupuncture, that the pain 'had to be' imaginary or psychogenic. However, someone may take this experience to mean that some pain can be controlled if the patient's psychology 'allows' it to happen. Well, perhaps, but only to a degree.

The sensation of pain is real. But it is subjective.

> "Wait, wait, wait! That's all wrong! It may subjective to you, but the pain is objective to me!"

Why might the suggestion be made that some people experience 'more pain more than ought to be'? The answer lies in the differences (1) in each person's chemistry, and (2) what, if any, psychological role does the pain play in the patient's life. The assumption of 'an emotional role for the pain' is one of the more prevalent themes in pain management.

> Her first intestinal and rectal illnesses appeared when she was 19 years old. She often stayed home rather than risk embarrassment. The pain was horrible, and caring doctors allowed her to use pain medications. But those same caring doctors did not know the extent of the dysfunctional aspects of her family, so the pain medications took on two roles: they successfully reduced both the physical *and* emotional pains in her life. Eventually her father called her an

addict and alleged that her pain was only psychosomatic. She was sent to a detoxification unit, when psychiatry was introduced into her life. A few years later she developed fibromyalgia. Not all her doctors believed in fibromyalgia. The intensity of the family issues lead many therapists to label her primarily as a drug addict escaping from her uneasy family life. Though this was ultimately found to be professionally short-sighted, the repeated allegations made her begin to doubt herself as well.

A series of psychotherapists unsuccessfully tried to figure her out; she said they were too focused on her medication needs and how she needed 'to learn to live' with her family. However, she eventually met a therapist who was comfortable with her medication needs but who also egged her into insight oriented therapy to the point where she began to see how some of her pain followed her emotional family environments. The psychotherapy was hard for her; it took time, and it bit into many of the agonizing issues about herself and family. She put it nicely when she realized that "I can now separate the 'psycho' from the 'somatic'." She was also lucky enough to have the money to pay for the better psychotherapy.

Interestingly, her father developed a temporary but painful medical condition. He suddenly became one of her allies. But when his condition resolved so too did his understanding. She saw that he merely went back to his 'pre-painful condition' personality. She, however, is now stronger and less influenced by his comments. Her pain signature had changed.

It is important to understand the *pain signature* concept.

> The styles, types, and qualities of any description used to communicate pain will always amalgamate into what is known as a 'pain signature.' When similar conditions are described by many people in similar ways, it sets up a common standard about what is generally observed. A woman in labor, a toothache, heartburn, or a broken bone—all are described by people in pretty much similar ways. How any one person relates their pain will develop into a person's personal 'pain signature'. Later stages of pain will further individualize the signature.
>
> Signatures are both physical and psychic. Part of the clinical challenge for the physician is to sort through all the items in the patient's report in order to find a signature that reliably represents the total problem. When the signature deviates from the usual one for similar situations, caution will appear: might the physical disease and the pain play no core role in the claimed problem? Doctors look at pathology and expect a signature that reflects the 'usual' complains associated with the pathology. But questions pop up if the patient signs a signature that is out of the ordinary. This is when the 'psychology of the condition' needs a careful exploration. However, and this is a key point, an

unusual presentation or an odd signature is not proof that real pain doesn't exist. The doctor has to learn to read what is veiled between the blatant signature lines.

Signatures evolve over time as experiences accumulate in a person's life. One patient mentioned that more and more cynicism began to flavor her signature. Likewise, patients may not be equally skilled in presenting themselves. A patient noted that "so then I began to see that my problem is my sloppy handwriting. No one could read my signature. No doctor seemed to understand me until a long time passed between us. I had to learn how to better write out my history, if ya know what I mean. I had to learn how to communicate. And the doc's had to see me in action over time. I guess for me the actions are better than my words."

Doctors need to contrast the psychic signature to the physical signature. This pain signature notion helps determine how much of the pain is psychological or physical. Engel says:

> "In general, the more complex the ideation and imagery involved in the pain description, the more complex are the psychic processes involved in the final pain experience."

He suggests that if the pain signature is crisp, "economical and relatively uncomplicated," then the pain is more likely to be real and not psychosomatic.

But he reverses this simplicity by saying that:

> "...we cannot conclude that the patient who gives us the more complex, the vague or the vivid type of description does not have a peripheral (physical) lesion. Such descriptions reflect the characteristics of the individual and if he is suffering from a peripheral lesion, the disordered patterns arising from it are subjected to the most complex psychic distortion and elaboration so that at times the peripheral qualities may be totally obscured."

Thank goodness for this counterpoint. It warns us not to be too glib or quick in coming to conclusions. One factor not adequately mentioned in Engel's thoughts is the effect of being in pain for years and years. Over such long time periods, patients learn new ways to describe their pain. They also become very sensitive to subtle differences in the pain which, to them, are tangible differences in their pain experiences. But a doctor may view these fine points as overly imagined or detailed. It is important to always remember that living with pain for a long time will change the signature.

Sometimes the patient's pain signature is correct but their hand writing is hard to read. So patients need to refine their 'handwriting'. Doctors may need to spend more time to understand what initially may be seen as illegible. Cultural and language barriers may be part of the hurdles in some of these cases.

It is important to also remember that doctors also transmit a signature as well. A 45 year old chronic patient, after being told about the notion of signatures, said he "learned real fast how to read a doctor's handwriting…..he didn't have to do much too tell me how he felt about me and my needs."

Pain can only be reported. This cannot be understated. Because of unequal language skills, great care must be taken not to give too much diagnostic power to subjective expressions. One difference between real and psychosomatic pain is the 'relish' a patient uses to make their pain signature. Real pain tends to be less dramatic and unchanging over time. A listener may feel pity for a horrible life story without the sense that the patient is asking for sympathy. The real patient's signature wants belief and understanding.

> The doctor may think: "this patient complains of pain. The physical signature is consistent with some real pain, but the psychic signature is much too much, and I am uncomfortable with it. She dramatically complains too much about the pain, as if the pain is her entire life, and that doesn't sit well with me. She asks me if I believe her pain. I want to. Yet I suspect there is a ploy to keep me off the real track. Even if I can't find enough real pain to warrant treatment, she is still overly complaining about it—so which signature do I believe? I'll believe the physical one and carefully see what happens."

Patients often ask "will you please believe me?" This may be taken as a request for mercy, pity, or as a plea for honest empathy. It takes time to know if the patient needs genuine mercy for an ailment, or if the plea is indeed a part of a deception (which might indicate a deeper psychological ailment).

Many people fear pain. Pain makes them catastrophize, which then sets up a whirlwind of uncontrolled emotions. This complicates, and thereby confuses, any separation of the relative influences of the physiological and psychological components that go into the final measure of pain.[217] Catastrophizing comes from the loss of self control and from the fear of future ruination.

> "After my accident, when the pain did not go completely away, all I could think of was my uncle who lives in horrible pain. I freaked out every time I got a twitch that was a little different because I painted it to mean that it was the start of an irreversible downhill course for me that would last for the rest of my life. I know this now 'cause I ran to a hundred doctors before a psychologist helped me get this perspective. But, and I gotta tell ya, it's slippery. I still get real scared if there is one inch of difference in the pain...."

A simple distinction is needed between the people who have pain versus the people who use pain. Psychologists work to find this diagnostic demarcation in their patients. The distinction lives in the life style of the patients and it can be seen in the nature of their signatures. The vast majority of people hate their pain. There is no secondary gain for this majority, though one patient did refer to his disability checks as his "gain-less, secondary gain. People think I gain some freedom because I get some money. They don't see that I am really under house arrest. I'd give the money back in a minute for lasting pain relief."

Engel notes the possibility that *'Pain is self-punishment'*. He concludes patients who feel this do not believe that they deserve success or happiness. A common statement is, "when I was having just regular hard times in life, I felt good because it was real life. But now, just when I should finally be able to enjoy myself, this terrible pain came to me like a depraved tax collector for a payback for something bad they say I did a long time ago. I wish I could convince myself this wasn't a punishment."

Some patients refer to pain as an 'old but bad friend' who offers them an excuse to be negative or unproductive. The diagnostic key here rests in what their behaviors and life style were like before the pain. It is so important to know about the pre-pain self. If they did not need excuses before the pain, then that is one personality make-up. If they secretly looked for ways to exculpate themselves from responsibility before the pain came into their lives, then that may speak to how they now use the pain in their lives. That is a different type of personality make-up. These are complex psychological issues.

One notion often bantered about in pain management is that of the self-defeating personality. [218] This diagnosis existed in the third but not in the fourth edition of the DSM.[219] This disorder is characterized by recurrent behaviors that lead to repeated failure or rejection. Some people believe that masochistic qualities live in the self-defeater. It is imperative that any suggestion of a self-defeating behavior, masochism, or any personality disorder come from only good psychodiagnosticians. These labels can be treacherously provocative, long lasting, and pejorative.

Self-defeating behaviors are thought to come from a background where the parents imposed grandiose and unreachable expectations on their kids. Such children grow up with a need to protect themselves from any real life tests that they might fail. This is a very complex psychodynamic and it should not be casually tossed about. It is often sloppily over-used to explain away complex and composite motivations.

Some self-defeating people may exploit pain as a means to avoid reality. Having pain really gives them an opportunity to avoid failure. Engel points out: "The patient who uses pain as a means of self-punishment and atonement almost always manifests other psychological and behavioral devices which serve the same purpose." This dysfunctional psychological process may have been dormant, only to come alive after the pain developed. This reinforces the importance of knowing what the person was like before the pain entered their lives; therein lies the real baseline and signature.

Speaking to other dynamics, Engel goes on to say: "We are often struck by the disparity between the intensity of the pain and suffering they describe and their general appearance of well-being. Their stoical behavior may express the need to see oneself and be seen as a martyr who tolerates suffering." Once again, this speaks to the nature of their signature.

Indeed, many chronic pain patients do their best to put on a good camouflage. They learn how to make a good presence because they do not want to be a person with only one dimension in life. One patient said: "there is no reason why I can't put on a pretty dress, wear makeup and smile, and still be in horrible pain."

Every now and then the word martyr is used in reference to some pain patients. This promptly opens up suspicion that doubts the legitimacy of the pain. The use of the term may emanate from people who look too quickly or narrowly at the patient. A martyr is too often thought only to be an attention seeker. Those who genuinely fit into the 'selfish' martyr category seek sympathy, usually want to avoid difficult or stressful endeavors, and are habitually less likely to skip pleasurable events. These people often have a histrionic, depressive or passive-aggressive quality to their personalities. Belonging to a genuine and 'honorable' martyr group is quite the converse: this noble person sacrifices, without publicity or need for pity, some pleasurable or safe aspect of himself to protect, honor, or save some other person or idea. True martyrdom grounds itself in how much the patient is willing to unselfishly sacrifice for the benefit of others.

The chapter on suffering mentioned that to suffer is to feel that one's future is endangered. This is a key psychological differential in what role pain plays in a patient's life, that is, this concept can help separate one who 'uses' pain from one who just has it. Consider and compare these two psychological signatures:

> The pain user will say: 'I can't work because it hurts too much'; little more background information will be added. But the pain non-user will say: 'I was a teacher, I loved teaching. What will I do now?'
>
> The *user gains a personality because of the pain; the non-user looses a personality because of the pain*. The user will never be bored with the pain; the non-user will abhor the idleness.

Engel continues this section with the statement that "treatments which are not painful or a hardship may be rejected." Again, there are some people who do this – this speaks to the user who gains a personality from the illness. But many mature chronic pain patients reject treatments simply because they see no utility in risking another procedure. As one woman put it, "why should I even try? Nothing has worked thus far and nothing will ever work. Now, give me something really new and tested and maybe I'll think about it...."

Engel suggests that the pain-prone patient experienced suffering and pain in his early family relationships. "This eagerness to tell of such distressing life experiences in itself of diagnostic value... and the manner of telling betrays the wish of the patient to present himself as long-suffering and abused."

This telling of one's past struggles is a prime example of the psychological signature concept. But Engel did not differentiate between the patient who, in a single diagnostic visit or in a brief office visit, has to get across to the doctor how he feels both physically and emotionally after living a very long time in chronic pain, versus the patient who may be only looking for chronic pity. A lot of professional time is needed to adequately look at, and get valid details, and study, and then to fully realize the amount of pain, anguish, tribulation, restraint, disillusionment, uncertainty, consternation, terror, and so on, that may live in what was once been a relatively content human being. Even someone from a horrific background may have been able to evolve into a functional life before the pain.

A psychological signature may come across as staged, but a dramatic presentation may also be more a function of the structure of the visit than of the patient's life. In other words, the type of signature given by the patient might be invalid (technically called a false positive) because the doctor doesn't give the person enough time or space to adequately write their signature.

Even noting that there had been some childhood or spousal abuse may precariously taint the 'perception' of the signature in the wrong direction. The real question to be asked is what the person did in response to the abuse.

> After being told about the concept of the 'pain signature', a woman retorted that many of her doctors made her 'sign my name with his pen'. Only afterwards did she also realize that the pen had just enough ink in it for half a signature. She went on to say: "After the injury I spoke to a psychologist. She asked if I was ever

assaulted. I told her how, in college, I had been date raped. But I really got over it. It was a long time ago in my past. Well, she wrote it down in my chart, and now every time a new doctor hears my complaints about the pain, that rape tag pops up. I can't get away from it because *they are hung up on it*. I'm not. I had all sorts of normal relationships with guys afterwards. But these doctors think it is the explanation for everything. They are the idiots. I am okay about the rape. I am not okay about my joint pain."

Engel made an honest and valuable study of certain types of pain patients. But his ideas have been too freely and sometimes inappropriately applied to too many patients with untreatable pain. His notions are used too frequently whenever a patient's pain defies medical explanation. (It's the old adage that patients hear doctors' say "Oh, you can't be in that much pain or need that much medication—you must be one of those pain-prone patients I learned about..."). The blame for the ailment is placed on the patient's psychology. Might the blame rest on a failure in the doctors' clinical and personal skills? How unfair and cruel this can all be on the patient. This is often part of the 'hunt' mentioned earlier in this book.

Friedman's 2008 New York *Times* article speaks to this very problem. Remember that Engel wrote his article in 1959, which is 49 years earlier. One would think this issue would have been resolved a long time ago. That the New York *Times* so recently published a piece about it says that the issue is far from resolved.

Much of Engel's article is about people who 'use' pain. This implies that the symptoms are not real (or less than 'what should be'). This rekindles the notion that doctors are loath to treat sham or exaggerated symptoms, although the label of 'sham' may really reflect no more than a lack of a diagnostic ability.

> "That doctor said I was faking it all. He implied I was bogus. But when I saw the next doctor, the cause was found! So the real sham was that the first doctor is even practicing medicine – I consider him to be faking his medical skills. I was never faking my pain."

When patients demand relief, which is often asking for a pain reducing medication, many doctors take this to mean that the medication is often more for psychological and less for physical reasons. This will commonly evoke the word 'addiction.' Constant requests for pain medications are then seen as an effort to 'maintain the deviancy' and mask an on-going somatoform disease. The somatoform notion is interesting.

The American Psychiatric Association publishes a diagnostic manual known as the DSM-IV-TR, a section of which addresses the concept of the somatoform pain disorder. Other references to this publication have already been made. The DSM-V is currently being written.

Psychiatry recognizes that emotional factors can cause or worsen pain. These conditions are called somatoform or psychogenic pain disorders. The essential ingredient is that pain complaints are present without a corresponding organic basis, or the degree of reported pain exceeds that of the level of organic problems. This category of disorders is in the same group as conversion disorders (once known as hysteria), hypochondriasis, body dysmorphic disorder, and the somatization disorder. These disorders have complaints that no physical finding can explain.

By definition, a somatoform pain disorder needs a preoccupation with pain for at least six months. The onset is usually in the 30-40 year old group. There is a great deal of incapacitation, even perhaps to the state of being an invalid. Often in this group are iatrogenic problems with medications and unnecessary surgeries. The illness can develop suddenly but can also exist for many years. It is twice as common in women as in men, and first degree relatives of these patients appear to have more pain, injuries, depression, and alcohol use than in the general population. Physical symptoms such as spasms or numbness may be seen. The person may refuse to consider even a partial psychological basis to the pain. This refusal can be a critical diagnostic point! Occasionally the pain has a symbolic meaning in that the pain keeps the patient from having to deal with some anxiety provoking problem. Some cases may initially present without any clear or possible role of psychological factors.[220]

The disproportionate report of pain when compared to the physical findings may not be so much the outgrowth of psychopathology but rather a reflection of the limitations of available or affordable medical techniques and skills. It is key to consider that the person may indeed also have some elements of a psychosomatic disorder, but their pain complaints could equally reflect just inadequate treatment. As with the notion of personality disorders (discussed elsewhere), applying this psychiatric label to a patient must be done with incredible caution, with lots of supporting background, and in consultation with a seasoned psychodiagnostician. Another basis to a psychosomatic diagnosis is that even though the 'origin' of the pain may be psychosomatic, it is still very objective to the patient. That in and of itself is a psychological condition which needs aggressive treatment.

> "Because most patients with pain are not evaluated by mental health professionals until long after the onset of the pain, the decision to use the diagnosis of somatoform pain disorder becomes even more difficult." This diagnosis does not apply itself well to chronic pain patients because many medical and psychiatric factors, complicated by long and unsuccessful treatments, are at play. The term somatoform suggests that the 'psychosomatic pain' is different from other pain, and this is not a valid argument.
>
> This dualistic view has often led to the belief that the pain associated with somatoform pain disorder is not 'real,' even through it is clear that the patient's perception of the pain is the same, and his or her suffering is just as real, as with pain of organic origin. This diagnosis.... may unfairly stigmatize the patients to whom it is applied." [221]

The DSM committee constantly considers revisions to the diagnostic criteria. So what is on the diagnostic list today may be re-modeled on tomorrow's list. Most people do not know that many diagnostic criterions transform as new science and new politics influence the compendium of definitions.

> "So I said to the doctor, ok, you claim you can't find the reason for the pain. Does that mean you know all there is to know about all of medicine, and that there is nothing more to learn? So how can you be so sure of yourself? What if tomorrow someone discovers a way to fix me?

Will I at least get an apology from you? All I really want from any doctor is an acknowledgement that while we still didn't know what to do, we will, as a team, keep looking...."

This story comes a doctor: "Years ago I treated a sincere man who complained of joint pain and fatigue. His insurance company said it was only psychosomatic. So a lawsuit followed. In court, the patient's lawyer asked the insurance company's doctor "how many diseases can a human being have?" The doctor guessed it was several thousand. The lawyer's next question was "Are there any diseases, cures, causes, situations, etc., that we may not yet know about?" The doctor had to say yes. The patient won."

The psychology of the pain patient is a critical topic. This subject matter has produced massive volumes of information, ideas, etc. Every pain patient has to be aware of how his psychology is being measured and judged by all those who treat, authorize, pay for, and live with them.

...Thought...

If a doctor honestly knows his patient, and if the patient works closely with the doctor, then appropriate pain relief can be given to almost anyone, be it medically real or suspected psychosomatic pain. The deciding and discriminating decision making slant often rests squarely on the doctor-patient relationship.

This brings up a critical proposition. Too often, after a psychosomatic diagnosis is offered, the pain meds are stopped because they are seen as unnecessary. This can be a big mistake. Instead why not carefully control and continue the medications to relieve the pain enough so that the person can focus on correcting his other problems? Hopefully the pain causing irritant will ultimately diminish such that the need for pain medication will also dissolve or lessen. This is maintenance plan with a goal.

> "Okay, yeah, I came to see that some of this pain controls the tension of living with my crazy Dad. But the doctor, when he heard the therapist tell him that, the doctor, he cut down my meds like I was a junkie! He said "you can't have these meds for that reason." He punished me. And I'll tell you, I changed doctors, and I kinda had to lie a bit to the new doctor, but I needed those meds. Now, over time, I got my head better together, and I do not need so much meds. But my first doctor – he wouldn't be reasonable, he didn't see how much I was getting better, he just punished me! I go to one of them walk-in clinics now, and it's kinda sleazy, but I get my pills and off I go."

The crux of any pain therapy in those with psychosomatic issues is always two pronged. The first goal is not to get them off the medications: that is the second goal. The first goal is to prepare and strengthen patients enough so they can leave, change, or reduce the need for the pain drug use.

Instead of beginning the treatment of resistant or difficult cases with a technical approach, one might begin with a moralistic one that does not punish the patient for his drug use or the life style that existed since the pain began. The patient's self-identity is at stake. The goal is to stabilize, if not improve, that identity. The first goal is to make the patient feel more secure and better about himself. Then the pain can be dealt with. Absolute rules and guidelines for any medication use, biofeedback, etc., are agreed upon between doctor and patient, but the sense must be of a real team work system, with defined boundaries. That even includes responsible but humanitarian plans about how to deal with slip ups, mistakes, etc. Imagine how good the patient would feel hearing this?

Sometimes a patient with an ill-defined pain signature gains the diagnosis of a psychosomatic disorder because a pain signature doesn't fit a standard clinical picture. The person feels a pain that doctors can't explain. That can make a person doubt themselves. When a patient is upset that they are not being believed, it leans against the reality of their complaints. "That doctor was wrong, I don't care that he doesn't believe me. I'll not waste my time here…" This situation demands a much deeper look into everyone's motives and psychological make-ups. The patient may be properly reacting to a malevolent doctor, or the doctor may be properly reacting to a suspicious presentation.

The stress of not being believed can increase the power and effect of the underlying physiological condition. If the patient agrees to look for any hidden psychological reasons for the treatment resistant pain, and the patient works hard to find something, but nothing can be found because there is no major psychological problem, then this effort becomes another negative event in his life. His efforts failed again! Nothing is fixing the pain. "I am a complete failure, useless, I must be defective. Something very hidden is wrong with me, what else would explain this pain. Maybe my life really should be over….."

The suggestion that a patient 'is not motivated enough to really work on the psychological problem' only adds further insult and defeat. This may intermingle another barrier to how the treatment community views the patient – the complaints of chronic pain are taken as negative, self-serving, and hooked to some secondary gain. The tensions from this situation can be explosive. In 1984, Hendler felt that the doctor-patient relationship can be destroyed if the doctor says to the patient that the pain is not genuine.[222] Too often this comment is the product of not finding an organic basis to the pain. But such disbelieving comments may also be used to rid a medical practice of a complex patient; it may be the doctor's means to redefine the patient's diagnosis to justify the discharge from the practice. When complex issues are at play, the proper shift is to get consultations to help with the problems. Pejoratively re-defining the diagnosis reflects back to the hunt which was mentioned before.

Doctor's words are a delicate but strong matter. The power of suggestibility can convert a slapdash comment into all sorts of pain. Misspoken or carelessly chosen words, or just the style of doctor patient interactions, can have very painful after effects.

> "I get two treatments from the doctor, his pills and his words. I get side effects from both."

The inclination in medicine is to be technically 'matter of fact with patients.' "Only absolute objectivity and neutrality in the observer, and the avoidance of personality and history in the patient are held to be valid. The patient's individual reality, as influencing his individual physiology, is not considered. The results are errors in diagnosis…these iatrogenic disturbances can be reduced by training medical students in biopsychosocial interrelations and by self experience courses for physicians." [223]

Patient's often take such 'honesty and conviction' as a reflection of the doctor's diminished sense of responsibility for the patient's well being. Doctors must always consider the patient's biopsychosocial world. Patients can usually handle almost any bad news if it is thoughtfully and benevolently attached to their biopsychosocial supports systems. Merging a clinical reality with the rest of a person's world is an essential activity. Doing so brings the "old fashioned art of humanness to modern scientific care." [224]

In 2001, a nursing study emphasized the importance of the patient's perspective of pain. Many patients come to specialists after long delays and a series of failed pain control trials. Patients want advice on how to help them cope with chronic pain.[225] They want something new, or if nothing is new, they want some help for their suffering.

A revealing but troubling paper appeared in 1997 about the role of iatrogenesis. This is 'doctor caused' pain. "We found that possible iatrogenic factors, such as over-investigation, inappropriate information and advice given to patients as well as misdiagnosis, over-treatment and inappropriate prescription of medication were common... we suggest that future studies should take account of the role of the doctors, as well as that of the patients, in the etiology, and hence prevention of chronic pain." [226]

Kleinbrink[227] wrote about the bioethical issues of insufficient medical work-ups in the Mensana Clinics study. He found that multidisciplinary approaches have "been largely utilized to simply manage chronic pain, instead of curing it." Kleinbrink makes this very perceptive comment: "If the underlying pathology of disease or existence of pain in general, is never addressed, the symptoms will most likely continue..." People frequently report feeling that little is being done to try to fix them, leaving them in the hopelessness that comes from forever living in limbo. One aspect of the psychology of being in pain is related to how long it takes to begin some vigorous pain treatment that might also have the potential of curative goals beyond mere pain management.

The quantity of human suffering that would be reduced is staggering if doctors would get to better know and trust their patients. Furthermore, doctors need to modify their treatments according to the patient's needs. Rarely do doctors modify their own personalities or styles according to their patient's needs. By the same token, patients may need to compromise and modify their personalities to meet their doctor's needs. Surviving chronic pain is an lifelong learning and diplomatic process.

...Thought...

> The priest said: "Good to see you, doctor. Do you have a few minutes?
>
> Ever since you invited me to sit in on the medical ethics committee last week, my mind has been reeling. This weekend my sermon will be called 'Thrice the pain' because I cannot empty my mind and heart of the pain patient's story.
>
> My thoughts are brief. Yes, there is a prejudice against pain patients. We treat them as if they have some mental illness, or as if they are very close to becoming mentally ill. You quoted someone, I apologize for not remembering who, but it went something like this: 'the problem is the widespread belief that mental illness is easily faked and doctors are frequently fooled by the illusion.' When you, in the meeting, dropped the words 'mental illness' and replaced it with 'pain', I was, honestly, struck down.
>
> But I should not have been surprised, for in my own profession we deal with the very basis of this same idea. In Samuel, Chapter 21, King David

is described as being: 'so afraid of Achish, the king of Gath. And he changed his behavior before them, and feigned himself mad in their hands, and scrabbled on the doors of the gate, and let his spittle fall down upon his beard.' In other words, he faked his symptoms.

First, these pain patients you talked about were the victims of triggering diseases or accidents. Then they became the victims of the system, insurance companies, medical delays, bad labels, losing jobs, money, etc. You used the phrase 'they are victims twice, once from the injurious event and once from the problems of putting themselves back together.' But I think there is also a further injury, let's call it a third victimization, and it is the on-going fear that if anything bad should happen again, then they additionally suffer from knowing of how it was to fight in the past, and will they be able to do all over again? Will they have the critical energies to get what they need to put their lives back together again? This fear is clearly another insult and it too causes a victimization. They don't fear another accident any more than anyone of us. It's just that they don't know if they can do it all over again. That's the part of the battle that you and don't know much about, but they are the experts. That's the third part of the victimization. Goodness, that's an uphill task..."

Let's end this chapter with a warning. Too many people do not separate us according to our inbuilt differences. We are indeed alike in many ways, yet we are also so different in an equal number of ways. Assuming we are all genetically and structurally equivalent is a misnomer.

> A lawyer made this point: "The legal world is at a historical cross-roads. People are not just bad or evil any more. Neuroscience can now show that a good portion of criminals have measureable abnormalities. The law is not supposed to prosecute if sick! But the law, until recently, did not have the developing science that could give us a brain scan which reflects an illness! Law was easier when we were unable to look into the brains of criminals. We have to work harder than ever to tease apart the causes of behaviors. The old rules were based on too much simplicity. The question is what do we do with someone who, because of an illness, commits a crime that society cannot allow? How do we prevent those crimes from happening? How do we know who are the sick people and who are the 'normal' criminals? And can there even be a psychologically 'normal' criminal? We have such a drug problem in our society. How do we know if a drug user is doing so to calm a psychological problem versus an untreated medical one? When do we vigorously prosecute, and when do we sympathetically hospitalize?"

These same questions apply to medication needing people in pain.

CHAPTER TWENTY
That word addiction

What does the word 'addiction' mean?

Where did it come from?

Why does it carry such a horrible connotation?

It's important to spend additional time on 'that word addiction.'

It's safe to assume that most pain patients have been called a drug addict at least once. Likewise, the doctor who prescribes narcotics will most likely be, at least once, accused of maintaining or encouraging addictions: the doctor is labeled as being a clinical fool or a simple mercenary; his accusers ask: doesn't he see that his patients are con artists?

Is any of this fair?

As a matter of reality, some doctors are indeed blind, naïve, or mercenaries. And some patients are con artists! But the very few must not represent the many. Medical professionals – and indeed all of us – need to know how to separate the few from the many. The heartbreaking product of those who don't know how to do this is that many people suffer.

The use of the word addict has become rampant in our society. We joke and even want to be called certain types of addicts. There are food addicts, work addicts, music addicts, drug addicts, movie addicts, gambling addicts, success addicts, television addicts, animal addicts, tobacco addicts, trivia addicts, religious addicts, sports addicts, idea addicts, sex addicts, history addicts, video game addicts, art addicts, war addicts, fashion addicts, and so on. There are as many types of addicts as there are nouns.

The National Institute on Drug Abuse [228] defines addiction as:

> "A chronic, relapsing brain disease that is characterized by compulsive drug seeking, despite harmful consequences. It is considered a brain disease because drugs change the brain—they change its structure and how it works. These changes can be long lasting, and can lead to harmful behaviors seen in people who abuse drugs....As with any other disease, vulnerability to addiction differs from person to person...and some estimate that genetic factors account for between 40 and 60 percent of a person's vulnerability to addiction, including environment on gene expression and function."

This definition sees addiction as a disease. Can someone accurately be called an addict if their troublesome behaviors stem from an established disease? What control do they have over the origin of the disease?

It's interesting to note how some definitions focus more on a different concept of abuse. For example:

The Drug Enforcement Agency (the DEA) considers abuse as the use of a drug in a manner or in an amount inconsistent with the prevailing medical or social pattern of a culture. The notion of use "beyond the scope of sound medical practice" has been used as well. But this 'sound medical practice' is a changing standard, and what is standard in one community may not be standard in another community. The DEA definition lacks reference to the clinical outcome. It appears the DEA (a law enforcement agency) focuses on abuse, and the National Institute on Drug Abuse (a medical research agency) focuses on disease/addiction.

The American Psychiatric Association (a medical society) considers abuse as a maladaptive pattern of behaviors that lead to a significant impairment or distress. Many psychiatrists must take the time to separate addictive from abuse patterns. These distinctions can be difficult to delineate and require a solid data base of background material.

When a vaccine or medical intervention finally exists that can stop drug addiction, the delineation will become clearer. We will be able to say that Mr. A used the drugs because of an uncontrollable disease, and Mr. B used the same drugs – maybe even in the same pattern – because of unsolvable psychological problems. The vast majority of pain patients will be in a third tier of people using the same drugs, because they fall into neither the addiction nor abuse categories. They are the medical users. What a remarkably different set of implications, value judgments, etc., will come to the table when we can make these separations; the politics will disappear as the science arrives.

A recent publication brings us face to face with the challenging issues between the amount of medication needed and used, the issues of addiction, the definitions of a proper dose, etc. This is the news report:

> **Genetic abnormalities in cytochrome P450 linked to quick opioid uptake.**
>
> "Chronic pain patients who require high doses of opioids may lead clinicians to suspect them as possible addicts or abusers." However, after assessing '15 chronic pain patients who required

1,000 mg or more of a morphine equivalent per day,' researchers discovered that "genetic abnormalities in cytochrome P450 may cause some patients to metabolize opioids at an accelerated rate, prompting the need for higher doses of medication to control pain." Lead author Forest Tennant, MD, "suspects that the abnormalities involve a 'lazy gene' that only responds to higher doses of a medication." [229]

The implications of this finding are profound. Now a genetic variant must be considered as part of any evaluation when a person needs higher than usual doses of medications. This possible genetic disease, per se, dilutes or removes some of the addiction allegations. Needless to say, though Tennant's exact findings are quite exciting, they need to be further tested. But look at the trend! The issue of slow and rapid metabolizers is not new to science, so reports like this make us re-think and mix new findings into the older concepts in order try to explain why something is occurring. Today, doctors have charts of the various P450 system interactions so they can anticipate how genetic variations can alter medication blood levels.

Consider this idea as a possible (yet overly simple) test for addiction versus non-addiction use: a chronic pain patient needing higher doses of medications does indeed test positive for the cytochrome P450 abnormality. A equally high dose user who does not have this same abnormality may then qualify as an addict. However, it is important to remember that other, still unknown variables may be the real cause of the high use in the person without the genetic abnormality. The key is to remember that once we did not have any genetic material to use as a centrifuge to separate the abnormal from the non-abnormal. What next discovery will help us do even better separations?

Addiction is still very much the outcome of entwined psychological and physiological workings.

Addiction has been referred to as a primary *disease* that manifests itself with behaviors that include a loss of control over drug use despite the reality that the use causes harm. The use is also compulsive, with a craving for additional drug use.

Dependence is a term slowly replacing addiction. It is a physical dependence resulting from the body's chronic exposure to some drug that results in a biological tolerance. A withdrawal syndrome follows if the drug is stopped too quickly. The psychiatric aspects of a dependence are the inability to reduce drug use, a preoccupation with drug-seeking behaviors, some compulsive use, and a vulnerability to relapse even after stopping the drugs. Interestingly, the majority of pain patients do not have a tendency towards relapse once the pain is gone. Any concern of with a pain patient's 'preoccupation with drug seeking behavior' is actually related to wanting to keep the pain under control. This speaks to pseudoaddiction and iatraddiction.

Is uncontrolled pain an environmental stressor that can lead to addiction? Here is the question: If the body fails to provide relief using its own inherent mechanisms, might someone who is biologically or psychologically predisposed to addiction be at a higher risk for addiction when they are thrown into the world of persistent pain? Remember, people come into the pain phase of their lives with all sorts of pre-pain characteristics. An important question to ask is how was it that a person avoided pain medication misuse through all the years before the pain started?

> "Man, I never needed stuff like morphine before this pain hit me. When the doctor gave it to me, something odd happened. The pain went away, but so did my uneasiness. Now the doctor wants to lower the morphine dose, and I know I can't do it. Maybe I was born to be an addict, but I was lucky that the pressures of life never hit me like it did. My brain didn't know what morphine could do for it....or how susceptible I would be to the morphine."

Or:

> "I never took a pain med in my life. But after the fall, and before the spinal surgery, I sure was using a lot of medication. One of the nurses in the hospital said I had turned into an addict. Baloney and balderdash! Two months after the surgery I was without both the pain and the pain meds. That nurse needs not to be so quick to assume...."

Some addictions are legal. Some are not. There is no categorical and clinical demarcation between the legal and non-legal addictions since any addiction (and it's not always a drug addiction) can be harmful to the addict and others involved in the addict's world. Consider how many success-addicts wreck havoc on others through their shady business deals or impassionate social concerns;

people whose addiction is for social power and success can destroy cultures and ruin entire civilizations! Tobacco and alcohol addiction is medically costly. Are these not socially dangerous addictions? A religious fanatic or unscrupulous politician can cause mayhem and despair.

Endless discussions exist amongst professionals about the actual definition of an addiction. It's like physicists who want to define dark energy – they know it's out there, yet it still defies definition.[230] Addictions occur without a certainty of what causes them. The last few decades have offered ideas that 'explain addictions', but in truth they are more likely to 'describe more than explain'. Strong programs like AA and NA control by teaching people how to resist the pull of the addictions; this suggests that the psychological aspects of addiction may even be stronger than the biological ones.

> "A growing number of researchers believe that the same processes lie behind all addictions, behavioral or chemical, whether it's gambling or shopping, computer gaming, love, work, exercise, pornography, eating or sex. They have more in common than different. It is said that as many as 10 percent of the US population will soon have a gambling problem....(and) there is no scientific consensus about how to define substance addictions, let alone behavioral ones...(yet) a key element is that addiction dominates people's lives.....and as time goes on, a greater dose is needed for the same effect....(and) there is a strong link underlying the vulnerability to drug addiction that increases vulnerability to compulsive behavior...(so) cravings can return by strong memories and drug taking locations."[231]

> Such highlights as these offer further points of separation between the pain patient and the addict. One of the key points in the above paragraph is how many drug abusers relapse once they go back near the places or people in which they once used the drugs – the memories themselves are terrible risk points.

The concern about addiction is so widespread that even non-scientific publications discuss it. In October 2008, *The Economist*,[232] ran a piece that "People are programmed for addiction." The reward pathways needed for survival can be subverted by chemicals and by certain behaviors, like gambling. It spoke of studies with GABA, NAC (N-acetylcysteine) and the fatty acid DHA, all of which are suggested as having an ability to reduce addictions. But treating addictions remains to be very difficult. The article goes on to report that the British National Treatment Agency "suggests that only 11% of those who start treatment complete it and are drug-free after 12 weeks."

But of course, these addicts were not pain patients. The typical path of the pain patient's entry into pain medication use is along other roads.

The word 'addict' comes from a sense of having to give something away or of having been taken over by some outside force. There is the sense of being attached to something bad. Maybe there is a sense that the devil or another evil force has taken control of the person. Regardless, the sneering upshot of the word is the assumption that the addict is a weak, lazy, childlike person who isn't taking responsibly for his behaviors. Addiction to drugs is often considered a sign of emotional irresponsibility and untrustworthiness. Of course, these implications will change if it is reclassified as a medical or neurological disease. If it remains to be a psychiatric disease, then it must gain the diagnostic confidence and status of a bipolar or schizophrenic condition.

Saunders and Cottler [233] provide some other key insights. It's interesting how the changes in the DSM paralleled the attitudinal changes towards the narcotic needing pain patient. Note also that the authors use the term 'use' and not 'abuse':

> "The first edition of DSM was published in 1952 and comprised a standardized nomenclature, definitions of disorders and statistical classification. Substance use disorders did not have a separate category. Instead they were grouped under the personality disorders. The statement that 'addiction is usually symptomatic of a personality disorder' reflected the view that there was a primary disorder of personality and that alcohol and drug issues were simply manifestations of this. This conceptualization continued until the third edition was published in 1980. In DSM-III (1987) substance use disorders were classified separately from other mental health conditions. A distinction was made between substance abuse and dependence. Substance abuse was defined as pathological use and impairment in social or occupational functioning. Dependence required pathological use and some impairment with evidence of tolerance or withdrawal. Subsequent revisions to DSM (III-R and IV) emphasized a broader-based concept of substance dependency."

The International Classification of Diseases (ICD) is another major medical diagnostic system. The ICD-10, published in 1992, has similar concepts of substance dependency to those in the DSM-IV, but the ICD added the term "harmful use." One of the differences between the ICD and DSM system is that the ICD does not admit social problems into its diagnosis criteria, which is the Axis IV category in the DSM system; this is the place to list issues with jobs, home, money, etc., that complicate and mitigate a patient's life. Some institutions and countries use the ICD coding systems. Other systems use the DSM manual. It can be confusing at times.

There are three central aspects to any substance use disorder: substance dependence, substance abuse, and/or harmful use. This triad model allows for people to be physiologically dependant but still properly functioning, which would be the case of a properly medicated pain patient. Clearly the universal and final definition of drug use, addiction, abuse, and harmful use is still unsettled.

Saunders and Cottler want to see the incorporation of the burgeoning knowledge about substance abuse into the diagnostic systems. "In particular, the present diagnostic terms and criteria reflect essentially clinical descriptions of cognitive symptoms, behavioral manifestations and physiological symptoms that were developed from the 1930's to the 1980's." The terms need to reflect the neurobiological and the sociocultural influences that condition an addiction. Finally they hope that updated terms will reflect the broader range of uncontrollable and obsessive behaviors, as well as mentioning the notion of salience (this is the giving up certain activities because of the dependency). The update should include the addition of gambling and computer games, as well as the full scope of non-substance using but still quite damaging and repetitive behaviors.

Drug or medication use that is 'out of the ordinary' is often considered as 'sufficient' criteria of addiction or abuse. This has been called 'aberrant medication-taking' behavior. Many physicians find it worrisome. Ballantyne and Mao believe aberrant medication taking behavior is a manifestation of addiction,[234] but this may be too limited because it doesn't include the notions of drug metabolic variance, pseudoaddiction, and iatraddiction. Out of the ordinary use does not necessarily mean bad. Again, the notion of addiction was, by and large, born from the 'non-pain patient' medication/drug users. An over inclusion of pain patients in this notion is inappropriate. And as noted above, cytochrome P450 variances may also play a central role in these definitions.

At the risk of being repetitive, the decisive issue is how to isolate those people who use these medications for pain reasons versus non-pain reasons. Some of the principal terms may themselves add to the confusion. For example, narcotics are known as pain relievers. So the press will often use a phrase similar to this: 'the non-medical use of pain relievers significantly increased in the last few years.' The inclusion of pain in that sentence is confusing and, by sloppy implication, mixes the pain patient user and the non-patient pain user into one group. Finding and sticking to the correct diagnosis, definition, or the motivation supporting the use of a narcotic is a key task for any narcotic prescriber. Many journalists need to do the same homework.

Many studies show the rates of addiction in chronic pain groups tend to be similar to the rates of addiction in the non-pain suffering general public.[235 236] Weaver and Schnoll wrote that because the incidence rates are so similar that "no firm conclusions can be drawn about the rate of addiction among patients with chronic nonmalignant pain that results in abuse of opioids."[237] This simply means that using narcotics for pain control does not increase the chance of addiction or abuse. Brown wrote that chronic nonmalignant pain may not be directly associated with a higher risk of addiction: he said that the risks reside in the presence of substance abuse that 'preceded the onset of the pain,' and that "chronic back pain did not connote special risk for current substance use disorders." [238]

> "I had it real emotionally bad after for a couple of years, and yeah, I did drugs then. But then I stopped them. But then I got hurt! And no doctor would give me enough medications because they said I would be using them like I did years ago. That was so wrong! So I went back to my old street drug sources. I hated doing that, but it worked. Anyway, I decided to find a doctor rather continue with my street suppliers. It took some time, but I did find one, and he worked with me, and I was real honest with him, and it took a lot of work and trust between us, and I needed a lot of meds to control the pain, but I am working again, and life is good again, and I learned a lot. So did I abuse pain pills earlier in my life? – yes. Was it wrong? – yes. Did I self medicate for a while after I was hurt? – yes. Was it wrong? – yes. But now my doctor says I'm a user, not an abuser, and that makes perfect sense to me and my family."

In 2007, ten years after the Brown paper, Martell said that "substance abuse disorders are common in patients taking opioids for back pain, and aberrant medication-taking behaviors occur in up to 24% of cases".[239] Needless to say, there is remains so much controversy in this field. The debate continues at full throttle. Great care must be used when accepting these numbers. Great care must be taken regarding how carefully these studies were done, etc.

Several problems exist with Martell's conclusion. Martell used a technique known as a meta-analysis, which means he used data and conclusions culled from other studies. That means all the strengths and weaknesses in those other studies were blended into his final conclusion; the conclusion assumes that there were no critical flaws in the studies they used. This is statistically treacherous. This type of meta-analysis project is best described by "you are what you eat." Let's look at some of the material carried into the conclusion. No clinical trial in the review evaluated the efficacy of opioid treatment for longer than 16 weeks – and we don't know if/how/when the patient was adequately treated in those 16 weeks. Then there is the statement that 24% of the patients showed aberrant behaviors. It leaves the careful analyst asking 'why did this happen?' Perhaps the aberrant behaviors resulted from inadequate dosing. Again, a study is only as good as the care and purity of the people being studied, the reliability and nature of the measuring tools, the personalities, consistencies and skills of the study coordinators, and so. We must not give more credit to any study than it strictly deserves.

It is still difficult for many people to think that addicted people can be dependable, trustworthy, and honest. Perhaps we need to coin separate words for each of these types of addictions, such as started by Weissman in 1987 with his new word 'pseudoaddiction'.

> Many years ago I needed to simplify the differences between pain patients and addicts. This is how I did it:
>
> **Addicts use drugs to escape the world, while pain patients use medications to re-join the world.**

The medical community has an on-going fear of missing or feeding an addiction. Weaver and Schnoll offer a first-rate paper to discuss this. [240] They also offer an algorithm to manage the opioid using, non-malignant pain patient. This excellent paper has the effect of converting the complex needs of a pain patient into simpler, and more effective, therapeutic encounters.

Unlike the stereotyped addict, the pain-patient 'addict' (if we must use the term) most often had a significant career and reasonably grounded relationships prior to the need for the pain medications. So the need for medications is not an effort to sustain an emotional deviancy. They are not lazy people. Their central concern is to return to the life that existed before the injury or disease. Compare this with the drug addicted person who loathes his life both before and after his addiction began.

One priceless diagnostic clue is to ask a patient or user if they would be pleased to go back to the psychological world that existed before the drug use began. The response to this question is an obvious window into their psychologies.

Tobacco is a very addicting drug, but it is not ranked and housed with the same degree of negative undertones as are the other traditional drugs of addiction, such as cocaine, oxycodone, or alcohol. It appears that some of this is related to the notion of the 'social burden.' This means that people do not rob or have automobile accidents because of tobacco use. The immediate cost to society for smoking too much is less than the cost of drinking too much beer. Other than second hand smoke, a smoker has little influence on other lives. Of course the impact of smoking on the medical side of things is unbelievably enormous, and so its eventual social cost is therefore much higher than the costs of the traditional addicting drugs. Tobacco and cocaine both kill, but they do it differently. Interestingly, the FDA just got the legal authority to oversee tobacco use. It is important to include in the operational aspects of the word addiction the notion of the social burden.

Another useful diagnostic tool to help identify an addiction is to know the 'rhythm' of a person's life. The rhythm is the clustering of all their good and bad days, thoughts, feelings, hopes, etc. Asking a person to describe the rhythm of their life can be illuminating. I often ask patients to try to put their lives into a poem. Even the non-poets like this offer. They then offer me words to describe their lives, and then I ask for them to overlay these words with their rhythms. "Ok, so you say you are too sensitive to others. How does that fit when you have a bad day fighting with your wife?" It is as if this project pulls back the curtains so light can enter the room. We can then see how an emotional response to an experience combines their words to their rhythms. This exercise picks up on the rhythm of a person's life, and it can be the one of best hints as to the person's psychological signature.

> "Hey, I met the doc today for the third time. I thought he was kinda silly caused last time he asked me to write a poem about myself on good days, and one about myself on bad days. Yeah, me writing a poem! I planned to just get my meds from him. But I wrote it anyway – felt silly too. But a neat thing happened. I kinda really told him how I feel. He laughed that my poem didn't rhyme too well. I laughed too. Then he told me to keep a diary and put my feelings down whenever I felt the need. He called them my rhythms. So here am me, the big tough football guy, writing poetry. But I think it worked, and I think I shared something about me that will make difference between him and me. No other doctor even got close to

> this....and then I asked if I could read some of his poetry. He said sure!"

The scientific problem with rhythms is that it is impossible to have complete knowledge of a person's rhythms. At any given moment a person has both a past and a future. The future has certain challenges. The observer, (who may be biased by his own history), uses a tiny spot of time and data from the patient to try to understand all of that person's life. The observer might then mix his own rhythm with that of the patients.

Psychotherapy devotes considerable effort to capture the nature and form of all these rhythms. The more rhythms explored, the better will be the understanding of why people choose to act in a particular way. Such insight in invaluable in the understanding of the 'if or why' of an addiction. It can also direct the therapy into the areas that need repair.

The word addiction connotes a sense that 'you are different from me' in a deviant or odd way. It can imply that 'Your rhythm is different than mine'. But in that implication is the allegation that '*your rhythm is bad* and *mine is good*' Consider that 'addiction', as a pigeonholing noun, often rests atop of speculations that tolerate premature verdicts because the conclusions are allowed to be based on too limited an exposure to the person's entire life. Too little time is spent looking for the bona fide motivations for what evolved into what may be called an addiction.

Anyone who has ever needed a drink to control anxiety knows that they are asking the alcohol to deal with the stress at hand. This is not necessarily a sign of being an addict. Yet many people consider asking for even a single alcoholic drink to calm themselves down is an addictive maneuver. On occasion the tossing onto a person the 'addictive label' is to suggest that the person has a 'fondness to giving over the responsibility of one's own life's decisions to someone or something else.' This separation from facing one's personal responsibilities is one basis of the Alcoholics Anonymous and other treatment protocols.

> Addiction, as a word, has been so misused that its real definition is hard to pin down. It has been called a scapegoat moral term for what society feels is unacceptable or unusual behavior. Obviously, the definitions of being 'unacceptable or unusual' are commonly fraught and burdened with more opinion than fact.
>
> Interestingly, the word addict was once an adjective, not a noun. It's said that Shakespeare was the first known writer to use it with the sense of a 'strong inclination.' In Henry V, the king was known to have an addiction to vanity:
>
> *"His addiction was to courses vain;*
> *His companies unletter'd, rude, and shallow;*
> *His hours fill'd up with riots, banquets, sports;*
> *And never noted in him any study,*
> *Any retirement, any sequestration*
> *From open haunts and popularity."* [241]
>
> The implication is, therefore, that an 'addiction' produces no valued or important activity. For many years there was also a sense that many addictive behaviors were harmless. Now it suggests either something is bad, or that the addict is a pathetically troubled person who lost of control over some significant aspect of life and who is not engaged in any socially sanctioned and productive activity.

For the many who seek spiritual or religious treatments for their addictions, more and more power must be handed over to a deity or other entities. This means that the older addictive self, which wasn't working right, is given the chance to be replaced by a better self. The old self is gladly lost. This is not the case with the vast majority of pain patients because their former selves were usually quite functional. They want the old back again.

> A 45 year old woman was in extraordinary pain. She hurt as much as she suffered. She had the choice of losing all self-identity in a sea of agony and being totally immobilized, or of loosing less self-identity when she used medications to reduce the pain. With less pain she could at least attend to some of her social activities, she could maintain a part-time job, and she could be a mother, etc. In agony she was forced into a total sick and dependant role; with less pain she functioned in a more normal role. Her doctor told her she needed a better attitude towards her life and the pain, and he recommended counseling with her minister. He also said he was worried about her desire to use medications.
>
> Her minister told her that she needs to hand her pain over to God. He suggested that her pain was in part due to several improper choices she made earlier in her life. But she didn't want to give up her prior self. She said there was no shame in what she did years ago. The minister said she was in denial, lest she would not be in as much pain. So she changed churches and later handed over her pain to a more aggressive

doctor. Interestingly, she was referred to the new doctor by the new minister. She got better spiritually and physically. She said she never realized how important it was that her doctor and minister be part of the same treatment team. "They know this in hospice and sometimes in the hospital, but hardly in out-patient care. By changing the doctor and the minister, I went from being considered a possible addict to not."

Most classic 'addicts' are troubled people who lack many social and emotional skills. Interestingly, using this definition means that most pain patients are not addicts since they have social skills and very much want to be productive and responsible. But these innocent victims of pain are made to feel guilty by an irreplaceable association with the narcotic molecule.

Feldman and Thielbar offer this definition of addiction: *"a distinct life style is evident when a single activity or interest pervades a person's other interests and unrelated activities—a drug addict is an extreme example."* [242]

Addiction has also been defined as 'a need repeatedly gratified by a substitution at the expense of something else.' This is a good descriptive definition because addiction, in its broadest sense, is always a compromise. But these definitions don't embrace the motivations for the addictive behaviors.

"I'm a physician with severe back pain. I hate to admit to it, but it's beyond anything I can control. And I take a lot of medications! My doctor keeps telling me that the dose is not as important as are the good effects, and little by little I'm learning that he is correct. One of my less enlightened old friends asked me if I'm addicted to the narcotic. Well, I knew I wasn't, but I had to prove it. So I started reading, and this is what I found. First, addiction is a chronic disorder, a brain disease. People who deal with addicts know that it is relapsing condition, and that continued abstinence is unlikely unless there is massive treatment. I started narcotic use only after the injury, so the addiction disease did not exist before the accident, so I don't have the brain disease. So I am not addicted! Isn't that a great thing to point out to people!

But I am surely physiologically dependant on an external source of opioids to do what my body cannot. I call myself a comorbid addict – the co-morbidity confuses people and makes them ask what I mean. I tell them that my co-morbid condition is pain. Take away the comorbid condition and the 'addiction' condition, to use their term, the 'addiction' will go away with it. It's all in the wording...."

Therefore, to understand addiction, one must ask this question:

What is the drug doing for the person that the person cannot do for himself?

This question has also been asked in a more philosophic voice:

It is not what a man does that distinguishes him, but how and why he does it.

One of the very finest comments about this came out during a talk between a nurse and a narcotic using pain patient. The nurse asked "What are you addicted to?" The patient answered "I'm addicted to no pain and to life. If and when you really get to know me, then you'd know that."

Too many think that addiction is one of the greatest health problems of our age. Wrong. The greatest problem is the pain. Were there be no pain, there would be no addiction. It is complicated because the pain can be emotional or physical. But really, need more be said?

Robert DuPont was the first director of the National Institute on Drug Abuse, and he was the "drug czar" under the Nixon, Ford, and Carter administrations. His excellent book, *The Selfish Brain,* outlines the theorized biological basis of addiction.[243] He talks about the neurohormone communication between various parts of the brain, and especially the ventral tegmental area and the nucleus accumbens, which are the sources of pleasure. Exposure to pleasure coming from these systems can produce an addiction. Part of the drive towards an *addiction* is towards the sense of euphoria.

> The pathophysiology of addiction is best described as a series of neurobiological changes following the exposure to opiates or other certain types of medications. We will limit this discussion to the opiates.
>
> The body's cells cease to function or degenerate, causing the user to be physically dependant on the external supply of opiates. We know, at a molecular level, that the opiates can alter the receptor kinetics and how signals are then sent from cell to cell. The tolerance to opiates can also be influenced by the environment

surrounding the user. If a person is around cues that were once associated with drug use, then these 'reminder cues' can induce drug craving. This seems to complicate the definition of addiction because the mere memory of a feeling can cause a desire. This can happen even long after a full detoxification is finished. This phenomenon emphasizes the intersection between a distorted chemical system, with some disease predisposition, and a top layer of an icing with psychological associations.

Every pain patient knows here is no euphoria from the use of pain medications. A confusion may appear because there is too little emphasis spent on the different responses that occur even though 'the same chemical systems' are being employed by both pain and non-pain of users. As a patient said "We and addicts both use Oxycontin® but for totally different reasons." It speaks once again to the fact that the traditional notions of addiction do not unanimously apply to pain patients. In fact, DuPont makes the distinction (page 127):

> "...the reason the addicted person is using alcohol or other drugs over a prolonged period of time can be traced to the person's love affair with getting high, not to the discomfort of a preexisting disease. People who are not vulnerable biologically to addiction, and who experience anxiety, depression, pain, and other uncomfortable feelings, do not become addicted to alcohol and other abused drugs, even if they are exposed to them and find some temporary relief from their discomfort as a result of their use of these substances."

A familiar problem is what to do when a person who is biologically vulnerable to addiction legitimately needs pain medications. This issue was also discussed thirty years ago (in 1967) by Petrie, [244] who noted that people differ in the intensity with which they modulate experiences; some reduce and some increase what is perceived. This is a genetically based difference which may apply to being biologically vulnerable to addiction. We cannot measure the genetic vulnerability, but we can monitor how a person responds to narcotic use, and often, with great care, the situation can be kept focused on pain control without it growing into the more nefarious forms of addiction. Also, what happens if a person discovers that his years of secret anxiety disappear when on pain medications following a legitimate illness? These are complex but central issues in the care of anyone needing pain management. These clinical situations are more difficult to manage, but they are definitely manageable.

One reason for the heavy focus on the euphoria associated with narcotic use stems from a 1959 work by Beecher.[245] He wrote that opiates work not on the pain impulse but on the psychological overlap of pain because they lower anxiety. This comment is a complex response, because the pain may indeed be less if the anxiety is less, and the anxiety may be less because the pain is being treated, so the suffering is less, and so it goes on and on and around and around. By and large, this manner of euphoria, as noted elsewhere, is not the pejorative flavored and intoxicated form of euphoria coming from escape, but is the celebratory form of euphoria coming from relief.

...Thought...

When suffering and tragedy strike without any explanation once, twice, and repeatedly, individuals in the community no longer know what kind of world they are living in. Like Job, they ask "Why do You hide Your face and treat me like an enemy?" (Job 13:24) [246]

"Pain, having no other locus but the conscious ego, is almost literally the price man pays for the possession of a conscious ego. Unless there is an awake and conscious organism, there is nothing one can sensibly refer to as pain." [247]

Suffering is a serious religious problem. It diminishes the covental passion for God. Theologians study the causes of suffering because it appears to be incompatible with a caring and benevolent God. The anthropologist, in contrast, re-forms this situation into a different question: he asks how one can maintain the continuity, stability and predictability of an on-going relationship with a God given all the shocks of life?

One answer is in the act of *mitzvah*, or 'good acts.' Doing *mitzvah* is an emphasis on one's behavior in this world, but it is based on an expectation to reap prosperity in the World to Come. The sense is that the current suffering is the tuition that must be paid to get a better afterlife.

> A deeply religious man told me: "When people strive to be righteous in this world, God's response is to inflict upon them suffering that will expiate their sins, so that they can enjoy complete bliss in the World to Come. Those who prefer iniquity are allowed to prosper in this world, because they have already ensured themselves punishment in the World to Come.
>
> But what of those of us without sin who want to give good thought and good bounty to this world, but because of our pain, we cannot do

that good. I am one such person. I did only a fraction of the good I wanted to do until I found the right doctor. One prior doctor said that he had to call me an addict because of amount of medication I needed. I believe I sinned by calling him crazy to his face! It made me think how I was enslaved to my pain and to the doctors whose pens could order me medications – I still look with amazement at the pen the doctor uses to write my prescriptions – that line of ink is a link to my sanity!

But the pain made me unable to do what I wanted to do. In that pondering, I came to realize that I am really addicted to life. I'm sure you've heard that before. I am gaining my entry tokens and points into heaven…that's nice. I can happily live with the medication if it allows me to maintain my addiction to life! But what is so interesting to me is how much my work with pain patients is quite different now when I go minister in the hospital and nursing homes.

Rabbis remind us to eliminate our expectations of any reward for good deeds done in this world, and to remember that the relationship with God does not end with death. People who suffer cannot be allowed to 'grow weary of God's covenant and despair of his love.' Moments of joy must become signs of divine approval. Through joyful occasions comes the strength to take life's disappointments in stride because joy is the pleasure of anticipating a future good. I'm working to keep myself addicted to that future of a good life here on earth. And

I work hard to share it with others. But my pain meds are the tires on my car – I need them to get around."

A wounded soldier in chronic pain said:

"My joy was stolen. The pain took it."

How do we address the suffering from a tragedy?

Rabbis ask after tragedies: 'What can we learn from this?' The suggestion that we should learn from a tragedy is a pittance of a response that for many does not befit the degree of suffering. But in a famous phrase, the notion exists that suffering is the product of one's incorrect ways. "If a man sees that painful sufferings visit him, let him examine his conduct. For it is said: 'Let us search and probe our ways, and return to the Lord.' (Lam 3:40) If he examines and finds nothing, let him attribute it to the neglect of the study of the Torah....If it did not attribute it [to that], and still did not find [anything amiss], let him be sure that these are chastenings of love." The question is if suffering comes from one's one choice versus that of a random accident, or from or by the design or sloppiness of other people.

It is hard for people to continually interpret suffering after a tragedy as an expression of God's love. The afterlife is a wonderful notion, and may indeed be a correct one. But when a young person anticipates that life will pass by without him being able to participate in the joys and activities of normal human experiences, then maintaining any comfort from those distant rewards redeemable in an afterlife can seriously lose their lure. If, however, suffering comes into a person's life long after they have achieved a mature relationship with life and with their God, then their established beliefs may sustain them. But if the suffering is too great, then even the time-honed beliefs may crumble.

Early death would be a logical route if someone feels that a sufficient down payment had already been made for an assured reward in eternity. Of course none of us knows exactly how much of a down payment is needed. And furthermore, it is difficult to accept why such misery and suffering is required by a loving God. It seems cruel. Perhaps the afterlife notion exists to offer a glimmer of hope and a reason d'être for people stuck in earthly pain. For many, this can challenge their basic faith. And thankfully, for many of them, the faith works.

> An honorable, but vociferous 72 year old man grew up in a deeply religious home. His cancer pain was incredible, but he did not yet qualify for hospice care. His medication needs were called by some as an addiction, which astonished and deeply wounded him that he could ever be so branded. He took it the same as being called a criminal, which in turn made him feel doubly bad because he felt he had been thrown into the leprosy camp of addicts. His own ego and soul could not understand why Got both let his pain be so horrific and why He allowed people to so label him in that way. His

insurance company also limited his pain prescriptions, so his family gave him financial assistance. All these united into a sense of despair, disgrace, and fear.

Because he was so religious, his suicide was quite a surprise. In one of our last visits, he jokingly quipped that he needed to "hurry up and get to God to get this all straightened out." He once said "So many suggest I am addicted to these medications. No, I am instead addicted to the notion that they don't work. I try so hard, but I can't accept the attitudes around me. I am addicted to God – soon it will be time to go home."

CHAPTER TWENTY-ONE
Pain in the dying versus pain in the living

"I'd get better care if I was dying."

No one seems to be upset when a dying person gets medication to control the pain. It is unarguably humane to die without pain and with some peace. But must a non-dying person, with severe pain, have to fight for pain medications? Shouldn't they be allowed to live in peace?

There is usually nothing to gain from death. Dying can't be faked. Death offers pain-lacking, hospitable fixtures. We end up trusting death more than we trust life because we know what the future holds after death – no more suffering.

So why is there a reluctance to adequately treat pain in the living? What topics need to be further understood in order to better care for those living with pain?

Ask about a doctor's attitudes towards giving narcotics to the dying: in the answer will be great insights into the doctor's psychological signature. Then ask about the doctor's attitudes about giving narcotics to non-malignant pain patients. Compare the two signatures.

Perhaps doctors fear their own deaths such that their treatment styles of the dying reflect these fears. Indeed, the doctor's own fear can affect how they view all of their patient's sufferings. Real pain management is more than the mere mechanical efforts to quell the physical chemistry of pain. Pain management attention must be allotted to the suffering caused by the pain.

Doctors know they will unlikely be prosecuted for giving 'narcotics as needed' to a dying patient. This can even elevate the doctor up to a hero level in the eyes of the patient's family. Impending deaths also limit the length of the treatment course, so it is also a shorter professional risk and emotional involvement for the doctor.

> "The doc gave us pretty much what my Dad needed. But the doc knew my father would be dead soon and no one would fault him for easing the pain of a dying old soldier."

Patients dying of cancer often suffer terrible pain. But patients living with cancer can also suffer equal pain, and thus the admonition that "No patient with cancer needs to live or die with unrelieved pain."[248] The United States Government has issued guidelines to deal with cancer pain.[249] When other treatments fail to control cancer pain, and narcotics must be started, then the government's publication states:

> "Opioid tolerance and physical dependence are expected with long term opioid treatment and should not be confused with psychological dependence ("addiction"), manifested as drug abuse behavior. The misunderstanding of these terms in relation to opioid use leads to ineffective practices in prescribing, administering, and dispensing opioids for cancer pain and contributes to the problem of under treatment. The presence of opioid tolerance and dependence does not equate with addiction."

Over time, some chronic pain conditions may need larger doses. Many fear giving extra pain meds to the non-terminal patients because of fear that an unruly pattern of escalating doses will follow. However, the same government publication states:

> "Increasing dose requirements are more consistently correlated with progressive disease which increases pain intensity. Patients with stable disease do not usually require increasing doses"

So a change in the needed dose may be actually signaling a change in the disease state, rather than it being a biological lessening of the response to the pain medications. This logic actually applies to any condition that is causing pain.

'Pseudotolerance' is another term that effectively stands for needing more medications. But this tolerance can come from more than a worsening in the disease state. It can come from doing more in life because the pain is under better control. It can even be a measure of how much the quality of live is improving. So pseudotolerance can exist either because things are getting better or worse.

> "When the doctor started me on meds, it was wonderful. I slept better, my mood wasn't as hopeless, I ate dinner with my family – it was great. But then I wanted to help shop, and stand up longer to make the salads, and even take short walks. That pushed the limits of what the pain meds could control, so I needed more meds. At first people just looked at my use and said I was going tolerant. Nope, I was growing intolerant of the former life style. It was really a pseudotolerance. We went up about 20% on the meds and that made it possible to go up

> 70% on my life...and my doc, he said that the only difference between me and a cancer patient was not the pain, but the absence of the lethal condition...then he said the suffering was my lethal condition – what a great doctor..."

A popular medical textbook advised physicians not to let people suffer. This is from the 1985 edition of Goodman and Gilman:

> "*Pain in Terminal Illness.* Although they are not requisite or even desirable in all cases of terminal illness, the euphoria, tranquility, and analgesia afforded by the use of opioids can make the final days far less distressing for the patient and his family. Some degree of physical dependence and tolerance develops whenever an opioid is given in therapeutic dosage several times a day over a prolonged period. In patients with painful terminal illnesses such considerations should not in any way prevent the physician from fulfilling his primary obligation to ease the patient's discomfort. The physician should not wait until the pain becomes agonizing; *no patient should ever wish for death because of his physician's reluctance to use adequate amounts of effective opioids* Such patients, while they may be physically dependent, are not considered "addicts" even they may need large doses on a regular basis; in states that require the reporting of addicts, patients with terminal illnesses should not be reported." [250]

There should be no suffering in the dying or in the living.

Narcotic use during pregnancy

It's a widespread and accepted caveat that a pregnant woman ought to use the least amount of medication possible. That includes narcotics. But what happens if legitimate pain patients on narcotics get pregnant? It is a difficult situation.

Narcotics are known to pass through the placenta to the fetus. So the baby is born addicted and will require detoxification and withdrawal. The other concern is the effect of the narcotics on the fetal development. This is a very specialized area of medicine, and if a narcotic using pain patient becomes pregnant, then a detailed series of explorations needs to follow. Hopefully this all happens in the planning phase before getting pregnant. But sometimes it is after the fact.

First, the obstetrician, working with the pain management doctor, must see if any available and less dangerous means of pain control is possible during the pregnancy. A careful withdrawal may be needed. If pain medications are needed to maintain the woman's quality of life, then the doctor must confer with a geneticist and other professions who monitor and know the latest literature about the effects of different medications on a developing fetus. Then all involved, the patient, the father, any other important people and key relatives, and the doctors, must have a risk-to-benefit meeting. It is from this that pain treatment decisions must be developed. Again, this is not an easy process in many ways. The best plan is usually to be off all medications during a pregnancy.

...Thought...

As a bit of history to illuminate –

In 1964, Helen Neal's brother complained of severe pain from his tongue cancer. Even her employer, the

National Institute of Health (NIH), near Washington, DC, had no one to help him. At the time, no NIH unit existed to study or treat pain.

Eventually she found Seattle surgeon Dr. John Bonica, who had been an advocate for better pain control for many years. In 1947 he established one of the very first pain clinics (in Tacoma, Washington). In 1953 he wrote one of the first books on pain control.[251] By the 1970's, he had helped form the International Association for the Study of Pain, which was a key in the fostering of better pain control efforts. The professional journal *Pain* was first established in 1975. Since then other professional journals have been born, and the literature is reporting more and more work about the control of pain. His work was one of the vital seeds leading to all these developments.

By the way, in 1978, Ms. Neal wrote *The Politics of Pain*, which became a pioneering book in its own right. [252] It is well worth reading.

Why did it take so long for the medical profession to embrace appropriate pain control? Why wasn't it seen as an obvious branch of medicine's tools? A quick history lesson will explain. Since the eighteenth century the fundamental aim of medicine has been to find the cause of disease and then produce a treatment thereof. Once curing meant 'to relieve' the symptoms, but over the years it came to mean the eradication of the cause; this is because some eradications became real possibilities. The clinical aim could go past the mere manipulation of the clinical signs and unwanted symptoms. Chronic pain management, however, is still largely symptom relief because most often pain management controls, but does not eradicate, the problem.

Pain was thought to grow from a 'broken process' in the organism, and the doctor was expected to fix the problem. This fit the tenor of the industrial revolution, but pain frustrated the process and hindered the belief that science and devices could magically transform the world. From Wall and Jones: [253]

> "...Such are the genuine triumphs of the shift to science. With the change of attitude, a new hierarchy was established in the medical profession. At the top of the heap were the new action men among the physicians and surgeons. If cancer was diagnosed, the patient and his doctor first seek a surgeon to cut it out and eliminate it. If the cancer is too widespread for surgical excision, the oncologist moves in with the magic bullets of radiation or chemicals that kill the dividing cells.
>
> Other specialties were rather less prestigious. Neurology developed intellectually impressive ways of diagnosing precisely what was wrong with the brain, but for a long time, it was unable to offer cures. Psychiatry contributed methods of interpretation which, by their nature, were less precise. Then came the physiotherapists, nurses, and social workers, who attempted neither diagnosis nor cure—they simply helped people. The phrase 'symptomatic medicine' became synonymous with 'bad medicine'. It was regarded as a concentration on signposts diverting doctors and patients from their logical progress along a road to a clear end. Coupled with the age of reason was a suspicion of pragmatic medicine. If something worked but lacked an evident rationale, it was condemned.

...It is becoming accepted that, while awaiting the definitive solution of diagnosis and cure, it is not contradictory to seek and even demand symptom control. People in pain and those who care for them are also rising up in revolt against their enforced passive waiting until a cure appears. One reaction is to search the classical folk remedies abandoned by modern medicine. Another reaction is to demand a better day-to-day care of the patient, which is another way of describing control of symptoms, principally pain. Until recently, such day to day care was left as it stood in the eighteenth century and took no part in the extraordinary advances since that time."

Wall and Jones offer an insightful note about the tone and tenor between these two questions: 'Why did he die?' versus 'How did he die?' The first is a clinical report of the cause of death. The second is a concern for the degree of suffering felt while dying. Knowing a death was painless offers immense solace to the grieving family.

Despite the many wonderful medical advances, far too many people still needlessly suffer. Old attitudes linger, and some of these may still be given more opinion weight than hard science. Pain patients know all too well about the struggle to be believed. When one is looking towards an impending death, then suffering will also soon end. When one is looking at on-going life, then suffering will not soon end.

Eppur Si Muove is Italian for *'and yet it moves'*. Galileo Galilei (1564–1642) uttered this phrase in 1633 after the Inquisition forced him to repudiate his conviction that Copernicus was correct in that the earth moved around the sun. Suggesting that the earth was not the center of God's universe was heresy. We use this example here to capture that same frustration, which is, and despite what many people may think, that far too many *normal* people needlessly suffer pain. A patient who heard me discuss *eppur si muove* rephrased it like this: "and yet we, the pain patients, unlike what so many people say about us – we want to live, and we are very normal! We really are! Galileo suffered for telling the truth. I can never forget that. I'm telling you the truth – I am normal, the pain is not! Don't make me suffer because of what the un-informed believe. You know what *eppur si muove* really means? It means I am right, you are wrong. But they have the power to make me suffer.....oh my....."

By the way, Galileo could have been sentenced to death for his belief. Instead he spent the last 11 years of his life in a permanent house arrest.

> "On December 7, 1938, the British Broadcasting Corporation (BBC) came to Sigmund Freud's Maresfield Gardens home in London to record a short message. By this time his cancer of the jaw was inoperable and incurable, making speech difficult and extremely painful. After his long struggle with cancer grew intolerable, Freud asked his physician for a fatal injection of morphine. He died on September 23, 1939." [254]

Was Freud's death act of understandable euthanasia?

We should all be shamefaced when we look at the extent of suffering that we impose on each other. Is there some flavor of danger that we detect in a sufferer such that we fear them or we walk away from them? What joy is there, or perhaps there is a lack conscience, in those who watch suffering?

We pity the dying yet deny the living.

CHAPTER TWENTY-TWO
The extended pain patient

"But what do I do while I'm waiting to see the specialist...?"

An ever increasing number of pain patients are finding relief. This is great. Earlier interventions after an injury, better surgical and interventional techniques, more aggressive physical therapy, new medications, the fact that pain centers exist and that research facilities are actively studying pain, the existence of narcotic pumps, internal stimulators, TENS units, a better understanding of the physiology of pain, and so on, all makes it a less painful world for many.

Yet for all of this, which is so good, a massive amount of work still remains because legions of people are still not being helped. Sometimes it is a matter of imperfect medical techniques, but at other times it is from an inappropriate attitude, having to wait, or having no access. "Sometimes it is no more a matter than I got no money." Often it is a combination of all of these.

There exists an intermediate group of patients between those with acute pain and those with chronic pain. I call this midway group the *extended pain patients*.

The *extended pain patient* is a working term for the sub-group of pain patients who are waiting to get adequate pain treatment. They may show all the signs of a chronic patient status but the gestalt of their situation separates them into this special sub-group. It is, so to speak, the 'wait your turn' group of pain patients. They may not actually qualily for the chronic pain label.

ME AND MY PAIN | 371

The reason is that, for this group, everything has not been yet tried. There may be delays in getting the patient to the appropriate specialist. A chronic pain patient label ought to apply to the clinical condition only after all means of intervention have been tried: being labeled as 'chronic' ought not to reflect how much time a person has been in pain as much as it should reflect the failure of aggressive attempts to reduce or remove the pain. Until all is tried, the 'chronic' label – which suggests some permanency given current technology – should be avoided.

Also, a subtle psychological difference exists between "extended" and "chronic" labels. The former has a sense of less permanency and speaks to the fact that on-going work is underway to correct the problem. Chronic pain has more of a long term, last ditch, palliative care only, quality. Chronic has come to mean permanent. But with ever new technology, old problems may become fixable.

> "I was a chronic pain patient with the first doctor because he did was keep me medicated. I became an extended pain patient with the new doctor because he medicated me as we went looking for a way to get rid of the neuropathy."

There is another notion that pain can bring on depression. This is a mixed truth. In all likelihood, the stress of undertreated pain will enormously increase the chance of depression. This is further enhanced if there is a history of depression in oneself or in a blood relative. Much talk exists amongst psychiatrists that major depression may not be inherited, per se, but rather there is a group 'risk genes' that become active when the person is under stress. Some genetically vulnerable circuits, when under stress, may break down, and if a large enough group of circuits fail, depression may follow. The key is to remove the stress of pain as soon as possible, and even if a depression develops, it cannot be treated only with psychiatric medications, but must have pain control interventions as well. But depression may actually be, at core, a despondency or despair or disappointment – and this may be the product of unsuccessful and fruitless looking pain management, return of security, etc., and it may not always respond just to antidepressant medications.

> "I told the doc I was crying all the time, I felt useless, nothing was working in my life, and the pain was like a daily abuser living in my life that I couldn't get rid of. So yeah, I felt I'd be better off dead. The insurance company kept delaying the surgery, and no doc was gusty enough to give me more meds, and I just felt it was the big signal for me to move on, away from life. I said I wanted to try one of those antidepressant pills I'd heard about. He said ok, but that wouldn't be enough. He said I need to see a counselor and get a new lawyer. He said it was bad because we'd not been able to do it all, and he said he was worried about increasing the pain med doses until the antidepressants and the counseling were tried. Ok, so I listened to him. He was right, especially about the counselor and new lawyer. Then he told me about this whole notion of being an extended pain patient. That made sense.
>
> By the way, my head got stronger too when my new lawyer took on the fight."

Here are some basic definitions of the traditional terms about pain:

'**Acute pain**' is that felt right after an injury, surgery or illness. It is expected to go away without much more than a short course of treatment. Toothaches, menstrual cramps, occasional migraines, pulled muscles or backaches after a strain, normal sunburns, bruises after a fall, and sutures after surgery are some examples of acute pain.

'**Chronic pain**' is produced by such things as unrelenting arthritis or bursitis, thalamic pain (from a stroke or injury), some cancers, persistent headaches, herniated disks, or joint pain from injury. It is a pain that won't go away. There is considerable debate about when to call a pain 'chronic;' a common number is that the pain must have existed for at least six months. But this group of patients is often improperly labeled because the word chronic suggests that things will never get better. In fact, things can still get better. That's why they should be labeled as extended pain patients.

Sometimes the condition causing the pain may not be treatable, but the resulting pain may be treatable. The pain source is unceasing, but the pain is not.

Chronic pain is usually divided into malignant and non-malignant pain. Palliative medicine (from *palliate*: to ease without curing) is defined as "the study and management of patients with active, progressive, far-advanced disease for whom the prognosis is limited and the focus of care is the quality of life."[255] This is essentially the long term treating of pain when no fix is possible. Palliative care has found much acceptance over the years because it is realistic and necessary, but hidden in the palliative term is an older, second connation suggestive of covering up something with excuses. Indeed, there is an old sense attached to the word 'palliate' that it 'hides sins'. So, in a subtle manner, to offer palliative care once carried a sense of hiding, which was, in a old sense, overlooking some sin or crime.[256] This connation is not, or is very rarely still suggested.

If being in pain is the product of a sin, then this older flavor must be understood because to 'palliate excuses' will not fix the sin. Treatment, therefore, adds to this bad situation because it further excuses the sin or crime that lead to the pain, and the treating doctor becomes party to continuation of some sin or weakness. This is another example of how the history of medical convictions can be so helpful since we still confront the spinoffs of these older attitudes in spite of our modern world.

The shift from an acute to chronic pain status involves a definite psychological transition called "mental deconditioning."[257] Typically, stage one of this process is related to the patient's perception of pain as it continues past the first 2-4 months. Stage two is marked by the development of psychological problems from the pain; it has been suggested that within this second stage is the beginning of some learned helplessness, and perhaps some onset of substance abuse, depression and somatization. Stage three sees the patient as developing a sick role. Naturally this overall progression has a reduction in physical activity as well, with a corresponding muscular atrophy, reductions in physical endurance, perhaps a loss of money, the upwelling of spiritual and social problems, and so on.[258] The character of this transition would surely vary with how adequately the pain is being controlled.

One subgroup of chronic pain patients are those for whom treatments once worked but do so no more. For example, a woman with a back injury had several neurosurgical procedures on her spinal cord. The first surgeries are successful, but scar tissue began to wrap around the nerve such that new pain developed. Subsequent surgeries trimmed away the new scar tissue but the scars returned. Eventually no surgeon would do more surgery, so now she stays in pain. Any further surgical treatment would require a new technology, so any of the usual pain treatments cannot adequately control the pain. The patient has to wait for a new treatment to come along. This patient is somewhere between the extended and chronic pain group, but leaning more to the chronic camp.

Pain management doctors must keep their extended pain patients adequately medicated until corrective therapy occurs. These people often complain that their doctors worry too much about addiction potential; the doctor ought to know enough about the reality of addictions so as to not make this a point of worry such that the patient unduly suffers. Patients who complain of uncontrolled pain while waiting often feel disbelieved (once again, those old words reappear: 'you can't be in that much pain!'). Extended patients may be seen as demanding, drug seeking, or as deserving some other pejorative badge. This is very unfair.

A few case examples will illustrate this quietly undercounted but very large group of people.

> A man suffered a crushed hip in an auto accident. The hip joint was replaced. Over time the joint began to fail, and his hip pain grew to be intolerable. Many medications were needed for him to be comfortable enough to even sleep. The surgeons refused to replace the hip, saying amputation would be needed. He was not psychologically sure if he was ready to lose his leg, so he preferred medications. Eventually he did have the leg amputated, and the pain was gone. But so was his leg. Until the leg was removed he was an extended pain patient.

Ten years ago a woman was in an auto accident. Her back was injured. One surgeon did surgery but she was immediately left with daily migraine headaches. She needed and demanded large quantities of pain medications. A second surgeon re-explored the injury/surgical site and found that a small puncture in the spinal cord was leaking spinal fluid. He plugged the hole and within days the headaches went away. She was an extended pain patient from the time of the onset of the headaches until the corrective surgery.

A woman suffered a facial injury. Several surgeons evaluated and tried some surgeries, but no one felt her pain was as bad as she was complaining. One surgeon even gestured to her that all the pain was imaginary. Her need for pain medications was great. She was told to learn how to be a chronic pain patient. Finally she located a surgeon who made the correct diagnosis and performed surgery. Since then there has been no need for pain medications. She was an extended pain patient from the accident until the right surgery.

A single mother developed bilateral carpal tunnel syndromes. She worked as a waitress, and it was her only source of income. Surgical correction was planned but no one would give her pain medications until the surgery. Yet without the pain medications she could not work. And she surely could not afford not to work. She could not understand why a doctor, who agreed that there was enough pain to warrant surgery would not give medications until the surgery occurred. She was an extended pain patient in between diagnosis and treatment.

Chronic implies permanency, and that takes away hope. At some time in the course of treatment, all available interventions may indeed have been tried but failed; the state of 'chronic' might then be declared. However, using the notion that the pain is merely being 'extended, but not chronic' delivers welcome psychological hope, which makes it worthwhile to get up in the morning. Hope is the antidote to suffering.

...Thought...

Many martyrs endured terrible suffering and death as part of their commitment to God. Suffering to them is good. It cleansed. It was a sign of being brave and not afraid. It raised one's moral statute. Many Christians use different levels of pain as one of the necessary ingredients in their quest for higher levels of spiritual spotlessness. In 1984, Pope Paul II said:

> "What we express with the word 'suffering' seems to be particularly essential to the nature of Man. Suffering seems to belong to Man's transcendence; it is one of those points at which Man is in a certain way 'destined' to overcome himself...Sharing in the sufferings of Christ is, at the same time, suffering for the Kingdom of God...Through their sufferings they, in a sense, pay back the boundless price of our redemption...Suffering contains, as it were, an appeal to Man's moral greatness and spiritual maturity."

Not everyone accepts this position, but it certainly influenced the cultural and spiritual environments of countless people.

A good number of people believe God assigns a purpose for human pain. Human commitments, so they believe, are tested with pain, and so it is through these tests that we can get closer to Him. This is not a limited notion: "The creation of the world is, then, the result of a blood sacrifice, and this archaic and widely disseminated religious idea justifies human sacrifice... In short, such a sacrifice (i.e., suffering) insures the renewal of the world, the regeneration of life, the cohesion of society" [259]

And yet, on reflection, suffering, though it may feel as if it comes from evil, does not. Consider the outcome of evil compared to the outcome of suffering. Something as robust as evil ought to keep us away from God rather than bring us closer. Suffering can teach, and so it may instead bring good. Suffering is not evil, but it is rough.

> "Even though the pain is because the idiot hit me after he ran a red light, I began to feel some evil force was after me. I needed to explain my suffering given that it was the result of someone else's stupidity. Then I wondered why God would let an evil force invade my life. I did nothing wrong that I knew of. What caused the suffering? I found no answer for this. When the therapist and I began to talk about my suffering, I thought the evil was to make me suffer, and then I would have to rise above the suffering to make the evil go away. So was the evil a seed to make me suffer, so I would get stronger? In that case, the evil was really not evil in the long run. Was the goal of the evil to bring me closer to God? So I played with the ideas, and then I felt that the evil was an agent of God. But I had always thought that evil ought to keep

me away from God. My preacher said God lets evil exist so it will push us closer to God. So if this suffering will make me stronger, that I'll give it a go. But I gotta tell you, I'm a lot stronger, but the pain is still here. Closer to God, yes; further from the pain, no. Something is not right yet."

A few questions arise. Phillips offers us much to think about: [260]

"How are evils compatible with the existence of an all good God? The theodicist will try to teach us how what appears to be evil to us has been sent out or created by God for the general good of mankind: a little evil does no one any harm and even the greatest evil, on closer examination, turns out to be worth the price."

A 61 year old pain patient offered some personal thoughts:

"Maybe I have the wrong impression of Him. Maybe God has no obligation to create the best of possible worlds for us. I often wonder what God would say if we challenged Him to explain why he allows us to suffer such pain. Why do we need to prove ourselves to Him? Is He insecure? I don't know other than I can't figure it out, and it is thinning my blanket of trust in Him, especially when I can't sleep at night because the pain is so bad."

This returns us to the task of finding a reason or purpose for suffering. Is it 'the down payment' for future rewards?

Some say yes, or at least they lean into the 'perhaps' side. John Hick offers some excellent thoughts:[261]

> "Man is an immature creature, undergoing further development which is spiritual rather than physical. Man is responsible for his own survival."

Might the admission that someone must use pain reducing medications in order to survive be seen as an embarrassing sin or as a sign of weakness? Taking medication takes away from the implied character-building properties of suffering and pain. So does cutting out the suffering in life limit the levels of possible new strengths that might come out of suffering? Yet the pain and suffering remove so much of life from a patient. What to do? Patients complain of being caught in this circular logic.

Let us continue with John Hick's thoughts:

> "The occurrence of moral evil is integral to the divine creative work. Man as a self-centered animal is the process of becoming a 'child of God' in accordance with God's purpose.
>
> ....man could not develop morally and spiritually in a paradise. The best of all possible worlds for his present comfort and pleasure might well be the worst of all possible worlds for his growth into a higher quality of existence. Moral and spiritual growth are not spontaneous but come in response to challenges, in the making of choices, in the facing of difficulties and problems, and through the experience of coping with setbacks and failures as well as enjoying success and achievement.

'Why do the wicked prosper and the righteous suffer?' is such a key question in the minds of us all.

All manner of accidents and misfortune strike randomly and therefore unjustly. But suppose that instead they occurred justly and therefore non-randomly, so that the evil were always punished and the virtuous rewarded. Such a system would not serve a person-making purpose. As Kant pointed out in the Critique of Practical Reason, it would undermine the moral life. In other words, moral responsibility and hence moral growth require a world in which there are genuine contingencies which distribute good and bad fortune not on the basis of desert. The other aspect of the problem concerns the degree of misfortune that can occur, the sheer intensity of human suffering. Is this not often too great to serve any constructive purpose? Yes indeed, sometimes, and indeed all too often, the effect of some crushing tragedy, as we see it in this life, is morally and spiritually destructive. But beyond this destruction there will be further creation, leading at last to the formation of a perfect being.

A world without pain would be one in which no one would be able to hurt someone else; there would be no such thing as a wrong action, or therefore a right action. There will be no caring or sympathy; ethical concepts would have no use and such a world would not serve any purpose of moral and spiritual person making. For

> there is, I suggest, a deep connection between morality and suffering such that a world without the possibility of real—and therefore unacceptable—suffering could not be inhabited by morally growing beings."

He continues to say that our transformation into the children of God does not stop at death, and we must see our lives as part of a greater process to be completed beyond this world.

> "For the justification of evil and suffering…is that it is a necessary part of the process whose end product is to be an infinite good—namely, the perfection and endless joy of all infinite life. This implies, in traditional Christian terms, universal salvation."

Yet how do we make sense of the day to day suffering that comes from chronic pain?

We cannot dispute that adversity can, at times, strengthen people, but perhaps the theological explanations of the role of evil and suffering in life weren't meant to deal with chronically unrelenting physical pain. It is awfully hard to sit with painful muscle spasms and believe that these spasms are steps on the ladder to an afterlife of salvation and ecstasy. But the notions still exist throughout our society that some suffering is 'good for you.'

> "How much suffering is actually needed to reach a state of sufficient and unblemished perfection suitable for a nice afterlife? No one has come back to tell me."

And what about suicide? It is the ultimate expression that intolerable suffering must end. Should a suicide following under-treated pain and awful suffering be seen as cowardice? No. Suicide is properly seen as a collapse. It is the result of an inability to continue to ward off some unchanging level of suffering. Suicide is often the end result of a distinctive penetrating moment in life when the person losses any hope that he may someday, while still alive, escape from the intolerable suffering and pain.

Like the hands of a doctor which might end or reduce suffering, so to do the hands of the suiciding patient also end suffering. Perhaps suicide, especially in pain patients, is the most honest statement one can make about the person's life. In many, but not all cultures, the act of the suicide act is strong enough to reject God's basic plan for how we should die.

But perhaps suicide is really a passionate pleading that God will understand and offer the soul a *serving of peace* in death that God did not provide while alive.

> One could argue that no patient ought to ever be labeled as chronic. To be chronic is to have no potential end to their suffering. Let them be labeled with a sense of hope that they are in the extended phase of their lives in the chapter of pain. It may be a matter of semantics for the scientific community, but it could be a matter of hope to the patient.

CHAPTER TWENTY-THREE
Pain patients have to be perfect people

These are the rules a patient must follow:

Pain patients can't have personality disorders; if they do then the pain is not quite as real.

Pain patients can't be depressed over their stations in life; if they weren't as depressed, then the pain would be less.

Pain patients can't be angry at, or want compensation from, those who wrongly injured them; if they do then the pain is not as quite as real, or it is amplified just so they can get a larger money settlement.

Pain patients can't have insomnia; the reason they can't sleep is because they have not learned enough self-hypnosis or haven't accepted their condition.

Pain patients can't have anxiety or phobic disorders requiring certain medications; they aren't allowed to have more than one curse in life needing treatment.

Pain patients can't have different or individual medication tolerances; if they do not fit within the normal dosing ranges, then they are addicts or placebo responders.

Pain patients can't have more pain than the doctor allows; if they do then they are manipulative.

Pain patients can't have good moods; they have to be miserable and complaining all the time.

Pain patients have to always be sick; they can't have good days and bad days.

Pain patients can't have a good day without everyone thinking the patient is finally learning to live with the pain, or that the pain is at last vanishing forever.

Pain patients can't disappoint people by having a bad day after a good day.

Pain patients can't look good; if they look good, then the pain can't be so disabling or menacing.

Pain patients can't respond to hope when they get good news; their demeanor cannot improve or change because to do so lessens the believability of the pain's intensity, constancy, intolerance, and presence.

Pain patients can't be skeptical; they aren't allowed to question new or proposed treatment decisions based on their real prior experiences as pain patients.

Pain patient's can't have other people steal their medications; being victimized, even one time, by a theft is too quickly considered as an indicator of the *patient's irresponsibility*, even for those who are generally very responsible patients.

Pain patients have to be average; if they are too smart then they are too 'pushy'.

Pain patients can't be normal like the rest of us; why should they find it easier to deal with pain, or even stop smoking cigarettes, than anyone else?

Pain patients can't believe in alternative life styles; if they do then they cannot be as trusted, or they might be considered as odd or eccentric. Such eclecticism can be initially spooky and uncomfortable for many who treat these patients.

Pain patients can't be diagnostic oddities; if their illness can't be labeled, then it's too quickly re-painted as psychosomatic.

Pain patients can't be picky; they aren't allowed to want other than second string doctors.

Pain patients can't take up too much of the doctor's time; if they do then they might become too erudite, insistent, or burdensome, and this may frighten the doctor away.

Pain patients can't shop, cook and clean; if they do then they are not in that much pain—but, by the way, who will do these chores for them?

Pain patients have to like everyone the insurance company sends to care for them; if they don't like everyone, then they are obviously non-cooperative and thankless.

Pain patients have to be meek; if they aren't, then they don't genuinely treasure all the good that others are trying to do for them.

Pain patients can't know their history better than their records; they aren't supposed to be upset when wrong or incomplete data and inaccurate conclusions are put into their medical records.

Pain patients can't feel the double bind: "if I tell him the other doctors were wrong then he'll think I'm too much of a smart ass, but if I don't tell him how the other doctors were wrong, then we may start with the wrong clinical impression of me, which is why I am here in the first place, to have a doctor get it right...."

Pain patients have to know magic; they are expected to take the cash won in a lawsuit, wrap it around the painful part of their bodies, and make the pain go away. They are the only people for whom money can buy happiness or cure pain.

Pain patients have to get better; if they don't, then doctors may not continue to treat them for the parts of the problem that don't get better.

Pain patients have to 'learn to get used to it'; this must be done with the same enthusiasm, gusto and savoir-faire of someone getting used to being poor.

Pain patients can't answer 'how are you?' with 'fine'; for to say 'fine' is thought to mean that they are better.

Pain patients can't choose to sacrifice; if they ever do something one day because of the emotional joy of doing it despite the pain penalty payable afterwards, then they can't obviously be in that much pain.

Pain patients have to perfect; I guess that means they can't be human.

...Thought...

"Good evening, ladies and gentlemen. I am Robert, an American by name and birth but Chinese by upbringing and heritage. As you can see, much of my life is now limited to this wheelchair. Before my accident I was a master in Chinese martial arts. I was trained in T'ai Chi Chum, which is most closely defined as the supreme and ultimate self-control in any situation. That was my goal in life, and in many ways I did achieve it. But what I really learned was a marriage of Eastern and Western philosophy. While I will give you my ideas towards suffering and how I manage life with it, I still suffer considerable pain. So the best comments available from me is how I live with pain. Please note those words: 'how I live with it.'

To live with your pain, you must live with yourself as well. That is the theme of this talk.

My philosophic ways go back to a prince in India, about 2500 years ago. He name was Gautama. He abandoned his wealth to find truth and a deeper meaning in life, and, fortunately, for us, he found it. He has since been known as the Enlightened One, or The Buddha, and he vowed not to be tranquil in his life until he shared his wisdom with all people. Many years later a monk named Tamo discovered that the health of those people around him was deteriorating, so he taught that the body and mind were united. He proposed that health could be achieved by the powers of the mind. He knew we all had flaws and he wanted us to be closer to perfection. He listed several disciplines, including those which would be known as the martial arts. But that aspect of his life is not what we are going to discuss tonight.

We are here looking at life, and the need to have a philosophy to make sense of it, and to give us direction. Let me, please, introduce to you a Taoist priest named Chang San-fang. Tao is a concept that means creation. It is some inner sense that can only be experienced. The I Ching says it is impossible to grasp it, for this ultimate meaning of Tao is the Spirit, the Divine, and the Unfathomable, which must be revered in silence. It is probably equivalent to what you might call God.

Tao is dualistic, what we call a yang and a yin. This is also called light and darkness, masculine and feminine, positive and negative, good and bad, life and death, sickness and health, and so on. It simply means that everything has both a form and essence. What we can see is the form. What cannot be seen or measured is the essence. Our bodies are our forms, but our spirits are our essences. The essence makes the form viable. The essence makes us function in life, as a unit or entity. Form without essence is dead. Perhaps we might also call this body and soul. Original essence, Tao, has no form and is called non-existence. Yin and yang are the basic make-up of Tao. I hope you can follow me.

I bring this all to you because Dr. Carl Jung, a Western psychiatrist, said that there is more to the Chinese way of thinking than meets the eye.

In the year 604 B.C., a great scholar was born by the name of Lao Tzu. He wrote a book known as the Tao Te Ching. Lao Tzu taught that when man contradicts the way of nature, the consequence is pain and suffering.

Man must be in accord with nature. Man and his universe become the yin and yang, and only by balancing do they revitalize one another. Man must give up the notion that he governs his world. Egotism must be relinquished. Now, follow this closely: being put into a state of non-action, or Wu Wei, opens up the person to experiencing the supernatural force of Tao. In other words, giving up one's old self, perhaps by going into a state of non-existence, is the way to rid oneself of pain and suffering and to feel revitalized. Some may see this as escapism or laziness, but it is not, for great discipline is needed to do this. One must not do anything which is contrary to the way of Tao. Man must learn to relax and, through stillness and meditation, then the correct thing will happen. The sense is that by allowing it to happen, it will happen. To fight nature is wrong; it is hard and tough. Hard and tough is death. Soft and tender is life. The position of the hard and tough in the universe is low while the position of the soft and tender is high.

Please, think, please. I know this may be confusing. So go slowly with me if you need to. Study all these ideas. Employing a good idea takes real work and some sacrifice. Our Western society says we must be tough and hard. It is how we achieve. It is how we measure ourselves. But when we hurt we must be sent both to those doctors who teach meditation and how to become accepting, and to those doctors who give us medications and perform surgeries. To give and seek a new existence that is so different, so alien, or so foreign to our surrounding cultural essence (i.e., to give in to suffering or become non-productive) is, well, to many it is a failure.

Yet to survive we must at times give in to the pain.

Do most Western doctors really know what they are saying to us? When they tell us to learn to live with the pain, do they also teach us how to do so? Doctors don't 'teach' as much as they 'do' – they 'do surgery' or they 'write' prescriptions. Do they understand how much of their work, that ' their doing,' is just mechanical? We need teaching. Do they know how we hunger for someone to teach and soothe our souls? Some do, but most don't.

It's wonderful when what they 'do' makes the problem go away. Often it doesn't go away; look at us, and look at me – I still need the wheelchair and I still hurt. So they tell us to learn to live with the suffering. I feel they tell us to do something that they themselves have never experienced. It's like a man editorializing about child-birth. We know, don't we, when we are given a memorized list of well-intended instructions.

We must learn to be strong and to be soft at the same time. The goal is Tao, which is the balance of all we seek in life. It is my job to convert the doctor's words — be they wintry or humane – into a philosophy that works for those of us living who live with the suffering of chronic pain. That's what I am trying to do with you now.

We are seeking Tao, a special, balanced state of mind and body. Most doctors don't know how to teach this. It's not that easy, I assure you. But it is not impossible! And I can assure you of that! It just takes work. It's the old sense that you must learn to how make yourself better rather than expect others to make you better. Others can guide, but you must do it. Too much of Western medicine relies on doctors doing the fixing. That is a limited expectation, and often short-sighted.

Tonight I really just want to set the stage for you to start your personal training.

It took spent years of preparing my mind and soul for this type of thinking. Too many who newly suffer pain find the pain experience to be something different from what might have been expected. The rules of being a pain patient seemed initially impossible to learn. It seems harder for chronic pain folk because it is so different. But it works.

One problem is that contemporary therapy teaches relaxation techniques without a relaxation philosophy. Stop for a moment to think about the differences.

To treat the psychological aspects of pain, we need to deal with the spirit. Spiritual exercises should become the good doctor's orders! But that is very unscientific, is it not? And how does a doctor bill for or prove the benefit of a spiritual enhancement to an insurance company? What is evidence based about a spiritual treatment protocol?

But think. Actually, most of life is a spiritual event. Consider love and passion. You know what I mean. My homework assignment for you is to look into your soul and feed your spirit. When you do this, all else in life is easier. But find a mentor, like a yoga master. Much of the success of yoga is that it is the product of thousands of years of countless human trials done by countless yogis, who now give us the legacy of their work. More trials of yoga exist than all the drug company studies put together, and yoga is still here – something must be good about yoga.

Another thought. We Chinese have great ways to foster inner strength, but we have never been so foolish to deny real and treatable pain. So we have Tao, *and* acupuncture, *and* massage, *and* moxibustion, *and* exercises, *and* a compendium of herbs to assist in healing. And modern Chinese doctors know about Western medications as well.

Because I have been called Kung Fu, which only means that I am a master, one might think I could weather my ailments without modern medications. Please, I take medications too. Medications are part of the Tao balance.

So do not think it odd that a doctor may someday refer you to me as part of your pain treatment program. I live with hope. It is never gone, though at times I struggle to hold on to it. Hope is having a perspective and being willing to work very hard to keep it alive. Working on hope itself can offer some healing.

We may change how we name things, but the I Ching has a wonderful saying about human needs:

> *The town may be changed,*
> *But the well cannot be changed.*

Live in China or New York, now or long ago – we are all people with a magical common spirit. The town may change, but the well feeding our basic thirsts cannot be altered."

CHAPTER TWENTY-FOUR
Insurance companies

For all the good that insurance companies do, they tend to lose their benevolence as time goes by. This is especially so if the patient remains ill for a long time, or if the cost of continuing care escalates.

Insurance companies are profit making or cost reduction organizations. This truth can never be ignored, overlooked, or diminished. It is as solid a fact as night follows day.

Insurance companies are usually big. Therefore they weld gigantic power. There is a collective sense that they have infinite resources and bevies of eager lawyers to protect them. Stories abound about insurance companies who are quick to drop coverage if a premium is late, yet this same standard does not apply if the company is late in issuing a payment or delays a treatment authorization to an insured or a vendor.

> "I know there must be a lot of good insurance stories, but the horror stories – there are just too many of them. The good doesn't remove the bad. I was told by an excellent billing clerk that we just need to know how to work with them because a lot of the minor rejections can be over turned. That's reassuring, but most of us regular people don't know how to do it. The clerk is like a lawyer who knows how to work the system. It's a whole new profession. Of course, then there are the big things that rarely get overturned, like when my son needed a follow up MRI and the adjustor said no, it was

> too early to repeat the test even though the doctor thought it needed. That type of thing should never be the basis of a battle. My wife and I paid for it ourselves because it was our kid. Now we battle the insurance company for the money. But then one adjustor told me that sometimes doctors order more tests so they can have move visits. I hope this isn't true, but it wouldn't surprise me. Doctors are businesses too. It's like a big check and balances system. My wife give it a different name – she calls it an un-checked and un-balanced system!"

There is no argument against the fact that insurance companies must protect themselves from fraud, but to most of their insured, the hint of this suggestion about them is an insult. The great majority of people are honest. Sadly, however, the insured patient soon sees what games must be played in their dealings with their insurance companies because of the games that the insurance companies play with the insured. Patients know the insurance companies constantly scan for any evidence that they can use to justify stopping or reducing payments. So patients, forced to 'insure' their own survival, develop their own protective tactics.

> Insurance companies develop formularies of medications. They go from inexpensive to expensive, in step-wise manner. Often they will reject a more expensive medication if a cheaper one will do the same thing. There is no argument with this because sometimes the new and more expensive medications are not that much better than the older ones. But, by the same token, sometimes they are therapeutically better, or

perhaps they produce fewer side effects. The process of getting these more expensive medications approved is a time consuming activity which has become a real burden to doctor's offices. The process includes contacting the insurance carrier, making the argument, sometimes writing letters, etc., to convince them that a clinical need exists to warrant the use of the newer or more expensive medication. Sometimes the prior authorization process is less burdensome, yet it is still an extra step for the doctor's office. There are staff costs involved in that process, be it quick or complicated. If the prior authorization request fails, then the doctor has to decide if he must insist on the medication being used even at the patient's out-of-pocket expense, supplement the patient with samples, or offer a different medication. That too involves clinical time and costs, and usually the doctor is not paid for this work. The typical modern office faces many prior authorization requests. It sounds harsh, but doctors see this process as efforts to get needed treatment, to save the patient money or argue on their behalf, etc., and so the doctors may have to charge for all this activity. Insurance traditionally does not cover for this aspect of the cost of medical care, but it is as key as is the direct clinical interaction with the doctor.

Sometimes people need higher than usual doses. But the insurance companies often reject this because the FDA did not approve the higher than usual dose. This is a sham argument because the FDA makes judgments based on the data provided to them by the medication manufacturer. And that data is often the minimal data needed to get the medication to market. The people who failed in the clinical trials may indeed have not failed because the drug didn't work. Indeed, the patient may have failed because the research limited the doses ranges to be used in the study. The patient may have gotten better if he had been allowed to use a higher dose. The study failed, not the drug. But the insurance companies consider the FDA approval as proof beyond debate. We all know of patients who need higher than standard doses. Getting them the needed medication doses is almost impossible with the insurance companies. (Many doctors supplement the patient's dose need by giving them samples.)

Sometimes a patient needs a medication or dose for which no formal study has been performed. This is called off-label use. The reason for the lack of the study is that the drug company chooses not to spend the money to seek another FDA approved indication. But the science is supportive and is usually reflected in the professional literature. Much talk exists about off-label use because it is so often necessary.

This is a key point. The doctor, who is the clinical scientist on the case, knows the biochemistry and physiology of the medication. With that knowledge, they apply it to their patient's needs. That is the art and science of a physician's training and experiences. Good doctors very often share among themselves their questions and experiences with off-label use. So, using this information, the doctor fashions a treatment for the patient. Interestingly, sometimes people only need very low doses of a medication. This too is technically off-label, but there is little argument against this use pattern. A low dose needing person may be accused of being a placebo responder; but this is unfair to the person; every doctor knows of patients who are low dose responders. People are so often too quick to make assumptions. The need for low, common or high dosing varies with the person's individual metabolic make-up and clinical history. This is why it may be critical for your doctor, in the appeals or prior authorization process, to speak to another physician or person with an equal scientific training; talking to lesser trained people can be unproductive.

"I work in a doctor's office. I initiate many of the prior authorizations. Sometimes I get a simple form back that asks if other meds have been tried, or if a disease really exists. It's a mixture of a bit of history and a sworn affidavit by the doctor. Then the authorization occurs. These seem to be a waste of time in so many ways. Sometimes getting the approval is a lot harder, and the key cost is how much of my time it takes. I wonder if that is deliberate, to dissuade us from going in that direction. Sometimes the doctor has to insist on talking to another doctor or pharmacist. It can be a lot of work. Sometimes nothing

> works, and so we go to samples, etc., but the costs can be high for patients. Sometimes the insurance company will not pay for as much med as the patient needs. It's kinda a diplomatic science that I'm learning. I think the insurance companies want us to prove the need. Once we had to call a Congressman to write to the insurance company on behalf of the patient – and we got it, we won, and it was for 2 pills a day, not one, and that story keeps going round and round, cause the patient was a lot better on 2 pills – I saw him in the office."

Most people simply do not realize that an FDA indication (that is, the approval for use) is based on a marketing strategy by the drug manufacturer. The FDA response is based on what the drug company presents to them. Insurance companies then limit their authorizations to the style of the FDA approval. Once any medication is on the market, however, smarter doctors begin to think about if it can be used in other ways that is consistent with the science of the drug. The market size for this off-label use may be too small to warrant the cost of seeking another FDA approval. Many a good drug never gets a formal approval for a new indication simply because there is not a large enough market for it. There is much talk in the medical profession about recognizing these off-label uses, especially when there are reasonable case reports, etc., that support the off-label use. Sometimes the lack of doing further studies which are aimed to get new approvals are more a matter that the drug is close to losing its patent protection.

Some drugs are so old that a formal FDA approval never existed, but insurance coverage exists. I've called it the 'common law' section of medicine. A separate civilization and society of regulations and conventions exists when it comes to coverage, availability, and so on. There has also been talk that the older medications should now be formally studied to prove their safety and effectiveness, despite that many of the older medications have decades of widespread clinical use and experience. This process would be very costly, and it might have the effect of turning older, currently generic, cheaper medications into 'branded' ones. Sometimes older medications are put into difference release vehicles (an immediate release version becomes an slow release version – the basic molecule is the same), and given a new name. Should the insurance company pay for the more expensive version? Perhaps, if there is some real clinical advantage to the new medication package. But sometimes the ultimate clinical difference is not that significant.

Some patient populations (and hence the potential markets) are very small, and so some orphan drugs (i.e., they have no active parent pharmaceutical company) saw that some schools of pharmacy would compound them on an as-needed basis. Insurance companies may not pay for these because they lack FDA approval, despite the presence of good science to support the clinical need for the medication.

> Orphan drugs are developed for rare diseases. The FDA has an office for orphan products development. [262] The 1983 US Orphan Drug Act says: because so few individuals are affected by any one rare disease or condition, a pharmaceutical company which develops an orphan drug may reasonably expect the drug to generate relatively small sales in comparison to the cost of developing the drug and consequently to incur a financial loss; there is reason to

believe that some promising orphan drugs will not be developed unless changes are made in the applicable Federal laws to reduce the costs of developing such drugs and to provide financial incentives to develop such drugs; and it is in the public interest to provide such changes and incentives for the development of orphan drugs. In the U.S., 47% of rare disorders affect fewer than 25,000 people. This is a good program. Insurance company polices may vary as to how much they will cover the care of a rare disease. Go to this website for more information: www.rarediseases.info.nih.gov

The National Organization for Rare Diseases (NORD) helps in many ways. "Since 1987, NORD has administered programs to assist uninsured or under-insured individuals in securing life-saving or life-sustaining medications. In addition to the estimated 50 million Americans who have no health insurance, an increasing number of insured individuals have policies that do not reimburse for prescription drugs. Others have policies with low annual caps on prescription drug expenditures." [263] NORD is at www.rarediseases.org

NORD will likely not be able to deal with issues of insurance problems for pain medications, but if the pain is the product of a rare disease, then it might be of help in treating the primary disease.

Sometimes, however, wide-ranging off-label use will find a new niche and use for the drug, so post-marketing research (meaning after the drug was initially released) may follow in order to get another FDA indication. This makes for an interesting point because what was once considered off-label can becomes on-label. What was once bad or not allowed becomes allowed and good. Yet too many patients suffer while the bureaucrats re-do the paperwork; clinicians and their patients may wait for the FDA formal approval before an insurance company will consider it, and the insurance companies may add additional delays because they may not quickly approve coverage for the new indication. There is a hot debate over the issue of an insurance company's responsibility to pay for off-label use of a medication. This is especially so if the medication is expensive. The insurance company may also deny it because, in their opinion, the new drug is not sufficiently different from existing ones, and so they see little or no reason to approve the use of the new one.

> For example, the medication Fentora®, which is a fentanyl formulation that dissolves in the mouth, was initially approved for cancer pain. However, clinicians thought it ought to work for back pain as well. It did. The potential market for such a new indication was big enough that the company did formal research and sought an FDA approval. Supportive research was published. After all, the medication is exactly the same molecule as is in the Duragesic® patch or the Actiq® lollipop, both of which are used for a wide range of pain conditions.
>
> Here is an example of the problems associated with this process:
>
> A patient could not wear the Duragesic® patch – his skin would not tolerate the 'glue'. The oral

lollipop Actiq® formulation had a disagreeable taste. The generic formulations were not as therapeutically reliable as the brand name. So when a chronic pain patient's physician asked the insurance company to authorize the Fentora® because a three time trial of it worked so nicely, (by the way, it was self-pay for those three prescriptions), it was rejected because it was not yet FDA approved for severe back pain. Interestingly, the FDA was actually in the midst of an approval for back pain, so the request was not uncorroborated. The patient said "that denial makes no sense at all – it's the exact same molecule. I know why they do this – it's because the drug is so expensive, and I can appreciate that part of it. But I cannot accept the other aspects – it worked for me, and I have no control over what it costs!"

This is a typical case of when a good clinician, using solid science, makes the type of decision that we expect a physician to make when about deciding to use a medication 'off-label.' The patient caught the theme when he called it "off label but on-science."

Nonetheless the insurance company will not pay for it. They base their decision on the line of reasoning that they only pay for FDA approved medications, doses, and indications. Time consuming and costly appeals may follow, but they are often futile.

Here are several common impressions of insurance companies: (a) that within the insurance industry is the assumption that far too many people are tempted to defraud in order to get a free ride, (b) that the average legitimate claim is a complex process in which the patient, and not the insurance company, has the greater financial risk, (c) that items thought to be covered for the insured are discovered not to be, and hence the insurance company is guilty of a type of hoax (the companies argue that the insured should have read the contract better), (d) that the 'friend' that the insurance company claimed it would be is actually a well defined and financially limited contractual relationship, (e) that no sense of ethical commitment exists to a customer, so that once benefits run out, the company, without so much of an iota of embarrassment or concern with the patient's health, protection or well-being, stops all payments for needed care, and (f) that insurance companies feel no hesitancy in raising their premiums if certain types of claims (for the very events which were insuring) are presented. These are some of the ever present and central issues in the on-going health care reform debates.

Some history will help:

> Insurance companies must estimate the risk of healthcare expenses. This is part of the underwriting process. With this information, they set up premiums to bring in enough money to pay for benefits specified in the insurance contracts. Insurance companies have reams of statistical data to help them decide on what risks they want to take, how much they expect any 'loosing of the risk' might influence their profits, and how much money they choose to charge for them to take those risks. My brother sells insurance. He keeps reminding me that "insurance companies are very good at math."

The not-for-profit insurance organizations, such as Medicare, also get premiums, per se, in the form of government funding. The not-for-profit's, however, do not include a corporate profit in their budgets.

Remember that the basic definition of an insurance contract is that 'if you get sick, we will pay for some or all of your care.' There are three parts to this contract: the nature and origin of the sickness, the limits of what will be paid, and the acceptance or rejection of your claimed needs for some types of care. In a practical manner, it comes to this: The insurance company may not pay for disease X, or if it does, the maximum total it will pay out is Y number of dollars, or they may claim that treatment Z is not covered by the policy.

The first ideas of health insurance go back to the late 1600's. By late 19th century, "accident insurance" was available. It was similar to disability insurance. For many years health insurance was actually referred to as disability insurance. The first accident insurance in the United States was by the Franklin Health Assurance Company of Massachusetts, and it insured against railroad and steamboat accidents. Sickness coverage first appeared in the late 1800's. [264]

Before there was sickness insurance, patients had to pay their health care costs out of their own pockets. This is known as the fee-for-service model. Eventually, throughout the 20th century, disability insurance slowly changed into our modern health insurance programs. These cover routine, preventive, and emergency health care procedures. Some policies also cover prescription drugs and other services.

In the first third of the 20th century, individual hospitals offered services on a pre-paid basis. This lead to the development of organizations such as the Blue Cross and Health Maintenance Organizations (HMO's). Unions fought for benefit packages that included tax-free, employer-sponsored health insurance. Government wage freezes during World War II accelerated group health care since employers, unable by law to draw new employees by offering higher pay, used better benefit packages, including adding health care, to get new workers. That is essentially how the structure of employer paid health care began.

The United States system has both profit and not-for-profit health insurance programs. The not-for profit programs provide coverage for most seniors citizens and for some low-income children and families who meet certain eligibility requirements. The principal programs are Medicare, which is a federal insurance program, and Medicaid, which is jointly funded by the states and the federal government, but Medicaid is administered at the state level, so there may be Medicaid differences from state to state. Medicaid insures very low income children and their families, as well as offering services to some disabled and to the elderly. Other federal-state partnerships serve children and families who may not qualify for a public program but who also cannot afford private coverage. Other large programs include Tricare and the Veterans Administration systems, which provide care for military personnel and families. And yet another program is the Indian Health Services. States may have additional programs to certain groups of people.

One of the on-going political issues about health care insurance is this: would people ask for as many health care interventions if they had to pay for them themselves? What would the market charge if people did not have someone else to pay for them? Does having insurance increase the cost of health care because more of it is used? But by the same token, how many people could realistically pay the costs of medical care? And of course, if more health care is used, is the product a healthier and more productive community? For example, how many people would be working and paying taxes as opposed to being in jail if really good community mental health services were available and affordable?

And, of course, one of the really big questions in any society is if health care should be a right or a privilege in our society.

Why do these concerns and experiences exist?

Insurance companies sell themselves as being a security blanket, if not even as a parent-like protector, but the extent of the 'caring parent' image is deceptive.

The biggest difference between an insurance company and a 'good' parent is that the insurance company 'has' to pay while a parent 'wants' to pay. A truly caring family will consider spending its last dollar to help a relative. And how many families have gone bankrupt because of medical bills? Many, sad to say. How many insurance companies would do the same? None that I know of.

CNN reported in June 2009 that 60% of all US bankruptcies occurred because of medical bills. [265]

The insurance company will argue that giving too much of its resources to only a few patients will deplete the resources needed for the many. Up to a point, no one can disagree with this position. Yet when someone is honestly sick, and legitimately needs help, will the insurance company lower its profits because of a moral or ethical concern for the patient? No. This is taken by the patient to mean that the company is more concerned with its own survival or of the survival of less expensive other cases than with himself. An insurance policy is therefore another version of the notion of the survival of the fittest. When a patient discovers that their insurance company, who once so caringly promised to help, now won't help, it means the insurance company chooses not to devote the money to the patient's needs. The demands for help are considered by the insurance company as either not legitimate or outside of the conditions of the policy. Hostility arises, lawyers are hired, and so on and so on.

> "When I got bought the policy, I never expected to be in an accident. Then when I was, I never expected to need more physical therapy than the policy allowed. Then I never expected that a file-reading-only doctor, who never saw me, would say my that doctor was wrong. Then when another second opinion doctor, paid by

the insurance company, agreed with the insurance company, and she said in effect that my personal doctor was also wrong, it was such a hammer hitting me in the head. I could go on. I never realized the amount of politics in the medical and insurance field. How could doctors be so different about the same clinical data? I don't understand this. My doctor was making real process with me, and we needed to go an extra step, so he asked for more PT. I was really benefitting!

It's like doctors expect other doctors to lie, or to make a misdiagnosis, etc., to make money for themselves. I told the second opinion doctor that my pain really decreased with the physical therapy. I guess that isn't important....I just don't know how to make sense of this. Explain this: One doctor looks at the x-ray and says "oh my, we have a problem here," and the other doctor looks at the same x-ray and says "nothing wrong.

There is no way that anyone could buy a policy knowing in advance what their real medical needs would be in a situation like mine. It's absurd. A friend told me it is because the insurance company 'averages' the needs. But like some people need more meds than the 'average', I shouldn't be punished because my needs are not average. I didn't expect this! I'd like to see a 'national read your insurance policy' day. Then if it's as full of holes as I discovered mine was, there should be millions of us stopping to buy those policies. They want our money and

I'd bet the market pressures would produce some real changes.

When I spoke to my lawyer about all this, he wasn't the slightest bit surprised. He said it is more common than many people realize. That's a sad commentary on our system.

When I spoke to another patient about my woes, she told me that she got her extra treatments. I wondered why there was such a difference. My husband thinks she had a more expensive policy. I wonder if she had a better lawyer or a more clinically eloquent doctor.

And by the way, being 'not average' doesn't mean I am any less legitimate."

Insurance companies employ people to rehabilitate the insured patient. This is an excellent move, and it provides beneficial care to many people. But as in the above example, what angers so many people is that when they buy an insurance policy they cannot exactly predict their later clinical needs. In fact, no one can.

A fear lives within the insurance industry that they must guard against the unnecessary use of health care resources. Deceit, fraud, or shams must certainly be avoided. But has this 'guard against fraud' mentality become the operating standard in the health care insurance industry? A 35 year back injury patient told me that "I suspect the insurance companies use this 'fear' as an excuse."

Apparently so. So many patients report, after some period of time being a patient, of implicit or explicit impeachments that their pain can't be as bad as is being reported, or that the pain is 'in actuality' related to some secondary gain or other non-pain process. This is especially so if the treatment is on-going, long-lasting, and more palliative than curative.

Now enter the lawyers. I've heard it said that insurance companies understand lawyers better than they understand doctors or patients.

> "Yeah, yeah, I know. I am a lawyer. I worked for an insurance company. I fought the real fraud. But now that I'm sick and on disability, I'm even sicker for what I did to some people. Here's my story. I never thought people could be as sick as I am. Hey, I saw so much real fraud, it became an expected part of so many contested claims, and so rampant fraud was real at that time of my professional life. But thinking 'fraud' became almost the norm for me in too many ways. So one day, after this illness of mine began to take hold, I went to get my meds. We were a self-insured company, but my medication was rejected. It needed a prior authorization. Okay, thought I, no big deal, it's expected. But I was rejected! My doctor had to appeal. Then the rejections happened a few more times. I couldn't believe it. One day I spoke to a vice president of the company about this. He said he would initiate an override on my behalf. That was certainly nice, but I said no. I was troubled that when I stood in line at the drug store, and I listened to other people in line with me, and I saw what they were going through, and then it hit me. I also listened to people in my doctor's waiting room. I never told them what my job was. Oh my God, it kept hitting me. These good

> people were being hassled for no fault of their own. I waited for good insurance stories, and when I heard one I almost wanted to shout out "See!" But so much of that I heard them talk about was how hard it was to get approvals, or about the delays, etc. There was too much bad in comparison to the amount of good.
>
> So I quit my job. Now, to be honest, I would probably have had to quit it anyway because I was getting very ill. But at the moment of my resignation, I quit partially out of secret embarrassment."

Many battles occur just over money because the facts are blatant enough to justify an uncontested settlement.

> A teenager was shot in the chest while working at an after school job. There was no doubt of her being the innocent victim of the robbery. The case got a lot of media coverage right after the shooting. However, one insurance company took the formal position that they were not responsible because she did not follow the employer's protocol on how to call the police. However, she never had a chance to do so – she was on the floor with a bullet in her chest. The case settled, in large part because her lawyers threatened to present the insurance company's arguments against her to the local media.

Once a lawyer is hired, the insurance company will also change its stance. Suddenly they are dealing with someone who knows how to read the insurance contract, who knows procedural and case law, and who is willing and able to take the insurance company to task. A patient without a lawyer is not a foe; with a lawyer the patient is a foe. How many times have people said: "My lawyer told me that I am entitled to this, that, and that! I never knew it."

> "The rehab nurse kept surprising me with new things. I thought they were being generous. Later my lawyer told me they were only offering what was in the policy; I did not know about those things."

Let's use the good parent analogy. The good parent looks at a sick relative and says "what else can I do to make you more comfortable?" Does an insurance company ever offer more than was asked for or that which may be out of the limits of the policy? One man called his insurance company "the equivalent of a dead beat parent who won't pay his child support unless you take him to court." It's a shame how many times a court must order an insurance company to assume it's due responsibility! One can only speculate that if a court finds the insurance company liable, then the liability existed in the first place.

The second major impact of having a lawyer side with a patient is that the insurance company knows that the clinical picture may be somewhat exaggerated. This sets in another level of distrust. The reason for this is simple: lawyers know how other lawyers think. The assumption is that the insurance lawyers look for ways to underplay the situation, and so the patient's lawyers may look for ways to highlight the injury to offset the lawyers on the other side. It becomes, at times, an amazing game of rouse, opposing experts, smoke, and mirrors. Yet so many times the facts of the case are so straightforward that these games should not even need to be played. A good lawyer works to keep only the real facts, and no smoke and mirrors, on the table.

There is another layer of problems with big insurance companies. The sheer size of some of them offers tremendous financial security, but the size removes the 'personal touch.' This indifference impedes the development of therapeutic relationships between the company and the patient. The standard of care becomes such that people need to fit insurance company formulas, and should they not fit, then a squabble ensues to get the needed coverage. A good permanent rehabilitation nurse, working and seeing the patient over a long period of time, might be the patient's best advocate. But the typical experience is that such nurses are not kept on the case for long enough. Perhaps this is the reason why.

Fortunately, many people's needs fit within an average range, and they get the financial help and guidance needed to get proper treatment. But these folks are not the subject of this book. "Those folks are the lucky ones," said one woman when we talked of the world of insurance, "and I never realized that my insurance policy said, between the lines, that if I am too sick, or I can't get better fast enough, then this policy is essentially null and void, and that they can hassle me. Hey, I didn't ask for this injury! But so far I fit in their guidelines, so I'm ok."

Sometimes insurance companies ask for second clinical opinions. These are the IME's, or the independent medical examinations. The IME doctors are selected by the insurance company. Patients often suspect they are selected because of a clinical bias against the type of conditions in the patients, or because of an allegiance with those who pay them for the examination. If you are involved in litigation, then your lawyer may ask you to be examined by one of his doctors as well.

Sometimes the IME doctor agrees with the patient. But sometimes not. It is an amazing moment for a patient to learn that an IME doctor doesn't believe that they are truly in pain or injured as badly as claimed. Sometimes the IME might even say an injury or illness exists, but that it is existed before the accident, which means that the insurance company might say they are not responsible to cover the cost of treatment for a pre-existing ailment.

> One patient addressed this chilling question: "I wonder what would have been the outcome if I had, by chance, first gone to that same IME doctor for my regular clinical care? In other words, what opinion of me would he have if my original connection to him would have been my asking him to be my treating doctor? Would he have told me, as a new patient, that there is nothing wrong with me and that I need to leave? I have to wonder."

Differing IME reports shift the battle zone. Often the combat zone will become full of more confusion and anger than peace and clarification. Patient's wonder how and why different doctors' arrive at such different conclusions given the same clinical history.

> "It makes me wonder how precise or capable docs are about agreeing on a diagnosis or procedure. What if I had a small tumor? One says yes surgery, another says no. I thought it was more scientific. This is so unsettling! Who do you trust? How can it be so different?
>
> I went to two IME doctors. One said I was malingering. The other said I was honest. The malin-

gering guy wrote a 60 page report. The honest guy wrote a five page report. So do you want to laugh? My lawyer found out that these two guys co-authored a paper on how to detect malingering. So in meditation my lawyer showed the publication to the other lawyers and said "what are we going to do about this?"

We won."

Lawyers gather in court to argue which doctor is right and which doctor is wrong. The stress of all this on a patient is incredible. Sleep, pain, mood, and confidence – these are so often shaken down into the patient's core. Patients may also loose insurance coverage until – and if – they win in court. The anger rises exponentially if the patient cannot afford a good enough lawyer or good enough expert-witness doctors. Many people believe these barriers, with the subsequent frustrations, are intentionally imposed by the insurance companies, or by the opposing lawyers, with the purpose of exhausting the patients so much so that they give up the fight. Much of the psychotherapy needed during the litigation phase of such situations is devoted to maintaining the patient's emotional grit and stamina.

The unexpected lack of insurance coverage, the allegations of malingering or of exaggerating one's complaints, or the unforeseen placement of severe limits on available care, can make people desperate. This is one of the background scenario's that lead to the phrase "going postal." It is very hard and very expensive to keep patients hopeful. The needed therapy is intensive. The therapist must not be shy about walking straight into the patient's world and soul. Then the insurance company may attack the therapist as well, alleging a prejudice or bias within the therapist that is not supported by their experts. The therapist may then have to become both a therapist and an advocate. Some therapists shy away from the advocate role.

It is tragic when there are no or limited funds to fix the primary problem. It is equally tragic when the secondary problems, such as the resulting psychological issues, can't be addressed. This is the notion of the second victimization. Following the original injury is a second injury that comes from the fight to get care for the first injury.

Finally there is the notion of the insurance company's medical panels. This is the list of doctors who are on the insurance panels as authorized treating professionals. This means that these doctors have contracted with the insurance company to take assignment or a reduced fee for patients under a particular insurance plan. Sometimes this is fine. The doctors are matched to the patients needs and things go along without a hitch. The problem, however, may germinate when there is no one on the doctor list who has the special skills needed for a particular situation. An appeal process may be needed to get an override. Sometimes it works, and sometimes it does not. The assumption that all doctors are clinically equal is a misnomer.

> "We nearly went crazy over this. The local doctors, nice enough people, but she wasn't getting better! So we went to a nearby medical school. That helped, but some specialized tests were needed. And they were expensive. Initially the insurance company said no, but we fought. We won a few of the battles. But it wasn't until we went up the list of medical school specialists that we finally got to one who knew what to do. He was doctor number 26 for us. Yes, number 26! The insurance company kept saying that their

local surgeons were just as qualified. Not true!! And when we told one of our local surgeons that the medical school professor was willing to do the surgery, he said: "Good, let's let the super specialist do it." It's was discouraging when another local, lesser skilled surgeon worked against us, saying he could do the same thing at the insurance rate – we dumped him, but his comments delayed getting the insurance approval. Finally the super specialist did the work, and we were lucky because it worked. He ultimately did some surgical technique that no local doctor had even considered. The insurance company paid only a small part of the bill. But that is okay because I have my wife back. That super doctor has since left the medical school, but every New Year we send him a heartfelt and spiritual thank you for fixing her life."

The next vignette is from William, a 56 year old accountant who was forced into disability by horrible rheumatoid arthritis in his fingers.

"For 55 years I liked things to be in order. I saw nothing wrong with making a profit. I loved my work, and vacations were more of an interference than a joy. But then the joints on my right hand began to swell. The pain was incredible. Holding a pencil was hard. Then typing was hard. When my doctor said it was rheumatoid arthritis I couldn't believe it. We tried so many meds – some worked a little, but the fingers took on angles and odd shapes – I thought I looked like some evil witch!

One day, a bad day, I threw up my hands and screamed to the world 'I can't do this anymore! I can't work. Look at me!' It was a combination of pressures to make me give up, but mostly because the wicked disease was stronger than me. I didn't know how to accept it. I'm still upset about it, but an accountant knows when something isn't working. I knew I wasn't working right. I know it was the end of so much of 'me.' The pain was so bad that my doctor referred me to a pain management doctor.

I also applied for disability. At first it went well. The insurance people made me fill out so many forms. They seemed to want to help. But then delays started. My checks would be delayed. They wanted more and more pre-authorizations from my doctors. Eventually they sent me to one of their doctors, who said that I wasn't as bad as I was claiming, but that it was my obsessive personality that ruled me more than anything. They felt I could still do some work. I was shocked.

I got a lawyer. He spoke to my pain doctor. Neither of them did much good, so I fired them both. I got a new rheumatologist who worked with a different pain clinic. This new doctor was not on my insurance plan, so it cost me. I got a new lawyer who actually spoke to the new doctor. They both told me I had to soften my Type A personality in order to learn to live with my disability, so they sent me to a super psychologist. I have to admit I was a bit miffed at first by seeing a shrink, but it really turned out to be a great move. And, to tell you the whole story, my wife endorsed the therapy as well – I never learned so much about me. The pain was just as bad, however. And the more my doctors got to know me, and my personality, the more they saw that regardless of my personality, the arthritis was the pivotal handicap blocking the resumption of work.

The lawyer had a ploy. He got records galore from all types of doctors, got literature, etc., and he sent to the 'team,' which was my several doctors, the psychologist, and the insurance adjustor. He asked for brief quarterly reports from the doctors – for many this was just the clinical notes that they put into their charts. Then, about every 3-4 months, he called the insurance adjustor and asked her what she thought of the information in the notes. That also tested whether or not she read the material. It kinda, really, put her on notice. He didn't want to set her up, but he did want to make sure that she had to address the information that all the doctors were writing about me. He told me he was humanizing me to the insurance company. We eventually got pretty much what we rightfully needed. When she sent me for an IME, he insisted that all my records be sent to the IME doctor as well. He told me that if we went to court and the IME doctor did not consider my big file as part of his report, then his report would be laughed at. He also asked that on occasion I speak to the adjustor with my own updates. I did so when things were good as much as when things were bad. I believe she saw that I was really trying to do as much as I could for myself and that I just needed their help. Given everything, things were ok. I still wished I could work, however.

After a few years I was told that my adjustor had been reassigned. The new one was hard as cold steel. Things stopped. My lawyer said I was becoming expensive for the insurance company. My feeling was that the new adjustor did not want to know me as a person. I remember the chill in me the first time I felt that. There was a rash of new IME's. There were, unbeknownst to us, also private IME record reviews (they did not actually examine me). They even did surveillance on me. So things got hot. My doctors spoke. The lawyer looked at the new developments in the law. And we went to a hearing.

My lawyer asked the insurance company why one adjustor was acting in one way, and the other was not. The other side's lawyers couldn't explain it, but they implied that the original adjustor had gotten soft with the facts of the case. But when my doctors proved that I was better, with fewer doctor office visits, etc., when under the care of the first adjustor, well, that too was hard for them to explain. We won.

But that was years ago. Since then, with each new adjustor, there were new challenges. It was as if the new ones do not read the full file before they try to change things. Some of them wanted to reduce the treatment costs with clever and ingenious new ways that no one other adjustor could find; I think they tried to win favor in their company's eyes. Eventually they brought back my original adjustor. I could tell she was different this time, but at least she knew the case. And some of the relationship she and I had from the past was still there. I know she had a job to do, and after all, she was an adjustor, not a defense disability lawyer. Remember who she worked for! But an element of humanity returned, for which I am so grateful. I am also grateful for an incredible team of a lawyer and doctors who worked with knowledge, warmth, and finesse.

My lawyer took a photograph of my hand, and each new adjustor got a letter of introduction from my lawyer that also had that photo attached. One adjustor suggested that it was not my real hand! So we have full body pictures available if needed. My lawyer, I think, went as close to nuts as possible on the day he was told that they doubted the veracity of that photo. I thought he was going to fly up there and do, well, I don't know what. He was angry and shocked, but not violent.

By the way, my fingers still hurt like hell. It's getting harder and harder to even hold a spoon. We're trying a new clinical research medication. I am scared. But my attitude is one-thousand times better than when this all started. And I am also getting closer to Medicare, which will be a relief in so many ways."

...Thought...

> "Death was never a wanted option for me. But death is surely able to do the one thing that no doctor could do—stop the pain. Don't people understand? Don't they understand how defeated I feel – no clinical means, always fighting with the insurance company, me going broke – just nothing is working."

Suicide as a result of uncontrolled pain does occur. But no huge body of absolute statistics supports the claim that the 'pain' was the spark that caused the death. Suicide customarily stems from depression's most pernicious colleague: hopelessness.

Depression, from the sense of feeling hopeless, is an existential one. It is based on the loss of hope for any echelon of passable pain control because an unending clinical, spiritual, or financial battle fighting against that echelon cannot be won. All things nice in one's life are seen as irreversibly gone or worsening. The ultimate and final decision about one's own death is based entirely on quality of life principles and options.

> "People don't understand the other side, which is the economics of being in pain, and the incredible costs of the medications. That is often as limiting as any other aspect of being in non-malignant chronic pain. Insurance companies see me as needing years and years of medications that cost them thousands of dollars per month.
>
> At times I feel like giving in to it all. How is it that my morphine costs that much too? It's such an

old drug. Why do the drug companies charge so much? And my insurance company will only pay for so many doses a month. How do they know how much I really need? I am not just an 'average' statistic. But I am, ain't I, just a statistic for them! They lose money on me. Sometimes, to be honest, death would be easier than life. God, I even hate when that thought goes through my mind. But I need a safe harbor with some freedom from nonstop strife.

I read a newspaper article about the number of people who die each year because they don't have any health insurance. I noticed no one did any research about the number who died with health insurance, because of the limitations from their health insurance. Not having it is one thing; not having it work for you is something else. My policy is effectively like having no insurance, so I am the 'insured uninsured'."

One study took a formal look at the risk of suicide in pain patients.[266] Other groups have looked at the same issues. Much is written on the relationship between misery and human self-destruction. Too often suicide is assigned to another diagnosis, such as co-morbid alcoholism, depression, personality disorders, or substance abuse. Actually, a very large number of the suicides in chronic pain patient groups represent failures of our society, insurances, and health professions to offer these people proper solace, care, or cure.

Let us take a brief look at some of the work about chronic pain and suicide after a comment about active, or doctor-assisted, euthanasia. This is a controversial topic, and it touches our religious, ethical and scientific roots.

One of the core differences about suicide is that a suicide is considered to be from something which is fixable, such as a depression. A doctor-assisted suicide or euthanasia carries the sense that the basic problem is not fixable, that is, it can be considered for terminally ill patients. As of January 2010, Oregon, Washington and Montana were the only US States that allowed doctor-assisted suicide. The Montana Supreme Court did not determine if the Montana Constitution guarantees the right for euthanasia. Instead it said that state law did not indicate that it was against public policy. Indeed, the 1997 Oregon law has been called the 'death with dignity' law. These legal and moral campaigns are far from resolved. As for pain patients, the issues are even more sticky because so much pain can be controlled. So before euthanasia is considered or any plan surveyed, there has to be an incredible history of all sorts and styles of failed pain management. Contemplating euthanasia demands the deepest consideration by the patient, the family, the doctor, and anyone else involved with the patient.

> The legalization of euthanasia has become a question for voters. The right to choose euthanasia is not accepted by many on moral grounds. A presumption against the taking of human life is embedded in the formative moral traditions of society. But the taking of a life is not the same as letting it go, especially if the condition is terminal and painful.
>
> It does not seem, in the United States at any rate, that all possible alternatives to affirm the control and dignity of the dying patient and to relieve pain and suffering, short of taking life, are exhausted. [267] How often would people

who are considering euthanasia drop the consideration if pain was not a problem for them?

Older white men have the highest suicide rate in the nation. Among the major problems leading to this are chronic sleep problems, pain, degenerative illness, or depression.[268] Drowning is a popular method of suicide in this group.[269] Fishbain found that all chronic pain patients have a significantly greater risk of suicide than those in the general population. While his study is small, he found that: white men are twice as likely to die as their counterparts in the general population, white women are three times as high, and white people on disability were also three times as high. [270][271] Hess, et al, reported that postherpetic neuralgia is the number one cause of intractable debilitating pain in the elderly, and it is the leading cause of suicide in chronic pain patients seventy years of age and over. [272]

Therefore, all medical professions, including emergency room staffs, need to consider that the presence of a chronic medical illness could increase the risk of suicide. [273][274] Appropriate pain management and psychological referrals, even if expensive, need to be considered. These are typically easier to get under Medicare than under private insurance programs.

One concern about suicide, with both pain and non-pain patients, is that the danger of suicide attempts rises when the patient feels he can no longer generate new ideas, new options, or new and reasonable alternatives to solve his situation. [275]

We cannot ignore chronic pain. Even the psychologically normal person can slowly drift into what many see as a pathological state of desperation and despondency when pain is not resolved. These patients speak of unspeakable suffering and loss of dignity. Kotarba offers some worthy thoughts on the topic:

> "The process of coping with chronic pain involves both the search for medical and non-medical cures, and the search for a meaning for the intractable suffering. [There is] great variability in the...ideas of death, the key elements extracted from belief systems...reflects the variable success in normalizing chronic pain. The paper [discusses] the issue of inevitability." [276]

> The need for an on-going access through which to a search for control, cure, and dealing with suffering are so important and of the essence to life.

The operative and most frightening word in the above section is *inevitability*. It means that no options exist with which to change a course. The synonyms for inevitability are these: uncertain, inescapable, predestined, obvious, fixed, and so on. This is a terrifying emotional state to be in. When the psychic finally gives in to the pain, then the struggle is over. It easy to understand how this emotional voyage may happen, but it is also downright unacceptable. It happens when hope vanishes. This suffering and torture is even more raw if some 'fix' exists but it is unaffordable, either due to insurance or personal financial limits. This frustration can heighten the state of affairs to unstable and explosively emotional levels.

Kopp says: "In modern society the reduction of creative ability and the capacity for work is caused primarily not by physical damage, but rather by states of depression and either anxiety and functional disorders arising as a result of the transitional or lasting failure of the psychological capacities to resolve conflicts, leading to such states as chronic pain syndrome." [277] It is this failure, which lives in the deep matrix of frustrations of psychological stalemate and incapacity, and which the naissance of suffering, that can lead to suicide.

Nonetheless, Kopp continues on to an optimistic note: "On the basis of the recent theoretical achievements, we are capable not only of treating the symptoms but also intervening in the causes. Psychotherapeutic methods and psychopharmacology supplement each other within this theoretical framework." The other satisfactory changes, though not yet as widespread as wanted, are the changing attitudes towards the reality of what is needed for proper chronic pain management.

It is amazing how much technology now exists which can better a person's life, but we are also so lenient and non-demanding when the access to it is denied because of money reasons. It is as if the lack of money is a suitable excuse to allow the treatment not to occur. "I would go to that doctor if I could afford her." Think about what this says about our society and what it does to the mindset of needy, un-insured, or poor patients or their families: Doctors don't treat, pharmacies won't dispense, physical therapists won't exercise, lawyers won't defend, therapists won't talk, and so on, unless someone will pay for it. Thank goodness for the many public clinics and charities who, despite many of their own financial limitations, at least try to offer some help outside of the 'who-is-going-to-pay-for-this' column.

"Okay, if I had to pay for the next surgery, well, I couldn't. I don't make enough money. When I had to stop working, the insurance soon ended. I could not afford COBRA. My brother offered to help, but he doesn't have $50,000 that I realistically could not pay back. I tried a public clinic, but these clinics are disappearing too. Right now I'm waiting for my Social Security application to be processed, but even if I get it – which would be good, I still have until the Medicare part starts 'cause I'm told the better docs around here don't take Medicaid. So I'd be dead, I'm sure, because the neck pain was intolerable and I am alive because I once had insurance to pay. Now its no money, no life; got money, got life. I don't know what I'm going to do now – the pain is coming back because I need part two of the surgery.

I met a guy in the pain clinic. He's really rich. He can get all the physical therapy he wants. His other doctors call him back because he bought into a boutique medical group. He can afford the more expensive medications that cause less side effects. He can pay for the weight control clinic. He speaks to a therapist once a week for a full hour. He could afford the expensive mattress for his back. He has people who clean his house for him. He's like a flower who has the luxury of good soil, good fertilizer, good weed control, and good sunlight. He represents what is possible. He once told me that he doesn't need insurance. He likes it, but he doesn't need it. Wow. Need I say more. And by the way, I met him the clinic that I went to when I had insurance. Now I go to one of those walk-in clinics.

But I have to say, too, he knows how lucky he is, and he is a good soul, and he helps a lot of people. Maybe he's got some charity fund or something."

CHAPTER TWENTY-FIVE
Epilogue and recommendations

We must always define a 'person' as the 'assembly of unique experiences and personalities' in the physical human body. When we see a sick human body, our empathies must go to the person within that body. An incredibly important soul exists within the person. If we stop at the body, then we miss the person and the soul.

> "One needs to talk of persons in order to understand humans, but not of humans to understand persons. A person does not include the properties that characterize humans as a biological species." [278]

Hence, we, as people, have existences bigger than our bodies.

Pain management is so complex. It involves social and cultural biases, money and the allocation of resources, an evolving technology, and even some rudimentary ethical decisions about what amount of medical care we elect to be a person's right or privilege. Pain management is also one of the medical specialties that must be better able to separate what is genuine and what is fake; as such, it's diagnostic process is akin to the mental health professionals. It's a sizeable challenge when a clinical condition is understandably a mixture of some real and some fake.

This is not a book about the usual clinical pain management protocols. Instead it is a book about the reaction to pain. This includes the nature of suffering, as well as how to test, push, change, improve, and enrich the many layers of systems that feed into unique world of pain management. It is, therefore, a book on the protocols needed to treat the suffering that comes from pain. Many of the social, insurance, and medical battles facing pain patients are the same as those facing psychiatric patients. Indeed, proper pain management is very nearly a branch of psychiatry in that the body and mind are its patients.

What can you do about your endless pain?

On-going levels of pain raise the question about the adequacy of treatment. If someone with real pain has tried most pain control interventions without relief, then it may be a case deserving of genuine empathy and sympathy. But within that empathy and sympathy there must never be the sense of giving up. Perhaps the source of the pain is out of the ordinary because it is not yet understood. Perhaps the first step is to get a new doctor or try a different specialized clinic. Keep looking. Indeed, never assume that any doctor, team, or clinic knows it all. The US National Institute of Health has an Undiagnosed Diseases Program to investigate patients with baffling symptoms. Talk about this with your doctor. And visit the NIH website at http://rarediseases.info.nih.gov/

Sometimes the lack of pain relief can make everything feel out of control to the point that death becomes an viable option. If this happens, call your doctor, a friend or family. Or call 911, go the emergency room, call the National Suicide Prevention Hotline (800-273-TALK), but do not be alone! Suicidal thinking episodes can be reversed.

Remember that death takes away all the future options for a cure or reduction to the pain. New methods develop or different doctors can be found. Medical changes occur so rapidly that the wait time for new developments may be shorter than anticipated. Sometimes the 'new development' for you is no more than getting into a more aggressive pain clinic or psychotherapy.

"My best friend had horrible depressions. Last week she spoke of wanting to die because her emotional pain would not stop. She told me that it's her reaction to the depression, not the depression itself, which causes the suicide. So I realized that it's the same with my back pain. It's how I react to it that counts. I finally got a good pain management doctor and a good psychotherapist and I'm better than ever, though the nasty pain is still pretty bad at times."

John Keats wrote in his "Ode to a Nightingale":

I have been half in love with easeful death... Now more than ever seems it rich to die. To cease upon the midnight with no pain.

We understand Keats. But the handle to hold onto is that which aims to continue to fight for life using whatever treatment necessary! Sometimes the treatment is physical, sometimes it is psychological, sometimes it is spiritual; often it is all three. And as trying, and challenging, and just as plain 'hard' as it may seem to be, there must always be the sense that relief will someday be possible. We know it can be so relentless and grueling at times. But keep in mind that so many conditions which were once considered as untreatable are now successfully treated.

Now a plan to help....

Many things can be done. They do overlap in places.

1 - **Test your own self honesty and personal self-awareness**

Stop and think about how much pain you can live with. What are your limits? Would you accept a 5 out of 10 level? Of course the goal is to lower the pain as much as possible. This may not be easily obtainable. This can be a hard bridge for many people to cross. It's a personal acceptance of an unwanted level and style of life that every pain patient has to make. Aiming for a 1 or 2 is an understandable, on-going, and required goal of the pain management team, but learning to accept a 5 or 6 may make daily living a bit easier. Remember that you, the patient, are an equally important pain management team member, so some of the team's outcome rests with what efforts you bring to the team.

Everyone waits for the time when universally successful treatments exist for all levels of pain. Until the time when such wonderful treatment proficiencies exists, you must think about where, in your world, is your balance between pain levels and your levels of functioning and levels of suffering? What is needed, at minimum, to keep a sense of yourself? Never lose sight of your goals, but never forget where you were.

Can you tolerate more pain? Can you honestly use less medication? Or do you need more medication? Where are your personal limits? Take a hard look at all the variables in your life, and measure what is being done by family, spiritual or philosophic grounds, by clinics, devices, medications, and psychological approaches, etc. In short, where is your life's perimeter? Learn to know yourself, but let someone be your life editor to keep yourself objective about yourself.

Where is your spiritual grounding? What helps you make sense out of your life? Though important to all people, with or without pain, it is more important for people with pain. It's hard to understand why pain became your perpetual, relentless, and demanding roommate. Your life becomes one of looking for a way to evict him! But if you cannot evict, can you at least find a way to ignore?

> "My pain is a bad roommate. But with the meds and re-thinking a lot about my life, I learned how to banish him, for several hours at a time, to his room and out of my moment to moment life."

Looking for psychospiritual grounding is a universal need. Meditation, a religious connection, or perhaps yoga, will not undo all the pain and discomfort, but it may help the suffering. It's been said that 20 minutes a day of meditation can reduce anxiety and stress, and over the period of a month or two, the meditation can strengthen emotional systems and tap into untapped potentials for change. But it takes time, consistent work, honesty, and of course, it is not a cure all. It does, however, address the science of your mind. One aspect of being in pain is that chronic, un-ending pain forces us to look at the rest of our lives. Interestingly, though the pain be a unwanted passenger in your vehicle, the journey and process of looking at oneself in new ways can be very enlightening and offer extra strength to fight the pain and all that it brought into your life. It is then easier to fight the pain, work towards cures, etc. It is also recommended that the journey not be made alone.

There frequently are concerns that secondary gains may exist to being a pain patient. Non-pain sufferers often imply this to be true about those in pain. Sometimes a secondary gain, so to speak, develops over time. Sometimes secondary gain is not a swindle. For example:

> "After the accident I kinda did ok, though the pain never stopped. I got the right amount of money from the insurance company, the driver who hit me is in jail for a long time, but my life is so limited now. So I think at times that I do make

a little excuse every now and then to make sure people remember that I cannot do what I used to do. I also need to make sure my wife doesn't forget me, and so the pain is one way to keep her attention. But really, that only accounts for about a 5% increase in my complaints of pain. My doctor looks at my x-rays and nods her head with disbelief about the massive damage inside me, so I'm lucky: the doc knows me for a long time, and doesn't question my pain.

But when I look at my whole life, I'm afraid my wife will get bored with me. Look, I'm not fun to be with anymore, to be sure. I can't even just walk through the streets at Christmas to look at the decorations – well, I can do it for maybe 30 minutes or so. And I know she loved to do that! And she wants to boat and ski and travel – and, I must admit, those were both our dreams. And I don't want her to think that if I do something unusual, like if I push myself to walk with her, that it means the pain isn't still here! She's really a great, thirty-one year old beautiful lady, who wants babies, etc., and I'm the albatross around her neck now. She said no, I am wrong, that she loves me, she knows the accident was not my fault, etc., but she's only human too. Hey, even sex is rough for me now. So I suspect other men will be able to do more for her than I can in so many different ways. And I want her to have the fullest life possible. So the secondary gain for me isn't about the money. It's my desperation and a game not to lose her.

> It's not very mature, is it? I need to work on it. Time to call both my minister and therapist."

What can you do, by yourself, to lessen the pain or the impact of the pain on your life? First, spend time learning to be more personally honest in such a way that will more maturely define you should someone ever challenge you about what you believe, what you report and feel, what you have learned, and so on. Too many times pain patients are seen as being somewhat less than honest about some aspect of their pain; it is as if there is some psychological ploy or weakness underscoring their need for medications or about their complaints of pain. Let these doubters know they can find nothing about your life as a pain patient that is immature, untested, fraudulent, undeclared, disbelieved or hidden; preparing for this challenge will also grow you into an improved you.

> A 54 year old woman developed very nasty, hard to explain abdominal pain. After numerous consultations, a doctor recommended a new type of surgery. Fortunately, much of the pain disappeared. But then it came back. This time nothing new or old worked. She was angry and frightened that she had developed an unknown, lethal disease. She agreed to enter psychotherapy, where it became evident that she never realized how much positive attention she got from her family while she was sick. That all disappeared once she got well. In time she realized that unconsciously she wanted some of the pain back, but at first the idea of her being psychosomatic was so sour to her that she rejected it over and over. Her physical illness brought out some help from the family, but

once her needs ended, the old family dynamics reappeared. It became much more complex because the family didn't believe her as much with the second round of pain as they did with the first round. She didn't realize how much she wanted the family to be as it was during the first 'helping her period.' She was also scared that if the pain remained, her family would quickly tire of her, and she would end up lonely and in pain.

This secondary gain embarrassed her. A long, intensive course of psychotherapy greatly helped strengthen her psyche. She eventually could talk about her old fears to her family, and that left them with as much surprise as respect for her. She and her family found all their relationships improve as she brought to light her concerns. The second course of pain complaints eventually disappeared. However, the physical cause of the original pain was quite real and was never questioned.

Be upfront with family and friends. Having a family member join you in some of the psychotherapy sessions can be a remarkably valuable experience. Pain may seem to be a two dimensional experience, being of both the body and the mind. That is then overlaid onto the world in which you live. So pain is really three dimensional – the body, the mind, and the surrounding world. All three domains need to be understood and mastered as much as possible. Perhaps you should also invite a family member to go with you for a few visits to the pain management doctor. The family member needs to sit in the actual meeting with the doctor!

The key is this: *You must develop a candid, painfully aboveboard, mature self-awareness and acceptance of what your life is currently about, with all its limitations, frustrations, and joys. Some facts or unwanted elements will just have to be accepted. Some unsettling elements or realities need to be shared. In some areas the anger coming from your situation may have to just be let go if doing so will give free up energy with which to grow.*

But giving up anger doesn't mean to give up a fight. It's just that some battles can't be won. Release them. There is not always justice in life. Sometimes bad people who do bad things go unpunished. Don't waste your tomorrows fighting yesterdays. Find that which is good in your life and move on. Build on the good as much as possible.

> In 2009, The American Headache Society published a report that a history of childhood neglect or abuse was found to be more prevalent in migraine patients, and that this same group of patients reported a greater number of other pain conditions than groups without the childhood maltreatment. [279] Needless to say, great care must be maintained not to over generalize the implications carried in such reports. But if you were maltreated, then any treatment resistance may be improperly proportioned and attributed – correctly or incorrectly – to the assumption that your current treatment problems are related more to your history of abuse than to the nature of your pain. This is such an important balance to keep properly aliened, and as such it may take the skill and diplomacy of a good psychotherapist both to help resolve it in your own world and to explain to others the

'real' nature and degree of impact it has on your life. The question is this: in your case, is the pain heightened or complicated by the history of abuse? For some, the prior abuse may have nothing to do with the current pain. Yet for some the two will be intertwined. You, however, are mandated to explore if this is a clinical issue with you because others may assume that the two are validly tied together. The danger is that once a history of abuse is noted in a chart – or even if it is only highly suspected – then those words may taint how all subsequent pain management teams approach you. Don't assume the professionals will have the moxie, skill, concern or desire to test the allegations.

"My car accident happened and the chronic pain began when I was 27 years old. I was giving my history to the pain clinic psychiatrist, who asked if there had ever been any sexual abuse. I wanted to be honest, so I said that I was on the fourth date with a guy who date raped me. Of course it was upsetting, and I wish such an event on no one. It was a date rape. But I truly got over it. I wasn't physically hurt, no diseases, no pregnancy – sure, it was an ugly time, the guy was a pig, but I put it into perspective and I was able to restart dating, etc. The doctor, however, wrote down that I was raped, and that label rose to the top of my chart like a cork in water. I was furious because it implied a mindset, a response, and a damage that I did not have. I know I got over the rape – but I don't think the doctor did. I guess he thought he

> found a smoking gun. Or maybe he had some crazy personal issue about sex.
>
> Well, I wrote a detailed entry that I insisted be put in my charts. I even saw two good psychotherapists, each for several months, to explore if I had some unconscious creature living in my psyche. They both agreed with me – a bad thing happened but I worked it out. They too wrote letters that we put into the charts. My hip still hurts from the car accident, but the date rape is long ago history. That doctor caused a lot of trouble. Let's keep things in perspective, please."

It would be nice to assume that all pain and suffering is 'fixable.' That is still, sadly, not realistic. But what is 'fixable' are our mind-sets towards our ailments and suffering.

> "I always called myself a chronic pain patient. Then I realized I was putting the pain before me. It was torturing me, like I was a political prisoner. So I flipped the words around. Now I refer to myself as a 'person who has pain.' That little word-flip makes me feel better. I am 'me' first, and I am learning to live around the pain, as if it is an expensive, nasty, uninvited rodent in my house that someday I will force to leave!"

2 - Get copies of all your medical records

Many states guarantee your right to your personal medical records. Get them. See what is being said about you. If something is wrong in the records, then ask the writer to make corrections. Speak to an attorney or the hospital risk management people if they resist making the corrections. You may be able to force a correction to be put into the record. Remember, many people judge you based solely on those written records. And remember too that those who write the records do not want to be regarded as foolish or sloppy, especially if they made a mistake. But also remember that charts are not court rooms, and arguing 'in the chart' is not the venue for debate. Try to settle things outside the chart, and then make a summary statement to correct the misinformation.

Be sure your primary pain control doctor has copies of all clinical records. Trust is not enhanced if your doctor feels you are keeping things away from him. If IME's occur, try to get copies of those reports. The more information, the better. Psychiatric and mental health records have different rules about confidentiality. Sometimes, for example, when in therapy, the patient may talk about 'a former drinking problem'. There may also be entries about such things as the patient's fantasy life, etc. (Don't hold back in therapy if you fear the record – doing so undermines the therapy.) These are legitimate entries into a mental health note if they reflect upon the patient's issues. When requested, it may be better to have a therapist merely provide summaries of the clinical care without all such details. The problem is that raw records could be too easily read by others, copied, moved about, etc. Federal and state rules protect against such a spread of information. Don't release information without knowing what doors will be opened. Sometimes a lawyer may be needed to oversee where, which, and how psychiatric records are released.

Sometimes a mental health treatment is kept secret. This is a complex situation, but the secrecy can be broken if another doctor notes in his medical chart that you are seeing a mental health professional. Likewise, pharmacy records will show the names of your medications (if any) and who prescribed them. So two points emerge – first, there should be, and often there is nothing, to hide, and second, it really is hard to hide all the records.

So, the first key is for you to know how to manage your own medical and psychiatric records. The second key to work honestly to get better, and so, should anyone read the file, they will see that you had a real problem and you are honestly doing your best to make things better; that position is hard to argue against. The third key is that sometimes parts of psychiatric records do need some filters. Legal protections and procedures exist to do just that. A lawyer may be needed to invoke those protections. But don't let the fear of what is in a record limit what you bring into therapy. The goal is a better you!

> "I was scared when the insurance company wanted to see all my psychotherapist's notes. I didn't want the whole world to come into the therapy room with me. I really open up a lot to my therapist, and the key was that I was safe doing that with her. I didn't need an adjustor reading about the problems I had with my Dad, of the lover's I'd had, or my fears, and so on. I started in the therapy to learn how to deal with the pain, and in the process we began to look much more at the rest of my life. And of course, the stronger I got in the rest of my life, the better able I was do deal with the pain. I spoke to my lawyer and therapist about the insurance company's request. She actually understood this process better than I expected, but I'd never had to ask her about this before. So she ended up writing summaries of my diagnosis, the psych meds I was taking, and how I was 'addressing, with incremental success, the issues

and psychiatric residue surrounding the accident, etc.' That worked! I think, however, they wanted to stop paying for the therapy. That's why I keep my lawyer in the loop as well. I see her therapy just as important to me as are the pain medications."

Buy an inexpensive scanner and make PDF files of your records. Also make copies of important insurance documents as well as copies of insurance payments, denials, court orders, medical records, police or accident reports if applicable, any other legal documents, wills, power of attorney papers, etc. Update them on a regular basis. Keep a copy disc in your underwear drawer. Give another copy to a friend, lawyer, or family member.

3 - Respect your doctor. Respect yourself

Be honest. Let the doctor see that you can be trusted. Try to customize your relationship with the doctor. Share successes and errors. Don't try to outwit – you will be caught. Remember, the tone of any working partnership is the product of repeated honest and vibrant communications that take place over time. These communications accumulate. The clinical system needs time to mature – it won't work any other way. If a medication or prescription is lost, admit to your role and your liability, but don't expect the doctor to be an open re-supply source to offset your errors. Show the doctor that you do learn from errors. Don't insist on paper prescriptions if the doctor wants to send them electronically or by direct fax to the pharmacy. If you need a paper prescription because you need to shop around for the lowest cost of the medications, then explain it to him. Ask for fewer pills on the new script. Go find the best price, and then ask that all new scripts be sent to that particular pharmacy.

If you are hospitalized, let the admitting doctor know about your pain control doctors; ask that they all talk together. Doctors hate to learn after the fact that their patient has undergone some other treatment without their knowledge, especially if during hospitalization some of the meds had to be changed. Give copies of the hospital discharge papers to the pain management doctor.

Don't expect every doctor to have the time and patience that 'you' would like top get from them. Attempt to understand the doctor's world; they aren't tirelessly forgiving, parent-like figures or friends. They do get tired, angry, annoyed, threatened, or uncomfortable with unusual behaviors or unrealistic demands. They are also unlikely to take on more than a very limited role as a psychotherapist or life coach.

Doctors live in very fragile and risky medical-legal environments. So the quickest way to destroy a relationship with your primary pain control doctor is to be unrealistically demanding or to be only partially honest about your history and activities; to do either of these will violate the confidence, reliance, and trust that nourishes and keeps a doctor-patient relationship healthy. It can also mislead the doctor away from the needed course of therapy. Don't be surprised if treatment ends should this trust be compromised. If you are doubted, then talk to the doctor about how to re-earn the trust. Outside psychological counseling might help with this as well. Sometimes eating a little crow will get you invited to the bigger table.

4 - Don't fear complicated looking medical terminology

Doctors understand medical concepts and terms because they study them. When you hear them used in reference to yourself, be patient. Ask what they mean. If needed, study the terms and concepts from 'good' resources. Internet web sites are not all accurate, so start with the major medical organizations, like the American

Medical Association. (www.ama.org). Getting information from several internet sites will highlight the good from the bad postings. Discuss any inconstancies in what you read with the doctor.

Many doctors have information packets available to give out. If a procedure is being recommended, be very careful about what other patients report because too many of them, especially on the internet, are reports from those who only have had poor outcomes. It is imperative that you also remember that these 'posting patients' may not report their entire stories. Furthermore, other people's medical conditions may not be fully equal to your case. This being said, the information in the condition specific support groups are invaluable, such as those found in the established diabetic, pain, psychiatric, or cancer groups. The key is not to rely on too small a selection of data sources. The more you read, the more you will see the real from the biased, the angry from the educating, etc. Keep in mind that with every publication, it is important to get a sense of what was editorially not included in the story.

Some basic science may need to be studied. Do your best. Then ask questions. Some doctors will not like this, but who cares. You have a right to know what is happening to you. Sometimes the best practical information comes from the nurses. Remember that 'you're the patient' in pain. You're the 'client.' It is nice to find a doctor who will comfortably, professionally, and aggressively work with you; but such a doctor may not be easily found, so...

5 - Doctor shop

Search for the doctor who works best with you. A doctor may not automatically give you what you want, which is okay if there is also genuine evidence that you will get bona fide and serious treatments.

Traditionally, doctor shopping implied treachery and deceit. These unsafe, 'shopped-for-doctors,' are usually discernible by their very limited doctor-patient interactions. These doctors basically give medications without insisting on other aspects of treatment. Some doctors, however, are just naïve or passive; this vulnerability is often exploited.

Before you shop for a new doctor, try as hard as possible to correct the problems and issues with your current doctor. It cannot be denied that doctors are not all the same in their clinical skills, creativity, points of view, humanity, psychological signatures, or sensitivity. The temperament of the doctor-patient relationship is often as predictive of therapeutic success as is the pattern of any set of prescriptions or interventions. So just as a different medication may be needed to reach success, so too might a different doctor be needed to achieve some therapeutic victory.

Look for the combination of technical skills and compassion that you need. Know your needs before you shop. Perhaps some counseling will clarify what those needs are. Be prepared to concede at times. All relationships need to be flexible. All relationships also need to learn and grow together. You're ideally shopping for an active collaborator and liaison who, as with you, is a student of science and life. You do not need an monotonously, emotionless prescriber.

Give a doctor enough time to make a difference. And compromise if the doctor's clinical skills are greater than his personality style.

It's also important to find a doctor who will not abandon you if there is no ready fix. Other patients and local nurses are rich sources of data to tell you who these doctors are.

If no technical skill exists to truly fix your problem, then stay with someone who compensates with compassion after the technical skills are exhausted. Modern medicine should not merely let you suffer just because it cannot fix the center problem. Explore how a doctor works with other treatment modalities, with set-backs, with new material you may bring to him, and with consultants. But again, as noted above, don't expect the doctor to be or do something that he is not or cannot do.

Doctor shopping is too often assumed to reflect a patient's desire to deceive a series of doctors in order to obtain multiple and duplicate prescriptions. Your doctor shopping is the opposite. You just want one good doctor or team to manage your pain in a forthright, hard-hitting, and interactive relationship.

6 - Within reason, try everything

If you are in a good treatment partnership with a doctor, then his experience should serve to guide and assess the relative risks of novel or untried treatments. Both you and the doctor should keep up with on-going reviews of research and new trends, ideas, devices, etc.

Psychotherapy can be extremely helpful if for no other reason than to get to know yourself better. It helps to work on emotional strategies to deal with the pain induced changes in your life. Being in psychotherapy may have nothing to do with any level of psychological abnormally. In fact, entering therapy can represent a higher echelon of good emotional health. Feel free to scorn anyone who quickly suggests that psychotherapy represents a weakness, or who says, without solid proof, that your pain is psychosomatic.

Good therapy can also help by using the adversity in your life to be a platform on which to build as much as can be done around the pain, to dilute out the pain with as much joy or insight as possible, and to develop growth producing projects using new understandings and wisdoms. Combining religious and psychotherapeutic efforts can be a powerful team for some people. Don't be afraid of making mistakes.

Don't feel you must always define or defend yourself to others. You should, however, be aware if you are asking for pity. Asking for understanding, and maybe some leniency, is fine, but it is not good if it reaches up to the point of asking for pity. Learn to ask for 'just and due' respect. Pain has limited the types of options available to you, so use those options that remain. Though it may be hard at times, focus on the good. John Stuart Mills said that "actions are right in proportion as they tend to promote happiness, (and) wrong as they tend to produce the reverse of happiness." [280]

Learn hypnosis and biofeedback. Study stress management. Exercise as much as can be safely done. Spend time outdoors. Learn to explore anything that catches your curiosity. Become philosophical. Use a psychotherapist, mentor, friends, family, and clergy to teach you how to do this. In this process is also the learning of why you may, at times in the past, have resisted asking for help.

Learn to pace yourself in life according to the pain, and then try to overcome each boundary in small but safe steps.

Try not to allow yourself to become bored.

7 - Maintain political and diplomatic skills, and don't hesitate to be vocal about pain

Tuberculosis was once treated by sending people to the mountains or the seashore. Once there were no effective treatments for diabetes or psychosis. For many years bleeding people was a common medical treatment, and the life spans of humans were much less than it is today. People scoffed at the idea of flying and at those who believed that sperm could be frozen until it was needed. Pain will meet its match because people are demanding good research and treatment.

Develop pain projects such as periodically writing the Congress about problems in the pain management world. Don't be intimidated – reach for the stars! Make yourself intimate with a project. Problems are not solved if we overlook them. Join groups, become political, write articles, start a blog, tell other doctors and family what pain is all about, help people on the internet, etc. The list of possible activities is long. The common point is not to be alone, and to do as much as you can. Find a reason to fight for something. And understand that those who really understand you will understand why the pain will make some days productive and some days not so productive.

I've often wished that pain management clinics had staff whose job was specifically to help patients become pain advocates and mentors.

8 – Never forget: we are composed of two parts, a body and a soul

Both the body and soul can hurt. Both need treatment, warmth, feeding, and solace.

> My mother taught me that if I found a dollar on the street, I should stretch myself to get it. Then I should spend half on a rose to feed my soul, and half on food to feed my body. She analogized the stretching to be the work we do in life, and from the real reaching out to get that dollar, often with pain and sacrifice, we feed our keepers in life: our bodies and our souls.

It is critical to be outspoken about these needs. The body and soul are our essences. Both are needed for us to survive and grow. The soul lives in the body. We must move our bodies as much as possible. Walk, swim, stretch, carry, push, throw, swing, punch – whatever you can safely do, move your body. The soul benefits from stretching muscles, so:

9 – Exercise your mind and body as much as possible

Ask your doctor and physical therapist about the safe types of exercises you can do. Daily physical activity will do wonders for your strength, sleep, and morale. Try to do the activities outside and away from your home. Be with other people when you exercise.

Learn about proper exercise. Here are two excellent websites which can give provide ideas and background: www.exerciseismedicine.org and www.instituteoflifestyle-medicine.org

Physical exercise is only half of the process. Mental exercise is equally as important. Take courses, watch TV that makes you think, have mental projects, etc. Try to do the mental therapy with groups, such as taking a course at a local religious organization or community center. At least sit in and listen if you don't want to formally take the course. All this overlaps with the recommendation to have an hobby.

Mental and physical therapy strengthen the mind and body. They also give you something to do every day. These two elements are vital to survival. It may take time to locate the styles, forms and places of these two therapies, but the effort of the search will be well worth it.

10 - If you smoke, stop

Smoking is more than not good for your lungs or that it raises the chance of cancer. It also reduces the ability for medications to get into your body. Smoking is simply 'not good for you.' We know it is hard to stop. Several treatments exist, and the pros and cons of these are worthy of a discussion with your physician. The American Lung Association is a good resource. Its web site is www.lungsusa.org

11 - Enhance your life—compromise on old feuds

Be the stronger person by giving in on some points so that you have open relationships with people. Life needs to be as uncomplicated as possible. (Life is never totally uncomplicated!) At least try. Speaking to clergy, a mentor, a friend, or a psychotherapist may help with this important task.

12 - Live near friends or family

Nothing replaces having a good family and friends. Being with then during holidays, etc., cannot be underrated. Phone calls, discussions about which color to paint a room, or who is spicy in current politics, maybe even a little gossip, are the emotional springs from which we feel coziness, security, and bonding. Enjoy and celebrate them.

Let your family and friends see you often so they can see the real borders and fences that the pain puts around you. Let them also see you as a person, and not just a pain patient. Don't ask for sympathy, but for knowledge. Be a part of their lives and your life will also improve. Talk and learn about them and not be over talkative about your pain. Working on their problems will refocus you away from the pain. It feels great to be part of a group. The goal is to share all your lives as a group. Family gatherings can be so therapeutic for all.

> "It all changed after I asked my sister what color dress she was wearing to the Bar Mitzvah. She

said it was one of the few times I didn't talk about my pain issues. Ok, there are tons of pain issues, but I guess I was exhausting her patience with me. I then realized my life would have extra dimensions if we went as sisters to buy her dress! So she knows I can't walk much, but we got a wheelchair, and I took some extra meds with me in case I needed them, and this is going to make me cry, but we spent the day like two teenage girls going from store to store in the mall, giggling, eating junk food, and it was wonderful."

13 - Eat a healthy diet

Sound nutrition plays a huge role in our lives. Bad eating habits are often from laziness. Take the time to eat better. Your body is made up entirely of what you eat. Talk to your doctor. Consult with a dietitian. Learn about proper nutrition and which supplements are being used for various conditions; sometimes these are called nutraceluticals. Learn to be skeptical of promises that are 'too wonderful.' If your doctor doesn't support this line of thinking, consult with one who does. The American Dietetic Association has many good ideas. Their web site is www.eatright.org

And yes, of course, there must always be time for a little junk food.

14 - Develop some connection to a religion or philosophy

This recommendation is also part of many of the other recommendations on this list.

All of us need to make sense out of our lives. So connections to a religion or philosophy help so very much. The process can also evolve into rewarding social, emotional, and intellectual activities, such as the taking of courses, joining a religious congregation, going to a lecture or concert, etc. Furthermore, pick an endeavor that can never be fully mastered, so there is always something new to explore or debate. One can never master all of history or science, and political events will always need monitoring.

Work towards trying to figure your life out. Don't laugh when we say that you might succeed!

Be wary and suspicious if your life becomes 'all for naught'. Seek professional help if this happens since it may be a depression. Depression is common enough among us, even in those who do not suffer pain. If you begin to think of suicide, call your doctor, clergy, friend, or one of the suicide hotlines, such as The National Suicide Prevention Lifeline at 1-800-273-TALK. They have a web site at www.suicidepreventionlifeline.org/

15 - Find someone to laugh with

Find someone to be your confidant and friend. Learn to laugh with and at them. Let them laugh with and at you. Laugh at life and fate and funny people. Laughing with a group is so therapeutic. Go into psychotherapy if you can't or don't know how to laugh.

16 - Develop at least two hobbies

Hobby #1. Become a specialist in a hobby. It may be limited by some physical or financial limitation, but find something. This is critical. It might open up a world that can never be fully explored. One patient was a former computer engineer — he used his home computer to communicate with other computer users who had problems that his special skills can solve. He said he is now so busy. Another patient always loved European history, so she began endlessly reading on the topic. She discovered that is a task that can never be finished! She always had something to do.

Hobby #2. Know your disease. Don't take it to the level of an obsession, but keep abreast of new developments, treatments, etc. Join a pain advocacy group. At least get on their mailing lists. Learn to use the internet to get new information. Beware and learn how to trust the internet. Trust the good sites. Beware of the self-declared experts or of people who promise too much. Always test an idea you get from the internet by seeing if it is supported by other groups. Don't afraid to bring new material to your doctor, but understand your doctor may not have the time to read large packets of material.

Remember that no one vets most web sites. The good ones get posted as easily as the bad ones. The Health On The Net Foundation, http://www.hon.ch/, seeks to insure the accuracy of medical information published on the internet. We tend to trust the major health organizations, but some of the smaller ones may not be as trustworthy.

It is interesting to see what clinical or other work is being done in other countries. One excellent site is the Karolinska Institute in Sweden at www.ki.se. Excellent treatments might exist in other countries. If something seems inviting, gather the data and bring it to your doctor. The United States is not the only location of significant treatment and research.

The major media frequently run updates about the science and the politics of pain. In the last several years, such articles appeared in the New York Times, www.nytimes.com. Learning how to use internet search engines, podcasts, and RSS feeds can bring much information to you; this is not as hard to do as it may first appear. Ask any teenager for help.

Ask friends to inform you if they see a news story about pain management. A doctor's name in that story could become a new clinical contact.

Explore the web site of the United States National Institute of Neurological Diseases. It is time well spent. www.ninds.nih.gov/disorders/chronic_pain/detail_chronic_pain.htm

Most conditions have specialty support groups. Type the name of your disorder into any search engine and begin learning. For example, TMJ suffers should go to www.tmj.org

The Dannemiller Memorial Educational Foundation was founded in 1984 in memory of Francis Joseph Dannemiller, MD. www.dannemiller.com. It offers an excellent web site devoted to pain. Also visit www.pain.com

The American Pain Foundation provides excellent information at www.painfoundation.org

Contact nearby medical schools and specialty hospitals. They may have a treatment or research program suited to you. Clinical trials are monitored and quite safe. Condition-specific research studies are posted at www.clinicaltials.gov

Hospice programs are quite good with many pain management issues. They may also be able to direct you to the better local pain management groups. Call your local hospice for information.

The US Federal Drug Administration (FDA) site is good for information about new and old medications, recalls, etc. It is at www.fda.gov

All drug and medical device companies have websites. Many of them have sections designed for patients.

The key is to read enough and talk enough to other people so you can learn without instantly believing everything you hear and read. Learn to be the expert about experts, and how to separate a clinician from a salesperson.

17 - Join a group or know other pain patients

At least have them to call on the phone. Maybe this could be someone you met at doctor's office. One pain patient lady called another pain patient after reading about her in a local paper; they because great phone friends.

Sometimes formal support groups are not beneficial for everyone. Yet for many people, these groups are fantastic sources of community data, social contacts, referrals, and so on. It isn't necessary to go to every meeting or join every project, but these activities should be known to you and you to them. These are also excellent sources of hard information about pain management issues in the news. It may help to join an advocacy group to foster better pain management laws. And as been said before, at least get onto the advocacy group's mailing lists.

18 - Don't be scared when things go bad

This is life. We wish bad times did not happen.

It's during these bad times that you need a viable support network. We know how hard it can be to live with pain, and having interludes of self-pity, fear, anger, etc., are acknowledged as events that are going to occur. But you must talk yourself (with help from your family and friends) through those bleak periods. Don't hesitate to ask for help. It's okay to be human, with all our fears and strengths.

Sometimes the days of a bad pain cycle overlap at the same time that something else bad happens, like an insurance company who begins to cause problems. This combination is nasty, to say the least, and it can usurp the self-confidence and fight right out of a person. This is when it is necessary to stop for a bit, take a big breath,

ME AND MY PAIN | 457

and re-compose. You may need your family or lawyer to help with that recomposing. It can be hard do this when the pain is in a full battle mode. Perhaps the below will soothe a little. You are not alone.

> Remember, we are all people whose human needs are quite similar. Pain patients are everyday people who happen to have pain.
>
> At times hope may seem thin and shallow, but hope does remain. When you are in one of these bad states, your life and its needs fall into one of the more central and controversial problems in medical ethics. It may not be a great honor to be in such a place.
>
> So many people are involved in the care you need and receive. When you are in such as crisis, it is more important than ever that the medical, governmental and other policy makers become your advocates. Use your crisis to educate them. They must become your partners in pain. Perhaps your family can speak for you when you are in a downward cycle. The facts of what is happening to you during your crisis are the very realities and insights needed to tutor those who pay for and control your pain treatment. This is especially so if your crisis is indeed brought on by a change in their policies. But even if the crisis is unrelated to their polices, their policies also have to provide mechanisms to help you through these innocent calamites. Your pain cannot go unnoticed.

In 1948, the World Medical Association produced the Declaration of Geneva as an extension of the Hippocratic Oath. The British Medical Association proposed that "The spirit of the Hippocratic Oath cannot change and enjoins the duty of curing, the greatest crime being co-operation in the destruction of life by murder, suicide and abortion." In 1968, the Declaration of Sydney revised the Geneva Declaration that: "The health of my patients will be my first consideration. I will maintain the utmost respect for human life from the time of conception." In 1973, this next powerful statement was published in the Journal of the British Medical Association: "The whole resources of an advanced medical service are currently deployed in the pursuit of the preservation of life... We should regard the prevention of suffering as our primary aim." [281]

So things do progress, and further progress will follow.

A pain patient said: "The hospice doctor wanted to really sedate my Dad because he was suffering so much. But my uncle said the pain meds would kill him. So we learned about the double effect. That means that his death – maybe sped up and partially caused by the meds – would be ethically offset by the effect of less pain, so maybe if we shorten his life by a week or so, we increase the quality of his remaining time. My emotions surrounding his death, now that he died, are actually easier to live with than the emotions of what it was like watching him suffer so much."

The prevention of suicide and human misery though the reduction of needless suffering is an honorable use of science. Don't be afraid to firmly but diplomatically bring a medical professional to this mandate. Ask for help when things fall apart. If your treatment team won't help, then look for another team.

Don't be ashamed of being confused about how to make sense of all this. Honest people admit to confusion. Almost every technical, social, financial, psychological, religious, and ethical issue has taken a role in your life now that you are a person in pain. The same can apply if you are taking care of a person in pain. Don't concede too many decisions to others, especially if their brand or position on how to live doesn't feel right to you. Remember, though you may be dealing with an illness, and the ravages of that illness has changed your approach to life, you are still normal. Scarred, a bit wiser, and scared, but normal.

> There is a wonderful adage, probably of Chinese origin: *Experience turns knowledge into wisdom and the scholar into a mystic.*

Let's end with a patient's chilling, cutting, and honest statement that, as Thomas Huxley said, "represents the intriguing collision of when a comfortable theory is faced with an inconvenient fact".

These are her words to me:

> "When the other doctor started by giving me narcotics to control the pain, he called them medications. But when he could no longer figure out why I still hurt, and why I still needed the narcotics, he started calling them drugs. His enthusiasm dwindled. He felt I should be better,

but his therapy just didn't work despite his insistence that it should have.

He was so happy when I moved on to a new doctor.

I'm the same person. My pain is the same, only the doctor is different now. What the first one so freely gave me when he thought it would help was suddenly relabeled as something bad. But the sad thing is that he also relabeled me as untrustworthy and somehow unsafe. My suffering grew to be as horrible as the pain.

He changed. I didn't."

      ....*Eppur Si Muove* ...

References

[1] Author Unknown. Copied from Unruh JD: The Plains Across: The Overland Emigrants and the Trans-Mississippi West, 1940–60, in Platt ed.: Respectfully Quoted. Library of Congress. Washington DC 1989, p 113

[2] Zautra AJ, Fasman R, Parish BP, et a. Daily fatigue in women with osteoarthritis, rheumatoid arthritis, and fibromyalgia. Pain. 2007;128(1–2):128–135

[3] Gracey RH, Petzke F, Wolf JM, et al. Functional magnetic resonance imaging evidence of augmented pain processing in fibromyalgia. Arthritis Rheum 2002;46(5):1333–1343

[4] Berrettini W. The dream of pharmacogenics. Psychiatric Annals, 2008 Jun;38(6):372–373

[5] Svenningsson P, Chergui K, Rachleff I. Alterations in 5-HT1b receptor function by p11 in depress-like states. Science 6 Jan 2006;311(5757):77–80

[6] D'Arcy Y. Pain management survey report. June. Nursing 2008;43–49

[7] Brody JE. Many Treatments Can Ease Chronic Pain. New York Times. November 20, 2007. Accessed via www.highbeam.com May 27, 2008

[8] Furrow BR. Pain Management and Provider Liability: No more excuses. Journal of Law, Medicine and Ethics, 29 (2001):28–51

[9] The Quiet Epidemic. Florida Medical Magazine, Fall 2008, page 17–22

[10] www.fbi.gov/publications/financial/fcs_report2007/financial_crime_2007.htm

[11] Rosenberg T. When Is a Pain Doctor a Drug Pusher. New York Times Magazine. June 17, 2007. Accessed via www.highbeam.com on May 27, 2008

[12] Roth-Isigheit A, Thyen U, Stoven H. Pain among children and adolescents. Restrictions in daily living and triggering factors. Pediatrics 2005 Feb;115(2):e52062

[13] Huguet A, Niro J. The severity of chronic pediatric pain. J Pain. 2008 Mar;9(3):226–236

[14] Catanese SP, Coakley RM, Deirdre E. Chronic pain in the classroom: teachers' attributions about the causes of chronic pain. J School Health, May 1, 2007 accessed via www.highbeam.com May 27, 2008

[15] Auret K, Schug SA. Underutilization of opioids in elderly patients with chronic pain: approaches to correcting the problem Drugs Aging. 2005;22(8):641–651

[16] Pergolizzi J, Buger RH, Budd K, et al. Opioids and the management of chronic severe pain in the elderly: consensus statement of an international expert panel with focus on the six clinically most often used WHO step III opioids. Pain Pract 2008 May 23

[17] Pediatric Pain Rehabilitation Program Restores Functionality. Mayo Clinic Psych Update, Vol 1, No 1, 2009 www.mayoclinic.org

[18] http://www.abajournal.com/news/family_files_claim_over_childs_death_from_dental_patch_medication_error/ Accessed October 1, 2009

[19] Schuster JL. Addressing Patient's Pain; Veterans Health Administration's addiction of fifth vital sign may have far-reaching effects. The Washington Post, Feb 2 1999. Access via www.highbeam.com June 5, 2008

[20] Lyons JS. California Court Issues Landmark Ruling for Patients with Pain. Knight Ridder/Tribune Business News, Aug 22, 2001. Accessed via www.highbeam.com, June 5, 2008

[21] http://www.ppmjournal.com/abstract.asp?articleid=P0803D09

[22] Staff writers. Pain Treatment is patient's right, agency rules. July 14, 1999. Accessed via www.highbeam.com June 5, 2008 Seattle Post-Intelligencer (Seattle WA).

[23] Conkin M, When the hurts 'trial' will warn doctors about inadequate treatment of pain. Denver Rocky Mountain News, Feb 13, 1998, accessed via www.highbeam.com June 4, 2008

[24] Okie S, Doctors duty to ease pain at issue in California lawsuit; physicians are wary in prescribing narcotics. The Washington Post, May 7, 2001. Accessed via www.highbeam.com June 4, 2008

[25] Phillips DM. JACHO pain management standards are unveiled. 2000 JAMA; 284:428–429

[26] http://www.jointcommission.org/NewsRoom/health_care_issues.htm#9

[27] Lipman L. New Medicare hospice rule would expand patient rights. Palm Beach Post. June 4, 2008. www.pbpost.com

[28] Conolly ME. Alternative to euthanasia: pain management. Issues in Law and Medicine. March 22, 1989. Accessed via www.highbeam.com June 5, 2008

[29] Chee W, Guevara E, Im EO. The pain experience of Hispanic patients with cancer in the United States. Oncology Nursing Forum, July 1, 2007. Accessed via www.highbeam.com on June 4 2008

30 Foley KM. "The Decriminalization of Cancer," in Advances in Pain Research and Therapy, Vol 11, Hills CD, Fields WS, eds. New York, Raven Press;1989:5

31 Alpers A, "Criminal Act or Palliative Care? Prosecutions Involving the Care of the Dying." Journal of Law, Medicine and Ethics, 26 (1988):308

32 The EPEC Project, 750 N Lake Shore Drive, Suite 601, Chicago, www.epec.net

33 http://www.fda.gov/cder/news/fda_cdc_partnership.htm, Accessed February 9, 2009

34 Elliott VS. FDA. CDC scrutiny follows surge in accidental opioid overdoses. AMANews, posted Feb 9, 2009. http://www.ama-assn.org/amednews/2009/02/09/hll20209.htm

35 Bates MS: Biocultural Dimensions of Chronic Pain. State University of New York Press. Albany, 1996, p 138

36 Peck SR: Quick, The Morphine, in Atlas of Facial Expressions. Oxford University Press, New York, 1987, p 138

37 Bruchmüller K, Meyer TD: Diagnostically irrelevant information can effect likelihood of diagnosis of bipolar disorder. J Affect Disorder 2008. doi.10.1016/j.jad.2008.11.018

38 Trescot AM, Helm S, Hansen H, et al: Opioids in the management of chronic non-cancer pain: an update of The American Society of Interventional Pain Physicians' Guidelines. Pain Physician. 2008 Mar;11(2 Suppl):S5–S62

39 Brodsky S, Heller P: Addressing the Perfect Phantom on the Witness Stand. J Am Acad Psychiatry Law 36:541–2, 2008

40 Grant JA, Rainville P: Pain Sensitivity and Analgesic Effects of Mindful States in Zen Meditators: A Cross-Sectional Study. Psychosomatic Medicine 2009; 71:106–144

41 Orsey, AD, Belasco JB, Ellenberg JH, et al: Variation in receipt of opioids by pediatric oncology patients who

died in children's hospitals. Pediatric Blood and Cancer. 2008: DOI 10.1002/pbc.21824

[42] Levin A: Adhering to Western Medicine May Limit Health Potential. Psychiatric News. August 21, 2009, page 9

[43] Surgeon General, US Department of Health and Human Services, (2001). Mental Health: Culture, Race, and Ethnicity. www.surgeongeneral.gov/library/mentalhealth/cre/

[44] Moore SL: Rational Suicide Among Older Adults. Archive of Psychiatric Nursing 1993;7(2):106–110

[45] Durkheim E: Suicide: A Study in Sociology. Free Press. New York. 1957.

[46] Illich I: Medical Nemesis: The Expropriation of Health. Pantheon Books, New York, 1976, p 153–154

[47] Proceedings of the National Academy of Sciences, DOI:10.1073/pnas.0813179106

[48] Siegel R. Intoxication: Life in pursuit of artificial paradise. 1989, Rochester VT, Park Street Press

[49] Miller L: Neuropsychological Concepts of Somatoform Disorders. Int J Psychiatry Med. 1984; 14:31.46

[50] Weissman D, Haddox JD: Pseudoaddiction – An Iatrogenic Syndrome. Pain. 1989; 36:363–366

[51] Marks RM, Sachar EJ: Under-treatment of Medical Impatiens with Narcotic Analgesics. Ann Intern Med 1973;78:173–181

[52] Amenta M, Bohnet N: Nursing Care of the Terminally Ill. 1986, Chapter 6

[53] Cecil-Loeb Textbook of Medicine. Beeson PB, McDermott W, eds., WB Saunders, Philadelphia. 1967, page 1473

[54] Wikler A: Conditioning Processes in Opioid Dependence and in Relapse: Mechanisms and Treatment. Plenum Press, New York. 1980, page 176

[55] DeQuincey T: Confessions of an English Opium Eater, 2003 London. Penguin Classics

[56] Portenoy RK: Chronic Opioid Therapy in Non Malignant Pain. J Pain and Symptom Management 1990; 5(1-Suppl)46–62

[57] Portenoy RK: Opioid Therapy for Chronic Nonmalignant Pain. Current Status, in Progress in Pain Research and Management. Vol. 1, Fields HL, Liebeskin JC, eds., ISAP Press, Seattle. 1994, p 247–279

[58] Portenoy RK: Opioid Therapy for Chronic Nonmalignant Pain: A Review of the Critical Issues. J Pain and Symptom Management 1996, 11(4):203–217

[59] Norton LL, Ferill MF, Omudhome O: The Use of Opioids in the Treatment of Nonmalignant Pain: Clinical Issues and Guidelines. Am J Pain Management. 1997;7(2):42–52

[60] Krames ES: Rational Use of Opioids for Nonmalignant Pain. J Pharmac Care in Pain and Symptoms Control 1997;5(3):3–15

[61] Martell BA, O'Conner PG, Kerns RD, et al. Systematic review: opioid treatment for chronic back pain: prevalence, efficacy and association with addiction. Ann Intern Med, 2007 Jan 16;146(2):116–127

[62] Fleming MF, Balousek SL, Klessig CL. Substance abuse disorders in a primary care sample receiving daily opioid therapy. J Pain 2007;8(7):573–582

[63] Kahan M, Srivastava A, Wilson L, et al. Misuse of and dependence on opioids: study of chronic pain patients. Can Fam Physician. 2006 . Sept;52(9):1081–1087

[64] Kahan M, Srivastava A, Wilson L, et al. Opioids for managing chronic non-malignant pain: safe and effective prescribing. Can Fam Physician 2006 Sept;52(9):1091–1096

[65] Deshpande A, Furlan A, Mailis-Gagnon A, et al. Opioids for chronic low-back pain. Cochraine Database Syst Rev. 2007 Jul 18;(3):CD004959

[66] Chou R, Huffman LH. Medications for Acute and Chronic Low Back Pain: A review of the evidence for an American Pain Society/American College of Physicians Clinical Practice Guideline. Ann Intern Med 2007 Oct 2, 147)7:505–514

[67] Fishbain DA, Cole BN, Lewis J, Rosomoff HL, Rosomoff RS. What percentage of chronic nonmalignant pain patients exposed to chronic opioid analgesic therapy develop abuse/addiction and/or aberrant drug related behaviors? A structured evidence-base review. Pain Med 2008 May-June;9(4);444–459

[68] Irick N: Pharmacologic and Nonpharmacologic Approaches to Pain. 1995 Annual Meeting – Focus on Scientific Symposia Highlights. Southern Medical Association, Birmingham 1996, p-3–4

[69] Miller L: Psychotherapeutic Approaches to Chronic Pain. Psychotherapy 1993;30(1):115–124

[70] Strauss A: Iatraddiction – A Diagnostic Term in Lieu of Pseudoaddiction. Practical Pain Management, April 2005, page 40–42

[71] Grafton A; New Worlds, Ancient Texts. Harvard University Press, Boston, 1992, page 1

[72] Taj RP: Practical Management of Pain. Year Book Medical Publishers, Inc, Chicago, 1986, p73

[73] Levine JD, Gorden NC, Fields HL: The Mechanism of Placebo Analgesia. Lancet 1878:2:654–657

74 Silber TJ: Placebo Therapy. JAMA 1979;242:245–246

75 Warfield CA: Principles and Practice of Pain Management. McGraw-Hill. New York, 1995

76 Fields HL, Price DD. "Toward a Neurobiology of placebo analgesia. In Harrington A, ed.: The Placebo effect: an interdisciplinary exploration. Cambridge. Harvard University Press, 1997;93–116

77 Scott DJ, Staler CS, Agnatic CM, et al. Placebo and nocebo effects are defined by opposite opioid and dopaminergic responses. Arch Gen Psych 2008 Feb;65(2):220–231

78 Journal of Neuroscience. DOI: 10,1523/JNEUROSCI.2534-08.2008

79 American Psychiatric Association: Diagnostic and Statistical Manual of Mental Disorders, 4th Edition, Text Revision. Washington DC, American Psychiatric Association, 2000, p 685

80 Institute of Medicine: Health Literacy: A Prescription to End Confusion. 2004. www.iom.edu or www.nap.edu

81 National Center for Cultural Competence, at www.georgetown.edu/research/gucchd/nccc

82 Plicta S: The Effects of Woman Abuse on Health Care Utilization and Health Status: A Literature Review. Women's Health Issues. 1992; 2(3):154–163

83 Rimsza ME, Berg RA, Locke C: Sexual Abuse: Somatic and Emotional Reactions. Child Abuse Negl. 1988; 12(2):201–208

84 Seidel JS, Elvik SL, Berkowitz CD, Day C: Presentation and Evaluation of Sexual Misuse in the Emergency Room. Pediatr Emerg Care 1986: 2(3):157–164

[85] Halpern S: Sister Sympathy. The New York Times Magazine May 9, 1993, p 28

[86] Bebbington PE: Monosymptomatic hypochondriasis. Abnormal Illness Behavior and Suicide. Br J Psychiatry. 1976; 128:475–478

[87] Chapman CB .Physicians Law and Ethics. New York University Press. 1984

[88] Insurance companies may not argue with the diagnosis or needed treatment, but rather deny based on what they are limits of the policy contract. "We don't deny the pain, but we are obligated by contract to pay only so much…"

[89] Henderson IJ: Physician and Patient as a Social System. N Engl J Med 1935;128:819–823

[90] Merril JM, Laux L, Thornby JL: Troublesome Aspects of the Patient-Physician Relationship – A Study of Human Factors. So Med J 1978;80:1211–1215

[91] McCaffery M, Ferell B,: How Would You Respond to these Patients in Pain? Nursing 91 June 1991, pp 34–37

[92] Cahill-Wright C: Managing Post-operative Pain. Nursing 91 December 1991, pp 43–45

[93] See S'Arcy June 2008

[94] Arendt J. Melatonin and human rhythms. Chronobiol Int, 2006;23(1–2):21–37

[95] http://www.nhlbi.nih.gov/about/ncsdr/index.htm

[96] Swift J: Battle of the Books, 2004, Whitefish MT, Kessinger Publishing. First published in 1704

[97] Treece C, Khantzian E: Psychodynamic Factors in the Development of Drug Dependency. Psych Clinics of N Amer. 1986;9:339–412

[98] Khantzian E, Mach SM: Self-preservation and the care of the self: Ego Instability Reconsidered. Psychoanalytic Study of the Child 1983:38:209–332

[99] Alexthymia is associated with difficulties recognizing and verbalizing feelings, with few dreams. It is associated with substance abuse. It is from the Greek for 'no words for feelings.'

[100] Beecher HK: Pain in Men Wounded in Battle. An Surg 1946, 123–96

[101] Bashbaum AI, Fields HL: Endogenous Pain Control Systems: Brainstem Pathways and Endorphin Circuitry. Ann Rev Neurosci 1984;7:309

[102] Warfield CA: Principles and Practice of Pain Management McGraw-Hill, New York, 1993; pp 358–359

[103] Roy S, Loh HH. Effects of opioids on the immune system. Neurochem Res 1996;21:1375–1386

[104] Daniell HW. Hypogonadism in men consuming sustained-action oral opioids. Pain 2002. 3:377–384

[105] Daniell HW: Opioid endrocrinopathy in women consuming prescribed sustained–action opioids for control of nonmalignant pain. J Pain. 2008 Jan;9)1):28–36

[106] Fishbain DA, Rosomoff HL, Rosomoff RS. Drug Abuse, dependence and addiction in chronic pain patients. Clin J Pain 1992;8:77–85

[107] Substance Abuse and Mental Health Services Administration, Office of Applied Studies. Results from the 2006 National Survey on Drug Use and Health: National Findings. Rockville, Md: Office of Applied Studies; 2007, NSDUH Series h-32, DHHS publication SMA 07-4293

[108] Elkashef A, Biswas J, Acri JB, et al: Biotechnology and the treatment of addictive disorders: new opportunities. BioDrugs. 2007;21:259–267

[109] Rutter JL. Symbiotic relationship of pharmacogenetics and drugs of abuse. AAPS J. 2003;160:323–333

[110] Wirz S, Klaschik E: Management of constipation in palliative care patients undergoing opioid therapy: Is polyethylene glycol an option. Am J of Hospice and Palliative Medicine. 2005;22(5):375381

[111] Hill CS: The Negative Influence of Licensing and Disciplinary Boards and Drug Enforcement Agencies on Pain Treatment with Opioid Analgesics. J Pharmacol Care in Pain and Symptom Control. 1993;1:43–62

[112] Thernstrom, M. Pain, The Disease. The New York Times. December 16, 2001. Accessed via www.highbeam.com June 4, 2008

[113] Scarry E. The Body in Pain: the making and unmaking of the world. Oxford. Oxford University Press, 1985

[114] Mersky H, el al. International Association for the study of pain classification of chronic pain. 2en ed. Seattle. ISAP Press, 1994

[115] Vanderah TW. Pathophysiology of pain. Med Clin of North Am, 2007 Jan;91(1):1–12

[116] Staud R, Rodriquez ME: Mechanisms of disease: pain in fibromyalgia syndrome. J Rehabil Med.2003;41(suppl):89–94

[117] Campbell JN, Meyer RA: Mechanisms of neuropathic pain. Neuron. 20067 October 5;52(1):77–92

[118] Bennett RM: Fibrositis: misnomer for a common rheumatic disorder. West J Med. 1981;134:405

[119] Burchkardt CS, Goldenberg D, Crofford L, et al. Guideline for the management of fibromyalgia syndrome pain in adults and children. APS Clinical Practice Guidelines Series, No 4, Glenview Ill: American Pain Society; 2005

[120] Davies KA, Macfarlane GJ, Nicholl BI, et al. Restorative sleep predicts the resolution of chronic widespread pain: results from the EPIFUND study. Rheumatology 2008;47:1809–1813

[121] Bar KJ, Boettger S, Wagner G, et al. Changes of pain perception, autonomic function, and endocrine parameters during treatment of anorectic adolescents. J Am Acad Child Adolesc Psychiatry. 2006;45(9):1068–1076

[122] Kato K, Sullivan PF, Evenbgard B, Pedersen NI: Chronic widespread pain and its co-morbidities: a population-based study. Arch Intern Med 2006;166(15):1649–1654

[123] Cook ND: The Brain Code. Methuen. London and New York. 1986

[124] Cao H, Zhang YQ. Spinal glial activation contributes to pathological pain states. Neurosci Biobehav Rev. 2008 Jul;32(5):972–83

[125] Watkins LR, Milligan ED, Maier SF. Glial proinflammatory cytokines mediate exaggerated pain states: Implications for clinical pain. Adv Exp Med Bio. 2003;521:1–21

[126] Lowenstein WR: Excitation and Inactivation in a Receptor Membrane. Ann NY Acad Sci, 1961;95:510

[127] Guyton AC, Hall JE. Textbook of medical physiology. WB Saunders Co., Philadelphia, 2000

[128] Cowen WM. The Development of the Brain. Sci Am 1979;241(3):37–

[129] Harris AC, Rothwell PE, Gerwirtz JC: Effects of the NMDA receptor antagonist memantine on the expression and

development of acute opiate dependence as assessed by withdrawal-potentiated startle and hyperalgesia. Psychopharmacology (Berl), 2008 Mar; 196(4):649–660

[130] Crockett MJ, Clark L, Tabibnia G, et al. Serotonin Modulates Behavioral Reactions to Unfairness. Science. June 5, 2008. Published online www.sciencemag.org

[131] Reisne T, Pasternak GW: opioid analgesics and antagonists. In: The Pharmacological Basis of Therapeutics. Hartman JG, Limbrid TS (eds). 1966 McGraw-Hill, New York, p 521–556

[132] Sudakiv SK, Rusakova IV, Trigub MM, et al. Self-administration of morphine by rates causes monoamine release in anterior cingulate cortex. Bull Exp Boil Med. 2007 Aug;144(2):210–203

[133] Zhu W, Cadet P, Baggerman G, et al. Human white blood white cells synthesize morphine. J Imm, 2005, 175:7357–7362

[134] Boettcher C, Fellermesier M, Boettcher C. Drager B, et al. How human neuroblastoma cells make morphine. Proc Natl Acad Sci USA 2005 June 14;102(24):8495–500

[135] Zhu W, Esch T, Kream RM, Stefano GB. Converging cellular processes for substances of abuse: endogenous morphine Neuro Endrocrinol Lett. 2008 Feb;29(1):63–66

[136] Enoch MA. The role of GABA(a) receptors in the development of alcoholism. Pharmacol Biochem. Behav 2008 March 15

[137] Manzanares J, Julian MD, Carrascosa A. Role of the cannabinoid system in pain control and therapeutic implications for the management of acute and chronic pain episodes. Curr Neuropharmacol 2006, 4:239–257

[138] Russo EB: Cannabinoids in the management of difficult to treat pain. Ther Clin Risk Manag. 2008 Feb;4(1):245–259

[139] Ashton J: Pro-drugs for indirect cannabinoids as therapeutic agents. Curr Drug Deliv. 2008 Oct;5(4):243–247

[140] Marx J. Marijuana receptor gene cloned. Science 1990;249:624–626

[141] Loopez-Moreno JA, Gonzalez-Cuevas G, Moreno G, Narvarro M. The pharmacology of the endocannabinoid system: functional and structural interactions with other neurotransmitters and their repercussions in behavioral medicine. Addict Biol 2008 Jun;13(2):160–187

[142] Hosking RD, Zajicek JP. Therapeutic potential of cannabis in pain medicine. Br J Anaesth 2008 May 28

[143] Smith PF. Symptomatic treatment of multiple sclerosis using cannabinoids: recent advances Expert Rev Neurother 2007 Sep;7(9):1157–1163

[144] McCarberg BH. Cannabinoids: their role in pain and palliation. J Pain Palliat Care Pharmacother. 2007;21(3):19–28

[145] http://www.helpforheadaches.com/articles/memantine8x11.pdf, accessed December 6 2008

[146] Bifal M, Rapoport A, Sheftell F, Tepper D, Tepper S: Memantine in the preventive treatment of refractory migraine. Headache, 2008 Oct;38(9);1337–42

[147] Cruccu G: Treatment of painful neuropathy. Curr Opin Neurol, 2007 Oct;20(5):531–5

[148] Mendez IA, Trukillo KA: NMDA receptor antagonists inhibit opiate antinociceptive tolerance and locomotor sensitization in rats. Psychopharmacology (Berl), 2008 Feb 2008;196(3):4597–509

[149] McPherson ML: Chronic Pain Management: A disease based approach. http://www.accp.com/docs/bookstore/psap/p5b8sample01.pdf, accessed December 6, 2008

[150] Sarchielle P, DiFilapp M, Nardi K, Calabresi P: Sensitization, glutamate, and the link between migraine and fibromyalgia. Curr Pain Headache Rep, 2007 Oct; 11(5):343–51

[151] Coderre TJ, Jumar N, Lefebvre CD, Yu JS: A comparison of the glutamate release inhibition and anti-allodynic effects of gabapentin, lamotrigine and riluzole in a model of neuropathic pain. J Neurochem, 2007 Mar;100(5):1289–1299

[152] Harris RE, Sundgren PC, Pan Y, Hsu M, et al: Dynamic levels of glutamate within the insula are associated with improvements in multiple pain domains in fibromyalgia. Arthritis Rheum, 2008 Mar;58(3):903–7

[153] Esch T, Stefano GB. The neurobiology of pleasure, reward processes, addiction and their health implications. Neuroendocrinol Lett 2004; 25:235–251

[154] Salamon E, Esch T, Stefano G. Pain and relaxation (review) Int J Molecul Med. 2006;18:456–470

[155] Marighi A, Salio C, Ghirri A, el al. BDNF as a pain modulator. Prog Neurobiol. 2008 Apr 26 (PubMed 18514997)

[156] Suter M, Yeong-Ray W, Decosterd I, Ru-Rong J. Do glial cells control pain? Neuron Glia Biol. 2007 Aug;3(3):225–268

[157] Kirby GE. Biosynthesis of the morphine alkaloids. Science. 1967 Jan 13;155(759):170–3

[158] http://content.karger.com/ProdukteDB/produkte.asp?doi=10.1159/000083036 Accessed January 2010

[159] Lasagna L. White House Conference on Narcotic and Drug Abuse. Pharmacol Rev. 1964, 16–47

[160] http://www.independent.co.uk/news/world/asia/doctors-propose-using-afghan-opium-as-nhs-painkiller-433429.html. Accessed January 2010

[161] Franz DN: Pharmacology of Analgesic Receptors. J Pharmacol Care in Pain and Symptom Control 1994; 2(3):37–58

[162] Galanter M, Kleber HD. Textbook of Substance Abuse Treatment. 2en Ed., Washington DC: The American Psychiatric Press; 1999

[163] Susuki T, Kishimoto Y, Ozaki S, Narita M. Mechanism of opioid dependence and interaction between opioid receptors. Eur J Pain, 2001;5: Suppl A:63–65

[164] He S, Li N, Grasing K. Long-term opiate effects on amphetamine-induced dopamine release in the nucleus accumbens core and conditioned place preference. Pharmacol Biochem Behav, 2004 Feb;77(2):327–335

[165] Dunlop BW, Nemeroff CGB. The role of dopamine in the pathophysiology of depression. Arch Gen Psych, Vol 64, Mar 2007, 327–337

[166] http://www.historicaldocuments.com/HarrisonNarcoticsTaxAct.htm Accessed June 8, 2008

[167] Narcocon. History of Opium. www.opiumaddiction.com/opiu-hisotry.htm

[168] www.usatoday.com/news/military/2008-10-20-pain-drugs.htm

[169] Musto D: The American Disease: Organs of Narcotic Control. In Foote C, Levy RJ, eds: Criminal Law – Cases and Materials. Little, Brown & Co. Boston. 1982, pp 891–906

[170] Flector Patch prescribing information. www.flectorpatch.com Accessed September 5, 2008

[171] Voltaren Gel prescribing information. www.voltarengel.com. Accessed September 5, 2008

172 Treede RD, Jensen TS, Campbell JN, et al.: Neuropathic pain: redefinition and a grading system for clinical and research purposes. Neurology, 2008 Apr 29;70(18):1630–1635

173 Maze M, Tranquilli W: Alpha-2 adrenoceptor agonists and anesthesia. Br J Anesthesia 1993;71:108–118

174 Vallejo RO, Leon C, Benyamin R. Opiate therapy and immunosuppression: a review. Am J Ther 2004 Sept-Oct;11(5):354–365

175 Whitten L. Morphine-Induced Immunospression, from Brain to Spleen. NIDA Notes 2008 June, 21(6). http://www/drugabuse.gov/NIDA-notes/NNvol121N6/morphine.html Accessed July 11, 2008

176 Office of Applied Studies. Substance Abuse and Mental Health Services Administration. National Household Survey on Drug Abuse, Washington DC: SAMHSA, 2001

177 http://dawninfo.samhsa.gov/

178 http://www.samhsa.gov/newsroom/advisories/0709043102.aspx. Accessed May 29, 2008

179 Prommer EE: Ziconotide: Can we use it in palliative care? Am J of Hospice and Palliative Medicine. 2005 (Sept–Oct) 22(5):375–381

180 Fink DJ, Mata M: HSV gene transfer in the treatment of chronic pain. Sheng Li Xue Bao 20008 Oct 25;60(5):610–616

181 Srinivasan R, Fink DJ, Glorioso JC: HSV vectors for gene therapy of chronic pain. Curr Opin Mol Ther, 20008 Oct;10(5):449–455

182 Melzack R, Wall PD. Pain mechanisms: a new theory. Science. 1965:150:971–979

[183] Melzack R: The Puzzle of Pain. 1973, New York. Basic Books, Inc., Chapter 6

[184] Khadilkar A, Odebiyi DO, Brosseau L, Wells GA: Transcutaneous electrical stimulation (TENS) versus placebo for chronic back pain. Cochrane Database Syst Rev. 2008 Oct 8(4):CD003008

[185] Buckalew N, Haut MW, Morrow L, Weiner D: Chronic pain is associated with brain volume loss in older adults: preliminary evidence. Pain Med. 2008 Mar;9(2):240–8

[186] Schweinhardt P, Kuchinad A, Pikall CF, Busnell MC. Increased gray matter density in young women with chronic vulvar pain. Pain 2008 Dec;140(3):411–419

[187] Geha PY, Baliki MN, Harden RN, Bauer WR, et al: The brain in chronic CRPS pain: abnormal gray-white matter interactions in emotional and autonomic regions. Neuron 2008 Nov 26;60(4):570–581

[188] Apkarian AV, Sosa Y, Sonty S, Levy R: Chronic back pain is associated with decreased prefrontal and thalamic gray matter density. J Neurosci. 2004 November 17;24(46):10410–10415

[189] Flor H: Cortical reorganization and chronic pain: implications for rehabilitation. J Rehabil Med 2003 May;(41 Suppl):66–72

[190] Witt CM, Jena S, Brinhaus B, et al. Acupuncture for patients with chronic back pain. Pain. 2006;125:98–106

[191] Weidenhammer W, Linde K, Steng A, et al. Acupuncture for chronic low back pain in routine care: a multicenter observational study. Clin J Pain. 2007;23:128–135

[192] Ellis A: Addictive Behaviors and Personality Disorders. Social Policy, December 22, 1998, accessed via www.highbeam.com, May 25, 2008

193 Bate MS: Biocultural Dimensions of Chronic Pain. State University of NY, Albany 1996, p 60

194 Hyman SE, Cassen NH: Pain, in Scientific American Consult – CD Version, 1990

195 Broodman S: Being Difficult. For Some Patients, It's a Coping Mechanism. The Washington Post, October 21, 2008. www.washpost.com

196 Friedman R: When All Else Fails, Blaming the Patient Often Comes Next. New York Times, October 21, 2008. www.nytimes.com

197 Peckamen J: When Your Doctor Doesn't Know: Don't Give up If Your Illness is a Mystery. Reader's Digest Pleasantville NY, November 1992

198 Dave, MK, Miceli KP, Modha P: Psychiatric Medicine. 2008; Philadelphia, Lippincott Williams and Wilkins, page 255

199 Hippocrates, "Art", in Reiser SJ, Dyck AJ, Curran WJ, eds.: Ethics in Medicine: Historical Perspectives and Contemporary Concerns. MIT Press. Cambridge 1977

200 Plato. Republic. Hackett, Indianapolis, 1974, pp 67–77

201 Steinberg A: Free Will Versus Determinism I Bioethics: Comparative Philosophical and Jewish Perspectives. Jewish Medical Ethics, Vol 2(1), January 1991, p 17–20

202 Marmer SS: Theories of the Mind and Psychopathology, in Talbott JA, et al, Textbook of Psychiatry. The American Psychiatric Press, Washington DC, 1988, pp 156–157

203 Ibid Steinberg 1991

204 Babylonian Talmud, Tractate Sabbath 31a

205 Mishnah Avoth 2:10

[206] Jerusalem Talmud Tractate Nedarim 9,4

[207] Ballantyne JC. Opioids for chronic non-terminal pain. So Med J. November 1, 2006. Accessed via www.highbeam.com, May 27, 2008

[208] Portney RK, Foley KM. Chronic use of opioid analgesics in non-malignant pain: report of 38 cases. Pain 1988;25:171–186

[209] Illich I: The Killing of Pain, in Medical Nemesis. Pantheon Books, New York, 1967, chapter 3

[210] Weizacher V: Arzt und Kranker. Kohler. Stuttgart 1949. Vol 1

[211] Good WJ: A Theory of Social Strain. Am J Soc 1960;25:483

[212] Ausubel DP: Drug Addiction: Physiological and Sociological Aspects. Random House. New York 1958

[213] Seltzer MD: Hostility as a Barriers to Therapy in Alcoholism. Psychiatric Quarterly. May 1957;31:301–305

[214] Imhof JE: Countertransference Issues in Alcoholism and Drug Addiction. Psychiatric Annals May 1991;21(5): 292–306

[215] Krystal H, Raskin HA: Self and Object Representation in Alcoholism and Other Drug Dependence: Implications for Therapy. In Blaine JD, Julisu DA, eds., Psychodynamics of Drug Dependence. Washington DC, National Institute on Drug Abuse. 1997, Monograph Number 12

[216] Engel GL: Psychogenic Pain and eh Pain Prone Patient. Am J Med 1959; June:889–918

[217] Hirsh AT, George SZ, Bialosky JE, Robinson ME. Fear of pain, pain catastrophizing, and acute pain perception: relative prediction and timing of assessment. J Pain. 2008 May 15

[218] Goleman D: New Research Illuminates Self-Defeating Behavior. The New York Times, September 1, 1987, accessed May 25, 2008 www.nytimes.com

[219] Colman A: A Dictionary of Psychology. Oxford University Press, Oxford, 2001

[220] American Psychiatric Association: Diagnostic and Statistical Manual of Mental Disorders, Fourth Edition, Text Revision. Washington DC, American Psychiatric Association, 2000

[221] King SA, Strain JJ: Revising the Category of Somatoform Pain Disorder. Hospital and Community Psychiatry. 1992;43(3):217–219

[222] Hendler NH. Depression caused by chronic pain. J Clin Psychiatry. 1984;45:30–38

[223] Adler RH. Are there psychological factors which lead to iatrogenic disorders? Schweiz Med Wochenschr. 1996 Apr 13;126(15):612–615

[224] Spiegel H. Nocebo: the power of suggestibility. Prev Med 1997 Sept-Oct;26(5 Pt 1):616–621

[225] McHugh G, Thomas G. Living with chronic pain: the patient's perspective. Nurs Stand 2001 Sept 12–18;15(52):33–37

[226] Kouyanou CE, Pither CE, Weesely S. Iatrogenic factors and chronic pain. Psychosomatic Med 1997;59(6):597–604

[227] Kleinbrink EL, Nikitin AG. Misdiagnosis of chronic pain: a bioethical problem. Michigan Academician, March 22, 2007. Accessed via www.highbeam.com, June 8, 2008

[228] National Institute on Drug Abuse: The Science of Addiction. National Institute of Health Publication Number 07-5605, April 2007

[229] Tennant F: Cytochrome P450 Gene Implicated in Need for High-Dose Pain Medication. American Academy

of Addiction Psychiatry (AAAP) 20th Annual Meeting & Symposium: Poster 5. Presented December 4, 2009. Accessed www.medscape.com/viewarticle/714030_print December 29, 2009

[230] Clark S: Cosmic enlightenment. The New Scientist. March 8, 2008, p 28–31

[231] Phillips H: Just can't get enough. The New Scientist, August 26, 2006, p 30–35

[232] Treatment on a plate: A dietary approach to treating addiction seems worth investigating. The Economist. October 18, 2008. www.economist.com/techview

[233] Saunders JB, Cottler LB: The development of the Diagnostic and Statistical Manual of Mental Disorders version V substance use disorders section: establishing the research framework. Current Opinion in Psychiatry. May 2007;20(3):208–211

[234] Ballantyne JC, Mao J: Opioid therapy for chronic pain. N Engl J Med. 2003;349:1943–1953

[235] Kouyanou A, Pither C, Wessely S. Medication misuse, abuse and dependence in chronic pain patients. J Psychosom Res. 1997;43:497–504

[236] Manchikanti L, Manchukonda R, Damrom K, el al. Does adherence monitoring reduce controlled substance abuse in chronic pain patients? Pain Physician 2006;9:57–60

[237] Weaver MF, Schnoll SH. Abuse liability in opioid therapy for pain treatment in patients with an addiction history. Clin J Pain 2002;18:S61–S69

[238] Brown RL, Patterson JJ, Rounds LA, et al. Substance use among patients with chronic back pain. J Fam Pract 1996;43:152–160

[239] Martell BA, O'Connor PG, Kerns RD, et al. Systematic review: opioid treatment for chronic back pain: prevalence, efficacy, and association with addiction. Ann Inter Med 207 Jan 16;146(2):116–127

[240] Weaver M, Schnoll S. Addiction issues in prescribing opioids for chronic nonmalignant pain. J Addict Med 1(1) March 2007;2–10

[241] http://www.allgreatquotes.com/shakespeareinsults220.shtml Accessed August 3, 2009

[242] Feldman S, Theilbar G, eds: Life Styles: Diversity in American Society. Little Brown & Co., Boston 1971

[243] DuPont R: The Selfish Brain: Learning from Addiction. American Psychiatric Press, Washington DC 1997, pp 93–133

[244] Petrie A: Individuality in Pain and Suffering. University of Chicago Press, Chicago, 1967

[245] Beecher HK: Measurement of Subjective Responses: Quantitative Effects of Drugs. Oxford University Press, New York, 1959

[246] Hartman D: "Suffering" in Cohen AA, Mendes-Flohr P: Contemporary Jewish Religious Thought. The Free Press, New York, 1972, pp 939–946

[247] Bakan D: Disease, Pain and Sacrifice: Towards a Psychology of Suffering. Beacon Press, Boston 1968

[248] Levy MH: Pharmacologic Treatment of Cancer Pain. N Eng J Med, 1996;335:1224–1132

[249] Agency for Health Care Policy and research, Public Health Service, US Department of Health and Human Services, Management of Cancer Pain, AHCPR Publication No-94-0592, March 1994, p 50–51

250 Goodman and Gilman: The Pharmacological Basis of Therapeutics – Seventh Edition, McMillian Publishing Co., New York, 1985, p 511

251 Bonica JJ: The Management of Pain. Lea and Febiger. Philadelphia 1953

252 Neal H: The Politics of Pain. McGraw-Hill, New York 1978

253 Wall PD, Jones M: Defeating Pain. The War Against a Silent Epidemic. Plenum Press. New York, 1991, page 19–20

254 www.psychking.net/id158.htm, and www.freud.org.uk Accessed December 20, 2009

255 Doyle, D, Hanks GWC, MacDonald N, eds. Oxford textbook of palliative medicine. Oxford. Oxford University Press, 1998: 3

256 Webster's Revised Unabridged Dictionary. MICRA, Inc., 29 Mar. 2009. http://dictionary.reference.com/browse/palliate

257 Gatchel RJ: Psychosocial assessment and disability management in the rehabilitation of painful spinal disorders. In: Mayer T, Mooney V, Gatchel R, eds. Contemporary Conservative Care for Painful Spinal Disorders. Philadelphia: lea & Febiger; 1991

258 Mayer TG, Gatchel RJ: Functional restoration for spinal disorders. The Sports Medicine Approach. Philadelphia. Lea & Febiger, 1988

259 Eliade M: A History of Religious Ideas. Vol 2, from Gautama Buddha to the Triumph of Christianity. University of Chicago Press. Chicago. 1982, p 156

260 Phillips DZ: The Problem of Evil II, in Reason and Religion. Brown SC, ed., Cornell University Press, Ithaca 1977, pp 104–107

[261] See Weizacher 1949

[262] www.fda.gov/ForIndustry/DevelopingProductsforRare-DiseasesConditions/default.htm

[263] www.rarediseases.org/programs/medication

[264] http://eh.net/encyclopedia/article/thomasson.insurance.health.us

[265] www.cnn.com/2009/HEALTH/06/05/bankruptcy.medical.bills/

[266] Fishbain DA, Goldberg M, Rosomoff RS, Rosmonoff H: Complete Suicide in Chronic Pain. Clin J of Pain Management 1991;7:29–36

[267] Capell CS: "aid-in-Dying" and the Taking of Human Life. J Med Ethics. Sept 1992; 18(3):128–134

[268] Melick E, Buckwalter KC, Stolley JM: Suicide Amount Elderly While Men: Development of a Profile. I Psychosoc Nurs Mental Health Serv 1992;30(2):29–34

[269] Copeland AR: Suicide by Drowning. Am J Forensic Meds Pathol 1987;8(1):18–22

[270] Fishbain DA, Goldberg M, Rosomoff RS, Rosomoff H: Homicide-Suicide and Chronic Pain. Clin J Pain 1989;5(3):275–277

[271] See Treece 1968

[272] Hess TM, Luitz LJ, Nauss LA, Lamer TJ: Treatment of Acute Herpetic Neuralgia. A Case Report and review of the Literature. Minn Med 1990;73(11);11–78

[273] Hofmann DF, Dubovsky SL: Depression and Suicide Risk. Emerg Med Clin North Am 1990;9(1):107–121

[274] Pary R, Lippman S, Tonias CD: A Preventive Approach to the Suicidal Patient. J Fam Pract 1988;26(2):185–189

[275] Bartfai A, Winborg IM, Nordstrom P, Asberg M: Suicidal Behavior and Cognitive Flexibility: Design and Verbal Fluency After Attempted Suicide. Suicide Life Threat Behav 1990;20(3):245–266

[276] Kotarba JA: Perceptions of Death, Belief Systems and the Process of Coping with Chronic Pain. Soc Sci Med 1983; 17(10):681–689

[277] Kopp M, Skranski HT: What Does The Legacy of Hans Seye and Franz Alexander Mean Today? Int J Psychophysiol 1989;8(2):299–105

[278] Engelhardt HT: Reason. In Vaux K: Powers That Make Us Human: The Foundation of Medical Ethics. University of Illinois Press, Urbana 1985, pp 90–91

[279] Tietjen F, Brandes B, Peterline L, et. al. Childhood Maltreatment and Migraine. Parts I,II,III, Headache; Published online January 6, 2009 (DOI:10.111/j.1526-4610-.2009.01556.x). Print issue Date January 2010

[280] Mills JS: Utilitarianism. Bobbs-Merrill, Indianapolis. 1975, page 10

[281] Mason JK: Human Life and Medical Practice. Edinburgh University Press, Edinburgh 1988, p 3

Index

A

AA and NA, 339
acedia and seven deadly sins, 55
acetaminophen, 116, 226, 250, 251
acetylcholine, 231
acupoints, 262
acupuncture, 79, 121, 262, 310, 391
acute pain, 370, 373
addicere, 111
addict, 111, 112, 114, 115, 135, 177, 178, 188, 249, 254, 265, 268, 271, 304, 311, 333, 334, 336, 338, 340, 345, 346, 348, 349, 351, 352, 364, 384
addiction, 96, 333
adrenal medulla, 231
adrenaline, 231
African American, 14, 60, 131, 248
alexthymia, 187
Alpers, 16
Alzheimer's disease, 227
American Academy of Pediatrics, 273
American Civil War, 246
American Dietetic Association, 452
American Headache Society, 438
American Indians, 70
American Lung Association, 451

American Medical Association, 445
American Pain Foundation, 455
American Pain Society, 455
American Psychiatric Association, 322, 335
amyotrophic lateral sclerosis, 254
ancient philosophers, 141
anger, 20, 21, 24, 69, 81, 101, 135, 157, 165, 169, 171, 176, 177, 195, 267, 409, 414, 415, 438, 456
Anslinger, 246
anticholinergic, 231
antidepressants, 72, 130, 223, 227, 228, 229, 232, 237, 253, 373
antihistamines, 226, 237
antispasmodic, 253, 254
anxiety, 87, 99, 104, 109, 137, 157, 176, 203, 206, 219, 220, 224, 242, 291, 323, 348, 354, 355, 384, 427, 434
Aristotle, 118
armodafinil (Nuvigil®), 208
Asians, 70, 131
aspirin, 189, 226, 249, 250, 251, 252

B

baclofen (Lioresal®), 254
Bacon, 283
Ballantyne, 294, 343
Bates, 283

Battle of the Books, 162
Bayer and heroin, 240
BDNF, See brain derived neurotropic factor
Beecher, 121, 193, 355
benzodiazepine, 116, 233, 254
beta endorphin, 230
beta lipotropin, 230
Bible, 85
bioavailability, 197
biofeedback, 24, 79, 133, 179, 193, 282, 327, 338
blame, 34, 117, 120, 135, 175, 274, 292, 321
blood brain barrier, 196, 200
body dysmorphic disorder, 322
Bonica, 366
Boodman, 273
borderline personality, 44, 75, 128
bradykinin, 225
brain code, 217, 221, 222, 224, 226, 228, 255
brain derived neurotrophic factor (BDNF), 5, 206, 207, 238
brain morphology and pain, 261
British Medical Association, 458
British National Treatment Agency, 340
Brown, 343
Buddha, 213, 274, 387

C

calcitonin gene-related peptide (CGRP), 238
calcium channel blockade, 256
California Intractable Pain Act, 12
Canada and Sativex®, 233
cancer pain, 14, 16, 233, 362
cannabinoids, 233, 235
cannabis sativa, 233
capsaicin, 231, 237
carbamazepine (Tegretol®), 253
catastrophizing, 72, 215, 316
Center for Medicare and Medicaid Services, 10, 13, 404, 405, 425
central nervous system, 5, 226, 229, 234, 239, 251, 258
central sensitization, 218, 237
Chapman, 141
cheating, 148
chemoreceptors, 223
childhood neglect or abuse, 438
children and pain, 65
cholecystokinin (CCK), 238
Christianity, 62, 85, 377, 382
chronic complex regional pain syndrome, 261
chronic low back pain, 294
chronic non-terminal pain, 294
chronic pain, 22, 102, 103, 191, 373
chronic vulvar pain, 261
chronic widespread pain (CWP), 219, 220
cigarette smoking, 199, 385
classical folk remedies, 368
clonazepam (Klonopin®), 254
clonidine (Catapres®), 254
coal tar analgesic, 251
Coca Cola and cocaine, 247

Conference for the Suppression of the Illegal Traffic in Dangerous Drugs of 1936, 246
constipation, 203, 208, 231, 239
conversion disorders, 322
cordotomy, 260
cortical reorganization in response to pain, 262
corticofugal inhibitory system, 99
corticotrophin-releasing factor (CRF), 206
Cottler, 341, 342
countertransference, 303, 304, 305, 306, 307
COX-1 and COX-2, 250
cravings, 339
Critique of Practical Reason, 381
cultural competency, 131
cyclooxygenase, 250, 251, 252
cytochrome P450, 335, 336, 343
cytokines, 238

D

Dannemiller Memorial Educational Foundation, 455
Dante and seven deadly sins, 56
de Quincey, 110, 111
death, 19, 54, 65, 67, 89, 193, 247, 281, 295, 357, 359, 361, 369, 377, 431
Declaration of Geneva, 458
Declaration of Sydney, 458
delta fibers, 258
delta-9-tetrahydrocannabinol (THC), 233
denial, 80, 183, 188, 407
depression, 4, 5, 20, 38, 55, 56, 63, 70, 71, 72, 101, 109, 123, 157, 178, 188, 203, 207, 208, 219, 220, 222, 223, 232, 244, 272, 323, 354, 371, 372, 374, 422, 423, 424, 425, 427, 453
diamorphine (heroin), 9, 120, 238, 240, 241
diazepam (Valium®), 199, 254
diclofenac (Voltarin®, others), 252
divinum est opus sedare tiolorum, 62
doctor shopping, 27, 265, 267, 268, 269, 272, 445
doctor's attitude, 40, 361
doctor-patient relationship, 11, 28, 33, 39, 143, 267, 269, 272, 297, 325, 328, 444, 446
dopamine, 295, 232, 233, 243, 244
dorsal column stimulators, 260
dorsal horn of the spinal cord, 218, 254
Drug Abuse Warning Network, 255
drug seeking, 10, 34, 59, 101, 130, 334, 337, 375
DSM-III, DSM-IV, DSM-III-TR, 341, 342
duloxetine (Cymbalta®), 4, 253
DuPont, 353, 354
Durkheim, 90
dying patient, 16, 17, 361, 424
dynorphins, 231
dysphoria, 109, 239, 243

E

eastern and western philosophy, 387
Ecclesiasticus, 84
Education in Palliative and End of Life Care, 17
ego, 75, 83, 133, 135, 149, 171, 174, 177, 306, 356, 398
egocentrism, 142
Egyptians, 85, 242
eighteenth century medicine, 366, 368
electromagnetic receptors, 223
elemental gold, 252
Ellis, 268
emotional anguish, 20, 110
emotional regression, 187
emotional role for the pain, 310
empathy, 21, 28, 192, 289, 291, 306, 319, 431
endocannabinboids, 234
endorphins, 97, 123, 229, 230, 231
Engel, 309, 313, 316, 318, 319, 320, 321
enkephalins, 121, 230, 231, 257
ennui, 90
environmental stressor, 219, 337
epinephrine, 231
eppur si muove, 368, 369, 460
ethnopsychopharmacology, 131
euphoria, 109, 230, 239, 243, 244, 246, 354, 355, 364
euthanasia, 13, 67, 369, 423, 424
evidence-based medicine, 71
evil, 49, 80, 85, 87, 120, 332, 340, 378, 379, 380, 381, 382
exercise, 157, 216, 339, 347, 391, 427, 448, 450
existentialists, 288, 289, 422
exorcism, 62, 284
extended pain patient, 370

F

facial expressions of pain, 39, 295
fatty acid DHA, 340
FDA accepted doses, 14
Federal Bureau of Investigation, 10
Federal Bureau of Narcotics, 246, 249
Federal Drug Administration, 455
fentanyl (Fentora®, Duragesic®, Actiq®), 196, 401
fibromyalgia, 4, 218, 219, 220, 237, 253, 262
fifth vital sign, 12
Fleming, 115
fraud, 9, 27, 142, 148, 174, 394, 409, 410, 436
free will, 92, 287, 288, 290, 292, 301
Freud's death, 369
Friedman, 273, 321

G

GABA, 232, 233, 340
gabapentin (Neurontin®), 16, 237
Galanin, 238
Galileo, 368, 369
gamma-aminobutyric acid, see GABA
gene therapy for pain, 257

generic medications, 197, 198
Geneva Convention to Limit the Manufacture and Regulate the Distribution of Narcotic Drugs of 1931, 245
Geneva Opium Convention of 1925, 245
giving up stage, 61
glaucoma, 233, 234
glial cells, 5, 222, 238
glutamate, 219, 222, 227, 236, 237, 254
glycine, 236
God, 56, 62, 65, 69, 79, 84, 85, 86, 88, 89, 126, 131, 151, 154, 175, 179, 185, 186, 195, 238, 242, 264, 286, 302, 350, 356, 357, 358, 359, 360, 368, 377, 378, 379, 380, 388, 410, 423
Goode, 300
Goodman and Gilman 1985, 364
G-protein, 256
Greek physicians, 278
Guatama, 274

H

Harrison Narcotic Tax Act, 245
Health Care Financing Administration, 13,
health literacy, 130
Health on the Net Foundation (www.hon.ch), 454
hell and the seven deadly sins, 55
Henderson, 143
Hendler, 328
heroin, 9, 120, 238, 240, 241

herpes simplex virus vectors, 257
Hick, 380
Hill, 208
Hippocrates and medicine 62, 86, 277, 280, 282, 284, 285, 458
hispanic patients, 13, 14
histamine, 225, 226, 237
Hoffman, 251
honor, 31, 40, 83, 103, 214, 318, 457, 459
hormones, 203, 207, 223, 231
hospice, 13, 15, 17, 66, 102, 113, 182, 351, 359, 455, 458
House Select Committee on Crime 1969, 249
hunt, the, 42, 43, 58, 328
Huxley, 459
Hyman, 272
hyperalgesia, 203, 225, 237, 250
hypnosis, 385, 448
hypochondria, 43, 137, 138, 144, 322
hypodermic needle, 246, 247
hysteria, 71, 322

I

I Ching, 388, 392
iatraddiction, 96, 113, 117, 205, 337, 343
iatrogenesis, 329
ibuprofen (Motrin®, Advil®, others) 68, 226, 250, 251, 252,
ICD-10, 341
Illich, 94
IME - independent medical examination, 413
immunological side effects, 255
incurable conditions, 277

inevitability, 54, 104, 426
infertility, 204
inflammation, 218, 225, 226, 234, 237, 249, 250, 251, 252
insurance, 2, 9, 16, 30, 45, 47, 48, 64, 65, 77, 85, 126, 142, 143, 148, 174, 192, 267, 281, 290, 292, 386, 391, 393, 431, 443
International Association for the Study of Pain, 253, 366
International Classification of Diseases, 341
intimacy, 364
intoxication, 69, 97, 98, 109, 157, 355
intractable pain, 12, 103, 105, 113
Iroquois, 118
it is divine to subdue pain, 62

J

Jefferson, 242
Jesuit Jose de Acosta, 118
Jesus, 85, 86, 87, 183
jiggery-pokery, 58, 267
Job 13:24, 356
Joint Commission on Accreditation of Healthcare Organizations - JCAHO, 13
joy, 26, 55, 61, 109, 123, 160, 161, 178, 194, 242, 264, 298, 357, 358, 359, 369, 382, 387, 438, 448
Judaism, 392
Jung, 388

K

Kahan, 115
Kant, 381

Karolinska Institute, 454
Keats, 432
kidney, 25, 196, 199
Kierkegaard, 288
King David, 330
Kingdom of God, 85, 377
Kleinbrink, 329
Kopp, 427
Kotarba, 426
Kung Fu, 391

L

lack of euphoria, 244
lamotrigine (Lamictal®), 237, 253
language barriers, 130, 314
Lao Tzu, 389
Latinos, 70
laudanum, 239
laugh and laughter, 146, 229, 264, 302, 415, 453
law and ethics, 141
lawyers, 24, 26, 43, 142, 332, 393, 407, 410, 412, 413, 415, 419, 427, 441, 442, 457
lazy gene and metabolizing, 336
legal sanctions, 16, 47
legal world for the chronic pain patient, 148
Leriche, 96
Leu enkephalin, 230
lidocaine patch, 252
limbic system, 231, 243, 257
lipid solubility, 200, 201, 240
liver enzymes, 131, 198
lofexidine, 254
loneliness, 54, 89, 90, 110, 176, 179, 264
lying, 40, 67, 89, 142, 158

M

maladaptive memory, 262
malignant pain, 202
malingering, 44, 174, 272, 415
Mao, 343
Marihuana Tax Act of 1937, 246
Marinol®(dronabinol), 233
Marks, 101
marriage, 24, 67, 183, 387
Martell, 344, 345
martyrdom, 319
mature pain patient, 45, 61, 77, 191
mechanoreceptors, 223
Medical Board of California, 12
medical charts, 419, 441
Medicare and Medicaid, 10, 13, 404, 405, 421, 425, 428
medication dependent secondary to untreatable or chronic pain, 42, 11
meditation, 63, 398, 434
memantine (Axura®- Ebixa®- Namenda®), 227, 236, 237
mental de-conditioning, 374
merperidine (Demerol®), 100, 241
Merril, 144
Mesopotamians, 85, 242
met enkephalin, 230
metabolic processes for medication, 196, 198, 343, 397
metaxalone (Skelaxin®), 254
migraine headache, 236, 373
Mills, 448
milnacipran (Savella®), 4
mind-body interactions, 123
misuse of prescription drugs, 113, 255

morphine, 113, 121, 122, 176, 189, 227, 229, 230, 232, 236, 238, 240, 241, 242, 246, 247, 248, 254, 255, 263, 336, 369
morphine and immune system, 203, 204, 245
moxibustion, 391
mu opiate receptors, 243
multiple sclerosis, 233, 234
myelin, 238, 258

N

n-acetylcysteine (NAC), 340
naloxone (Narcan®), 230, 260
narcosis, 111, 215
narcotic, 10, 17, 27, 30, 72, 96, 98, 99, 107, 108, 109, 110, 111, 112, 114, 115, 121, 135, 136, 147, 215, 227, 230, 231, 245, 246, 247, 272, 275, 281m 285m 333, 341, 343, 351, 355, 362
narcotic addiction (see also addictions), 136, 172, 205, 246
narcotic craving, 126
narcotics to the dying, 16, 361
narcotism, 111
National Association for Rural Mental Health, 70
National Institute on Drug Abuse, 243
National Organization for Rare Diseases (NORD), 400
National Pain Care Policy Act of 2008 , 18
Neal, 365
Neapolitan evil, 120
nerve block, 259, 282

nervous system, 5, 217, 221, 226, 229, 234, 238, 239, 251, 253, 257, 261
neuroimaging, 4
neuron code, 217, 221, 224, 228, 255
neuropathic pain, 113, 233, 234, 253, 262
neuroplastic effect, 218
neurotrophin, 206
New York Times, 7, 11, 18, 214, 273, 321, 454
Nietzsche, 213, 288
nitrous oxide, 225, 237
N-methyl-d-aspartate receptors (NMDA), 227, 236, 237, 254
nocebo, 121, 122
nociceptors, 217, 223, 225
non-malignant pain, 346, 361
non-steroidal anti-inflammatory drugs (NSAID), 226, 249, 250
norepinephrine, 231, 232, 254
nursing attitudes, 145
nutraceluticals, 452
nutrition, 200, 238, 452

O

observer shift, 144, 176
Ode to a Nightingale, 432
off-label medication use, 396, 397, 398, 400, 401, 402
opioid - definition, 239
opioids - general, 4, 9, 16, 17, 19, 65, 100, 101, 113, 114, 115, 116, 117, 120, 145, 202, 203, 208, 227, 231, 233, 236, 253, 254, 336, 344, 345, 364

opioid induced constipation, 203, 208, 239
opioid induced hyperalgesia, 203, 237
opioid receptors, 243. 256
opioid tolerance, 256, 335, 362
opioidphobia, 16
opium, 238, 239, 241, 242, 245, 248
Opium Wars, 242
orphan drugs, 399, 400
oxycodone related emergency room visits, 255

P

p11, 5, 229
pain amplification, 192, 223
pain as exaggerations, 67, 142, 145, 148, 149, 223, 226
pain as punishment, 61, 62, 84, 85, 124, 316, 317, 318
pain in terminal illness, 364
pain in the elderly, 425
pain intensity, 37, 145, 192, 363
pain in 'excess' of the pathology, 29
pain patient signature, 37, 40, 77, 298, 312, 314, 315, 316, 318, 319, 320, 327, 347, 446
Pain Patient's Bill of Rights, 12
pain perception, 256, 260, 261
pain receptors, 196
pain threshold tolerances, 37, 220
painful neuropathy, 4, 26, 113, 218, 233, 234, 236, 253, 262, 305

palliate, the word, 112, 373
palliative medicine, 373
papaver somniferum, 239, 242
parataxic distortion, 290, 291, 292, 306, 309
Parkinson's Disease, 232
Pekkanen, 274
peptides, 218, 257, 258
peripheral nervous system, 218, 257, 258
personality changes and pain, 67
personality disorders, 129. 134, 268, 323, 341, 384, 434
Petrie, 355
phantom 'perfect' patients, 58
pharmacogenetics, 51
phenacetin, 251
philosophy, 14, 16, 41, 46, 60, 76, 90, 111, 118, 141, 214, 220, 277, 278, 287, 288, 387, 388, 390, 391, 433, 448, 452
physiological dependence, 207
physiotherapists, 367
placebo, 113, 121, 384, 397
Plato, 277
pleasure, 29, 97, 98, 110, 205, 206, 217, 232, 298, 353, 380
polyethylene glycol 3350/electrolyte, 208
Pope Paul II, 377
poppy seeds & juice (opium), 2, 239, 243
Portenoy, 113, 114, 115, 294
positive reinforcer, 109
post-operative pain, 146
pragmatic medicine, 367

pregabalin (Lyrica®), 4, 253
pregnancy, pain med use during, 365
President Kennedy's 1962 Ad Hoc Panel on Narcotic and Drug Abuse, 249
pro-nociceptive positive feedback loop, 218
propoxyphene (Darvon®), 241
prostaglandin, 225, 226, 250, 251
protein binding, 199
pseudoaddiction, 96, 337, 343, 345, 363,
pseudotolerance and tolerance, 139, 284, 322, 367, 431
psychiatry, 139, 284, 322, 367, 431
psychoanalytic theory, 186
psychogenic pain, 99, 309, 310, 322
pain prone patient, 104, 309, 319, 321
psychological significance of the injury, 83
psychopharmacolgists, 131, 229, 427
psychosomatic disorder, 323, 327
psychosomatic pain, 138 313, 315, 233, 324, 325, 326, 385, 436, 447
psychotherapy, 24, 36, 45, 62, 70, 72, 79, 80, 83, 133, 135, 139, 174, 296, 301, 307, 348, 415, 427, 431, 437, 444, 447, 448, 451, 453
pushy patients, 76

Q

quality of life, 2, 23, 203, 295, 365, 373, 422

R

Rabbis, 131, 192, 195, 357
rapid metabolizer, 197, 240, 336
rare diseases, 399, 400
religion, 185, 195, 288, 293, 452
resting default mode network (DMN), 262
rhizotomy, 259
riluzole (Rilutek®), 237, 254
risk genes, 371
risk-benefit ratio of treatment, 203
Robiquet, 241
role strain, 300
Rose, 12

S

Sachar, 101
sacrifice, 62, 318, 319, 378, 387, 389, 449
Sartre, 289
Saunders, 341, 342
Scarry, 215
Schnoll, 343, 345
Schopenhauer, 90
second victimization, 416,
secondary gain, 29, 172, 173, 174, 316, 328, 410, 434, 435, 437
self-defeating personality, 81, 317
Selzer, 304
sensitivity training, 307
sensory receptors, 223
serotonin, 123, 225, 227, 228, 229, 237, 259
Sertüner, 238, 239
side effects to medications, 17, 49, 130, 131, 203, 231, 239, 243, 250, 251, 254, 257, 259, 328, 395, 428
Siegel, 98
signologists, 8, 9
sin, 55, 62, 84, 85, 278, 356, 373, 380
sin causing pain, 374
Sister Helen Prejean, 137
sleep, 156
sleep hygiene, 157
sloth, 55, 56, 57
snail toxin (Conus Magus), 256
social burden, 346, 347
social workers, 35, 52, 95, 367
soldiers, 83, 193, 246, 358, 362
somatoform pain disorder, 322, 323, 324
somatosensory cortex, 257, 261
soon-to-rain pain, 24
soul, 14, 22, 26, 62, 96, 281, 282, 296, 359, 383, 388, 390, 391, 415, 429, 430, 449, 450
Spanish pox, 120
spinothalamic tract, 260
spiritual deprivation and depression, 71
standard of care, 47, 48, 49, 413
step-wise protocol of medication use, 17, 394
stigma, 63, 71, 160, 324
stress management, 124, 448
substance abusers who need pain medications, 136, 144

substance P, 259
suffering, 295
suggestibility, 328
suicide, 283, 360, 422, 423, 424, 425, 427, 459
Suicide Prevention Hotline (800-273-TALK), 431, 453
Sukkot, 298
Sullivan, 290
US Surgeon General Report of 2001, 71
Swift, 162
symptomatic medicine, 367
synapse, 221, 222, 226, 232, 253

T

Talmud, 292
Tamo, 388
transcranial magnetic stimulation (TMS), 4
Tao, 388
Tao Te Ching, 389
tapentadol (Nucynta®), 4
TENS units, 74, 79, 259, 260, 282, 370
thalamus, 257, 260, 373
The New Testament, 140
theodicist, 379
thermoreceptors, 223
Thielbar, 351
third victimization, 331
thyrotropin releasing hormone (TRH), 238
tikkun, 2
transcutaneous electrical nerve stimulation (TENS), 259
treatment failure, 28, 34, 42, 43, 82, 220

treatment response, 39
treatment standards, 13
trephination, 279
tristitia, 55, 56
trust, 8, 11, 30, 31, 32, 53, 74, 78, 100, 117, 125, 140, 145, 147, 161, 175, 178, 291, 306, 330, 340, 345, 361, 414, 441, 443, 444, 445
Tylenol® (acetaminophen), 116, 239, 250, 251
type A Delta fibers, 258
type C fibers, 258
types of pain, 191, 253, 258, 321
tyrosine, 239

U

U.S. National Institute of Neurological Diseases, 455
Undiagnosed Diseases Program (NIH), 431

V

valproic acid (Depakote®), 253
vasoactive intestinal peptide (VIP), 238
velleity, 15, 267
Veterans Administration, 12, 406

W

Wall and Jones, 367, 368
Warfield, 201
Weaver, 343, 345
Weissman, 100, 101, 345

when modern medicine fails, 62
Wikler, 109
will to live, 89, 91
wisdom, 41, 77, 244, 293, 387, 448, 459
World Health Organization, 17
World Medical Association, 438
Wright, 240
www.ama.org, 445
www.clinicaltrials.gov, 455
www.eatright.org, 452
www.exerciseismedicine.org, 450
www.fda.gov, 455
www.instituteoflifestylemedicine.org, 450
www.ki.se, 454
www.lungsusa.org, 451
www.ninds.nih.gov/disorders/chronic_pain/detail_chronic_pain.htm, 255
www.nytimes.com, 454
www.pain.com, 455
www.painfoundation.org, 455
www.suicidepreventionlifeline.org, 453
www.thinkculturalhealth.org, 141
www.tmj.org, 455

Y

yin and yang, 388, 398

Z

Zen, 63
ziconotide (Prialt®), 4, 256

Made in the USA
Las Vegas, NV
23 January 2024

84793747R00282